Kai Leichsenring, Andy M. Alaszewski (Eds.)

Providing Integrated Health and Social Care for Older Persons

A European Overview of Issues at Stake

ASHGATE

Published by

Ashgate Publishing Limited
Gower House
Croft Road
Aldershot
Hants GU11 3HR
England

Ashgate Publishing Company
Suite 420
101 Cherry Street
Burlington, VT 05401-4405
USA

This publication was co-sponsored by:

THE EUROPEAN COMMISSION
THE 5TH FRAMEWORK PROGRAMME
QUALITY OF LIFE AND
MANAGEMENT OF LIVING RESOURCES
Key Action :: The Ageing Population and Disabilities
Contract No. QLK6-CT-2002-00227

Copy-editing and DTP: Willem Stamatiou
European Centre for Social Welfare Policy and Research
Berggasse 17, 1090 Vienna, Austria

British Library Cataloguing-in-Publication Data. A catalogue record for this book is available from the British Library.

ISBN 0-7546-4196-1

Printed by Facultas Verlags- und Buchhandels AG, Vienna, Austria

Contents

Introduction

Providing Integrated Health and Social Care for Older Persons – A European Overview

Kai Leichsenring

Preface

9

Doing research on long-term care with a focus on the interfaces between health and social care, between institutional and community care and between primary and secondary health care calls for a broad scope of experience and perspectives that often go beyond classic scholarly divisions. This is especially true when it comes to transnational projects with the aim of comparative perspectives. Even though interdisciplinarity has increased it cannot be denied that the social and health divide is still reflected by different approaches, thus duplicating or reflecting the reality of organisational structures, policies and professional cultures.

"Providing Integrated Health and Social Care for Older Persons" (PROCARE) is an international research project co-financed by the European Union's Fifth Framework Programme (Quality of Life and Management of Living Resources, The Ageing Population and Disabilities). The challenge for PROCARE – and thus also of this first European overview – consists in taking into account the different professional and organisational backgrounds of individual researchers in the different national teams, most of them social gerontologists, some with a special focus on social policies, some more public health oriented, with psychological or social work training; in addition, there are also some economists and nursing professionals. Together we are to explore the realm of integrated care in Europe, to find out about different approaches towards what has been described as one of the most prominent shortcomings in European health and welfare systems – the improvement of service delivery at the interface between the health system on the one hand and the system of social care for older persons on the other. Despite the variation between cultures, and the diversity of health and social care systems studied, the PROCARE national reports suggest that the last 20 years have brought partial success in integrated working and some clear examples of innovative practice, yet overall there appears to be evidence of a failure to sustain cooperation between the organisations that are involved.

The idea for this project was born as new challenges and changing political and economic contexts in EU member states call for a new effort to define the concept of an integrated health and social care for older persons in need of care and to contribute to the provision of a sustainable model of this type of service by comparing and evaluating different modes of care delivery. The PROCARE project work has been undertaken within the context of a number of parallel initiatives,[1] and the opportunity to draw upon this existing expertise helps us to fulfil our aim of finding ways to increase the quality of life of older persons in need of care. Nevertheless, PROCARE is one of the first attempts to map the relatively weakly documented area of integration in health and social care for the older client group.

The following overview is a first attempt to draw together information from nine national reports that were produced by the teams from Austria, Denmark, Finland, France, Germany, Greece, Italy, the Netherlands, and the UK participating in the project. As coordinator and author of the European overview I owe all my knowledge and findings to my colleagues who provided both their inputs and their comments (special thanks also to Kirstie Coxon who cared for the linguistic editing) to complete this first stage of a project that will go on to carry out detailed case-studies on model ways of working in the participating countries.

1 Introduction: A Common Agenda in spite of Diverse Health and Welfare Systems in Europe?

Comparative approaches of European health and welfare systems are a most fascinating attempt to compare apples and oranges. Both general comparisons (Flora, 1986) and the ensuing attempt to categorise different systems

(Esping-Andersen, 1990), specific areas of social policies (Cichon et al., 1998), health policies (Freeman, 2000), and detailed studies on long-term care systems for older persons (Pacolet et al., 1999; Jacobzone, 1999; Tester, 1999) have elaborated on these differences and thus enriched the scientific and political debate. Also the development of the European Union has contributed to an ever-increasing interest in comparing social policies and trying to find common traits as a basis of a "European Model".

Focusing on the interface between health and social care services and potential coordination and integration mechanisms seems to be even more fascinating as we address an area that is influenced by all the above-mentioned differences between but in particular within the single countries. As we are dealing with personal social services, the local often becomes more important than the national or the European context. Still, we have to take into account national frameworks and their differences, in particular with respect to financing, systemic development, professionalisation and professional cultures, basic societal values (family ethics), and political approaches.

There is no need to underline that health care expenditure is decreasing across Europe from Northern to Southern European countries. Even knowing that the level of GDP does not necessarily reflect the level of health care services in a given country, it still provides an illustration of the relative importance of these services within the different countries (Kanavos/ Mossialo, 1996). On the other hand, not even this kind of a measure or indicator is available for all EU Member States if it comes to expenditures for long-term care. As these expenditures are usually dispersed between various budget lines of the social assistance systems, between regional and local budgets or simply subsumed to health expenditures, data must be interpreted with caution. As the Economic Policy Committee (2001) has undertaken research intended to overcome this problem,[2] we propose to offer a brief overview of their findings as a basis for discussion (see Table 1).

It remains to be seen whether countries with low levels of expenditure will really be able to keep their public investment in this sector as low as predicted by the EPC study. In any case one can say that social care services are by far less funded and less privileged than health care services. This leads to a first question that will be addressed in this overview:

- To what extent can an integrated health and social care system give space to social care as part and parcel of this type of care delivery? Could coordination be a first step to integration in order to prevent social services from losing their autonomy?

11

Table 1: Total Public Expenditure on Health Care and Long-term Care as a Percentage of GDP in EU Member States

	Total health and long-term care		Health care		Long-term care	
	2000	Range of increase in % of GDP 2000-2050	2000	Range of increase in % of GDP 2000-2050	2000	Range of increase in % of GDP 2000-2050
B	6.1%	2.1-2.4	5.3%	1.3-1.5	0.8%	0.8
DK	8.0%	2.7-3.5	5.1%	0.7-1.1	3.0%	2.1-2.5
D			5.7%	1.4-2.1		
EL (1) (4)			4.8%	1.6-1.7		
E (1)			5.0%	1.5-1.7		
F	6.9%	1.7-2.5	6.2%	1.2-1.9	0.7%	0.5-0.6
IRL (2)	6.6%	2.5	5.9%	2.3	0.7%	0.2
I	5.5%	1.9-2.1	4.9%	1.5-1.7	0.6%	0.4
NL	7.2%	3.2-3.8	4.7%	1.0-1.3	2.5%	2.2-2.5
A (4)	5.8%	2.8-3.1	5.1%	1.7-2.0	0.7%	1.0-1.1
P (1)			5.4%	0.8-1.3		
FIN	6.2%	2.8-3.9	4.6%	1.2-1.8	1.6%	1.7-2.1
S	8.8%	3.0-3.3	6.0%	1.0-1.2	2.8%	2.0-2.1
UK	6.3%	1.8-2.5	4.6%	1.0-1.4	1.7%	0.8-1.0
EU (3)	6.6%	2.2-2.7	5.3%	1.3-1.7	1.3%	0.9-1.0

Notes: (1) Results for public expenditure on long-term care are not yet available for a number of Member States; (2) Results for Ireland are expressed as a share of GNP; (3) Weighted average; weights are calculated according to the Member States for which results are available, Therefore for health care it is a weight for the EU-14, and for long-term care, and total expenditure on health and long-term care, the average is for 10 Member States; (4) The expenditure estimates for Greece and Austria, unlike for the other Member States, project only those parts of expenditures which vary according to age, Therefore, both the projected expenditure levels in the base year and in al projection years underestimate the total public expenditure on health and long-term care in those countries.

Source: Economic Policy Committee, 2001: 44 (central demographic variant).

In all countries, social care service systems are characterised by a definitely shorter history than health care systems. We can observe different traditions and states of systemic development in the context of a general North-South gap. On the one hand, the Nordic countries started to develop specific so-cial services already during the 1950s, thus undergoing a marked differen-tiation between different types of services and institutions, and respective professional concepts and approaches. On the other hand, in Southern Eu-

rope we experience a general scarcity of social services that present themselves still in a "pioneering phase" with respective difficulties concerning
funding and staffing. This is in sharp contrast to the general health care
system, which is – despite all differences concerning their extent and quality – characterised by quite well-defined medical professions, differentiated
competences and values.

These differences between and within countries may be highlighted
by the simple fact that, while medicine and – in many countries – also nursing studies are approved university studies, social service professions are
often lacking even national regulations, not to mention international ac-
knowledgements (Badelt/Leichsenring, 1998). Furthermore, the different
status of social and health professions may be gathered from the income gaps
and deteriorating general working conditions the more "social" a service is
defined. Finally, research expenditures with respect to social care are far
behind spending on medical research.

- A main question for this European overview and for PROCARE in
  general will therefore be how joint working and integrated modes of
  care delivery can be promoted in spite of these differences to improve
  the quality of life for the users of these services.

Another general feature that has to be considered in relation to long-term
care systems is concerning societal values and respective political approaches
to face the growing challenge of meeting long-term care needs in an ageing
society.

- To what extent is long-term care a task of the family and in how far are
  family carers capable and/or prepared to deliver long-term care? What
  is the role of the family in evolving coordinated or integrated service
  schemes? How can family or informal care be included as a partner in
  long-term care delivery?

These complex problems co-exist alongside additional economic, demographic and societal developments that, at first sight, do not seem to favour
innovation and investment in social care issues. However, PROCARE will
elaborate on opportunities that could be used to further promote the concept of integrated service delivery, i.e. to develop proactive strategies towards
comprehensive care provision, rather than to carry on with a reactive "mud-
dling-through" in organising support for people in need of long-term care.
The optimism underpinning this approach is based on evidence that integrated modes of care delivery contribute to preventative policies and help
to:

13

- avoid a further decline of social capabilities of older persons in need of care,
- to increase their quality of life and their level of social inclusion, and to
- reduce inadequate and more expensive medical care.

However, the tasks of gathering evidence to increase the existing knowledge base, and disseminating new knowledge to practitioners and policy-makers remains. The PROCARE strategy for achieving this includes the development of a web site (http://www.euro.centre.org/procare) and the formation of "National Project Committees" in each participating country, to act as forums for dissemination and provide access to practitioners and policy-makers.

One of those aspects is the surprisingly similar agenda in terms of health and social reforms, in particular in the area of long-term care. This is why we would like to take up the discourse on coordination and integration in the new context of attempts to increase care at home, to raise the quality of services and the quality of working conditions towards a European model of social well-being.

In the following, the understanding of integrated care in the different countries will be illustrated. As we try to reflect on the definitions and approaches described in the national reports and in the general debate on integrated care, this discourse will be carried on in the following chapter by Alaszewski, Billings and Coxon to lead to a more common understanding of integrated care as a contribution to develop a theory and a definition of integrated care.

The task of the present overview is then to draw attention to most interesting features from the practice of integrated care and/or coordination efforts in the realm of health and social care for older persons. All national reports reflect a wealth of experience from both model projects and mainstream ways of working.

These concepts, methods, strengths but also weaknesses should be taken as a basis for further policy developments and for evaluation methods of such ways of working. Still, we have to be aware that we are confronted with completely different national contexts that we shall outline in section 4, also drawing on current debates and the role of different stakeholders. The overview will end with some reflections on perspectives and necessary debates for the desired improvement of integrated care delivery.

2   Different Understandings of Integrated Care

Integrated Care is a concept of providing care services in which the single units act in a coordinated way and which aims at ensuring cost-effectiveness, improving the quality and increasing the level of satisfaction of both users and providers of care. Means to this end include the reduction of inefficiency within the systems, the enhancement of continuity, tailoring services within the process of care provision and the empowerment of service users.

In this context the term "unit" can have a multitude of meanings, for example care providers, strategies of care provision or care services. The process of integration can aim at linking parts within a single level of care, e.g. the creation of multiprofessional teams (horizontal integration) or the linking between different levels of care, e.g. primary, secondary and tertiary care (vertical integration). Those links can work in one direction or include a feedback-mechanism. The concept of integrated care can be found in various countries and under various names, e.g. seamless care, transmural care, case management, care management and networking (Gröne/ Garcia-Barbero, 2001; Delnoij et al., 2002; Kodner/Spreeuwenberg, 2002; Komp et al., 2002; Wistow et al., 2002).

Integration within and between care services is especially important when it comes to service provision for elderly people. Elderly patients tend to be chronically ill and being subject to multi-morbidity. Hence a broad spectrum of needs has to be met over a long period of time. To fulfil this task there is a vast number of possibilities to choose from: health and social care, formal and informal care providers, *domiciliary service as opposed to residential, hospital or clinic based services* ("intra- and extramural services" as it was put in some national reports) and many more (Ewers/Schaeffer, 2000: 8f.; Steiner-Hummel, 1991: 162; Wendt, 2001: 166f.). Considering this scenario, both the necessity of integration and the diversity of approaches towards achieving integration become inevitable.

In general, we can observe two larger streams within the integrated care discourse. On the one hand, there have been developments starting within the health care realm, on the other hand there is a broader approach putting increasing emphasis on social services and social integration.

In particular public health scholars and health management literature explore "managed care" and other forms of integrated care, and are based much more on a health care perspective. Also the WHO has taken up this approach, not least by the implementation of a "European Office for Integrated Health Care Services" in Barcelona. This institution suggested the following as a working definition of integrated care:

> "… a concept bringing together inputs, delivery, management and organisation of services related to diagnosis, treatment, care, rehabilitation and health promotion. Integration is a means to improve the services in relation to access, quality, user satisfaction and efficiency" (Gröne/Garcia-Barbero, 2001: 10).

Also Kodner/Spreeuwenberg (2002), who have made an important contribution to the definition exercise, can be located in this stream of thought as they take a "patient-centric view on integrated care", though taking into account the "provision of health care, social services and related supports (e.g., housing) at the right time and place" (Kodner/Spreeuwenberg, 2002: 3).

It is exactly this broader approach that most national reports of PROCARE have looked at, in view of opportunities to create a more equal inclusion of the social services realm in the integration discourse. As within most concepts, we still can find a variety of meanings, approaches, theories and practices in the participating countries of PROCARE. In a geographic perspective, the approach might be interpreted as "Northern European" as Niskanen (2002: 1f.) put it:

> "Integrated care includes the methods and strategies for linking and coordinating the various aspects of care delivered by different care levels, of primary and secondary care. In Finland the concept of integration applies also to the social services, since especially long term care patients need support, which is a duty of the social sector as well."

Pragmatically, the Danish report illustrates this approach as follows:

> "The integration of health and social services implies that the services are provided to all elderly – independent of where they live – by integrated teams of home-helpers, home nurses etc. Each older person in need of support has a case manager in the municipality, who is the individual counsellor of the older person applying for support. The case manager coordinates the services and calls them off when the client is hospitalised, on vacation or when s/he is visiting relatives. The decision for support is made on request from GP's, hospitals, the elderly or relatives." (Colmorten et al., in this book)

The Finnish report (Salonen/Haverinen, in this book) refers to integrated care as seamless service chains, i.e. as "an operating model, where the social welfare and health care services received by a client are integrated into a flexible entity which will satisfy the client's needs regardless of which operating unit provides or implements the services (Ranta, 2001: 274, 275).

This definition is very close to the Dutch notion that, both in theory and in policy-making, is tending towards the construction of "demand-driven" care systems that, in summary, are promoting integrated care delivery:

> "Demand-driven care simultaneously means integrated care for, when the requests and needs which the client may experience in various areas are met, integrated care is provided. From a client perspective, integration is realised when (s)he can expect to receive the right kind of care, and the right amount of care at the right moment in time." (Ex et al., in this book)

This concept draws on the individual as the point of departure and tries to de-medicalise long-term care, focusing on the interface between independent housing and care ("transmural care"; see also van der Linden et al., 2001), inter-sectoral joint working and the development of service-networks to guarantee older persons' participation in society.

In Austria, the scientific discourse on integrated care is mainly influenced by the "Public Health" approach (integration between primary and secondary care) but it was extended with a view to both the vertical and the horizontal level, and to social service delivery. The definition of integrated care given in the Austrian report (Grilz-Wolf et al., in this book) is thus clearly in line with those described hitherto. The idea of integration refers to a process aiming at guaranteeing demand-orientation, a continuity of provision and a high standard of quality (Grundböck et al., 1997; Kain, 1994; LBI, 2000). At the centre of attention is in particular the hospital/community care interface. This focus is comparable with the German one: also in this country transition from hospital to subsequent care is the area where, for instance, a high number of model projects have been carried out, very close to what has been called "intermediate care" in the UK, i.e. a range of services to "facilitate the transition from hospital to home, and from medical dependence to functional independence, where the objectives of care are not primarily medical, the patient's discharge destination is anticipated, and a clinical outcome of recovery (or restoration of health) is desired" (Steiner, 1997: 18).

In the UK, a variety of similar terms have been used to describe integrated care, including "joint working", "partnership" and "collaboration", but the actual meaning of "integrated care" has never been clearly defined within policy documents – there is a sense that understanding of this and other related terms is taken for granted or assumed. The UK report (Coxon et al., in this book) refers to a recent definition provided by the Audit Commission which has developed a "systems model" of organisational partnership. According to this definition "whole system working takes place when services are organised around the user, all of the players recognise that they are interdependent and understand that action in one part of the system has an impact elsewhere" (Audit Commission, 2002: Section 1.2). Users should thus experience services as "seamless" and providers share "vision, objectives, action (including redesigning services), resources and risk" (op. cit.). This concept is surely most remarkable, though its translation into practice will call for major efforts concerning organisational development and communication between players. This definition as such could in any case help to create a shared vision between scientists, policy analysts and practitioners.

The question remains whether this definition really means "integration", rather than "coordination" or "networking". As the French national report suggests, "integrated services are a set of services made available for a specific population group over a given geographical area, or for the population of a given geographical area, by a single company or organisation, grouped together under a single decision-making authority" (Frossard et al., in this book). For "real integration" to occur, a stable organisation providing for the complete coverage of health care needs of a given population must be created, and this would probably be within the health system. An attendant concern is that social services would either lose their identity and autonomy or would become further "medicalised". Due to the existing fragmentation of health and social care systems the different units would barely be ready to accept a unique, vertically integrated decision-making authority. This is why, in France, the concept of integration in the form of a "Consolidated Direct Service Model" (Zawadski, 1983; Davies, 1992) is rather undesirable. Instead, we can observe in this country a long history in theory and practice of "gerontological coordination" and networking:

> "Network or coordination means a voluntary organisation of professional people (which may include voluntary workers) who pool their means and resources to develop information, social and health care, and prevention services designed to resolve complex or urgent problems, which have been identified as priorities over a given geographical area, according to criteria decided in advance on a consultation basis (...) a temporary or permanent collaboration between different organisations working towards a specific objective." (Frossard et al., in this book)

A triad of *coordination, cooperation and networking* is commonly found within the national reports. The three terms refer to ways of working together, within as well as between different sectors. The difference between the three expressions is the extent of working together, which increases from coordination over cooperation up to networking: While coordination might still imply the existence of a hierarchy, cooperation hints somewhat more to working together on an equal level, whereas networking additionally requires a certain closeness and continuity (Block/Skrobacz, 2002: 21; Mutschler, 1998: 49).

Given the above definitions, in particular the Audit Commission's "systems model" and the "client-centred approach", it appears, however, that neither "seamless care" nor "client centred" approaches are heading towards an "unfriendly take-over" of the social sector by the health system. It is just the use of different terms that seems to create confusion, while the meaning is more or less compatible. Coordination, too, aims at a certain level of structural integration (e.g. a front-office or "one-stop-window" where clients may go and address their questions), a process of joint working and learning to work together, and person-centred, seamless care as a result (see also Coxon et al., in this book).

Apart from the Nordic countries, there is only one country where we can find clearly defined legal guidelines towards integrated care. Indeed, Italy as a "latecomer" in the development of European welfare states, offers a range of interesting experiences concerning the integration of health and social services. When the National Health System was eventually installed in 1978, the "Local Health Units" were designed as "Local Health and Social Service Units", with the organisation of social services being delegated by most municipalities. Thus a kind of consolidated direct service model was founded by law – with the result that, aside from various implementation problems, municipalities were generally dissatisfied with the standards, the quantitative and qualitative level of services that they had delegated to the "Local Health Companies" (ASL) as they were renamed during the 1990s.

Whilst Italy continues to experience compulsory standardisation in the health sector, the parallel development within the social sector is still characterised by a vast regional and local variety of operative models, professionals, approaches and methods of intervention. In 2000, a reform was proposed in response to these cultural, financial, dimensional and organisational distortions. The "Framework law for an integrated system of interventions and social services" defined the process of integration between health and social care stemming from the cooperation and coordination among different territorial levels of governance and among public and private actors. Particular attention is given to older persons with care needs for whom the creation of a local integrated network of services is foreseen. Furthermore, the process of provision (geriatric assessment, personalised individual care plans, coordination of different government levels and governance of public and private actors), and fundamental principles (individual right to welfare, anti-discrimination, universality) are defined (see Nesti et al., in this book).

Greece is known as another "latecomer" in social welfare development, with care for the elderly being "a family affair" (Sissouras et al., in this book). Two distinct mechanisms – the National Health System (NHS) and the National Social Care System (NSCS) – have contributed to a soundly segregated service delivery. Two developments have improved the situation during the past few years, also contributing to a definition of integrated service provision. On the one hand, the "Open Care Centres" (KAPI) for older persons have introduced preventive health services and psycho-social support to older persons under one roof in local communities (Sissouras et al., 1998; Emke-Poulopoulou, 1999). The Open Care Centres are staffed by teams comprising social workers, medical staff, visiting nurses, occupational and physical therapists and family assistants.

On the other hand, the Greek report (Sissouras et al., in this book) underlines another aspect of integration, which is the integration of different types of providers, an issue that has been discussed in most countries with respect to different "welfare mixes" (Evers/Wintersberger, 1990; Evers/Olk, 1996). This development is particularly evident in those countries where market mechanisms and choice are part of the equation (e.g. Austria, Germany, increasingly Italy), and there is a strong argument that the numerous different types of providers are just adding more complexity to a realm that has already been described as being "among the most complex and interdependent entities known to society" (Kodner/Spreeuwenberg, 2002: 2). Indeed, steering mechanisms with respect to the Third Sector and other private providers, have been developing during the past few years, in particular where these new providers have only started to blossom (e.g. Italy; see Nesti et al., in this book).

In Table 2 we undertake the – scientifically – risky experiment of classifying the relative importance of different concepts in the participating countries. Obviously, this classification only builds on the subjective experience of the participating researchers and evidence given in the national reports (see also the brief descriptions of model ways of working in the respective annexes) but it might help to gain some insight into the different concepts at stake.

Table 2:   Main Concepts of Integrated Care in Selected EU Member States

Key concepts of integrated care	A	D	DK	EL	F	FIN	I	NL	UK
Public health discourse	**	**	**			*	**		**
Managed care (health system)	**	**	*		*	*	*	*	***
Horizontal integration (provider mix)	**	**		**	*	*	*	*	*
Vertical integration						**	**		**
Seamless care/transmural care	*					***		**	*
Gerontological coordination/ networking	*	*			***		*		
Whole system approach									**
Person-centred approach			***			**		***	**

Denotation: ***) most important concept being followed and implemented in mainstream provision; **) important concept followed (partly implemented); *) concept being discussed and tried out in experimental (model) projects.

Source: PROCARE National Reports;

The single concepts described above have deliberately not been construed in a mutually exclusive way although, for instance, it seems logical that a person-centred approach includes horizontal integration (that is, integration across organisational boundaries and across professions) and "transmural care" (that is, integration across residential and domiciliary services). It may be that implementing horizontal integration is the first step in the process of developing a system that supports person-centred care. Furthermore, there might be additional and/or alternative pathways towards integrated care, for instance by developing "gerontological coordination". In brief, Table 2 should be read as an attempt to provide indicators on the level of integration in the individual countries: we are not trying to propose single "best" strategies of integration here. In fact, there are variations both within and between countries in methods of service organisation. As a result, the above table should be considered generally representative of the country in question, as opposed to an accurate representation of the "status quo" country-wide.

As a corollary of this section we may, notwithstanding the existing different approaches, consider the term "integrated care" as a helpful concept to describe coordination, cooperation and networking between health and social care services with the aim of improving services and quality of life from a user's perspective (for a further analysis, see Alaszewski et al. in Chapter 2; see also Kodner/Spreeuwenberg, 2002: 4). Still, it depends on single strategies and the specific mix of methods or instruments used to achieve these objectives. Some key innovations in this respect are outlined in the following section.

3 Different Approaches towards Integration: Strategies, Methods and Instruments

As Delnoij et al. (2001) suggested, it makes sense to distinguish different levels of integration. His typology includes clinical integration as a first level, i.e. the micro-level of the primary process, "chains of care" and transmural care. Secondly, professional integration between different kinds of professionals (and between them and the institutions they work for) has to be taken into consideration. Another level is concerning organisational integration, which can take place with respect to the specific welfare mix of a country, by creating networks or even by mergers of different organisations. And finally, functional integration can be described as a continuum of cure, care, and prevention.

Policies and strategies to reach integration may then try to use different forms of leverage and diverse starting points to strive towards the creation of integrated care systems. Kodner and Spreeuwenberg (2002) have suggested a continuum of strategies towards integrated care, addressing the problems that we have mentioned above in five interdependent domains: funding, administrative, organisational, service delivery, and clinical.

Again, in trying to further "de-medicalise" the discourse, we would like to emphasise those methods and strategies that concern the various "interfaces" between the health care and the social care realms, and the structures and processes that are to overcome these bottlenecks.

3.1 Case and Care Management

The most genuine method within the integrated care discourse is probably what has been described as case and care management, a technique deriving from the social care sector, which aims at matching supply and demand for persons in complex situations. The idea is to build up a network of services (resources) over time and across services and to empower the patient and his/her relatives to use it self-reliantly. The methods used are client- and therefore demand-oriented. It should be noted that in this context the term "case" refers to the situation the person is in, not to the person itself (Davies, 1992; 1996; Wendt 1991; 2001; Ewers/Schaeffer, 2000). This approach was also taken up in other domains such as, in particular, the health sector where it is more known under the heading of *care management* or "managed care" which is mainly to introduce steering mechanisms and economic think- ing in medical care (Haubrock et al., 2000). The idea is to maximise the ben- efits derived from a given amount of money. This aim is reached by means of coordination of the care delivery, thus avoiding loss of information and double treatments and – eventually – leading to a cut-back of the utilisation of care services. It is currently uncertain whether this strategy even leads to a cut-back of the use of necessary but expensive services (Barr, 1996; Huntington, 1997; Seng, 1997). A further definition problem concerns the term "care management" that, referring to German sources (Roth/Reichert, in this book), denotes the coordination of help and networks of service pro- viders at the general level in a care region, while in other contexts it means the management of the individual care process.

In any case, most national reports make reference to case and care management. The instrument is used in most countries, though with differ- ent interpretations. While in the UK, the Netherlands, and the Nordic coun- tries case managers might be characterised as a mainstream service, in Ger- many, Austria, Italy and France case management is mainly provided in model projects. Differences concern objectives, funding and the organisa- tional setting. For instance, in the UK case managers also fulfil a gate-keep- ing function. The GP performs this function with respect to health care, and social services employed "care managers" to purchase social care on behalf of clients following an assessment of a "social" need. In Austria and Ger- many, case managers are mainly working in projects at the interface between hospital and community care.

In theory, case managers should follow the client's situation from the initial moment the person in need of care is asking for support. Thus, "one- stop-windows" and information centres have been developed in some coun- tries, mostly on a project basis in different organisational settings (munici- pality, health care centre, old-age home).

As with other instruments of integrated care, a key issue relates to who the "case and care managers" are, which professional background they have (nursing rather than social work?), which kind of training they get and whether they are given the real means and competences to "steer" the processes and to act as an "advocate" of the client – in Dutch, the "ouderenadviseur" (consultant of the elderly) is a widespread service (see also the role of the "omtinker" mentioned in one of the Dutch projects; Ex et al., in this book). Other questions with respect to care management concern the role as "gate-keepers" and/or the dedication to individual care planning and the monitoring of outcomes: How should case management be organised? Should case management remain a public responsibility? Could target setting serve as a mode of steering case managers? How and by involving whom should the role of case managers be developed?

3.2 Intermediate Care Strategies: The Hospital/Community Care Interface

As the need for care often occurs unexpectedly (mostly in relation to a dismissal from hospital), and as frail older people (and their family) often do not know where to turn to, rapid intervention and quick, unbureaucratic support is an important factor to obtain client-orientation and thus an indicator for quality assurance. At this interface, rapid response teams (see UK report: Coxon et al., in this book) may be an instrument to prevent unnecessary hospital admissions and/or request for a place in a nursing home. This method is part of a whole range of interventions with respect to "intermediate care" that could be complemented by intensive rehabilitation services (situated in hospitals or people's homes) to help older people regain their health and independence, recuperative facilities (short-term care in a nursing home or other special accommodation to ease the passage), and quick information exchange (transition forms).

While these instruments are part of the UK government's strategy for improving health and social care services for older people (Coxon et al., in this book), they can also be found in other countries. In Denmark, preventative visits at the home of all older persons have been introduced. Furthermore, early warning systems, contracts between municipalities and hospitals about discharge procedures, meetings between home nurses and hospital staff, and geriatric teams that are following-up the older persons in their own homes are part of the Danish strategy to increase integration between hospitals and community care (Colmorten et al., in this book).

Of course, care managers situated in hospitals can also contribute to a better preparation of hospital discharge if they are able to create a decent network around the client's needs (see, for instance, the Austrian report: Grilz-Wolf et al., in this book).

Also Wistow et al. (2002: 44) underline the necessity "to conceive of intermediate care in terms of a service system which is built around the needs and aspirations of older people for valued lifestyles (…) in ways which enhance their capacity to meet their social and psychological needs as well as their optimal level of physical functioning". It cannot be taken for granted that the different environments (hospital/community) are recognised, or that working in partnership between health and social care agencies is always successful.

3.3 The Beginning of A Complex Relationship: Needs Assessment and Joint Planning

If it is important to provide a single point of reference for persons who have become chronically ill and/or care-dependent, it is at least equally important to cater for an assessment of needs that considers both social and medical aspects, both psychological, mental and physical factors, i.e. an interdisciplinary and multidimensional team. In order to provide integrated care it seems only logical that from the very moment a person is taken in charge by a service-providing agency, his/her general needs should be assessed and matched with the existing resources. If needs are assessed only in relation to medical requirements, it is most probable that only medical remedies will be prescribed (home nursing, medicines etc), and vice versa, if only social needs are assessed, social care interventions will be used. Furthermore, if needs are not assessed correctly, clients/patients could tend to make use of the most expensive but perhaps less efficient and less satisfying service – major underlying problems could thus be missed.

Many countries have introduced interdisciplinary assessment teams and/or agencies responsible to guide the citizen through the "jungle" of service providers. The multidimensional "geriatric assessment units" within the Italian health system (Nesti et al., in this book) are one example but in reality they often only start their activity when older persons are applying for a place in a residential setting. In the Netherlands (Ex et al., in this book), the Regional Assessment Boards (RIOs) are a most important starting point for integrated care strategies: their interdisciplinary members decide to what kind of care, facilities or support the person is entitled. A similar function is given to the Community Assessment and Rehabilitation Teams (CART) in the UK and the "Centres Locaux d'Information et de Coordination" (CLICs) in France. In most other countries, the assessment process remains quite medicalised and fragmented. For instance, in Austria and Germany specially trained medical doctors are carrying out the assessment of needs, i.e. to check entitlement rights for the LTCI (Germany) and the Austrian long-term care allowance. Thus, entitled persons who choose services as a support to family care often have to undergo a further, "duplicating" assessment concerning service needs and individual planning. An integrated approach, i.e. a "single assessment process" could serve to reduce this kind of "parallel actions".[3]

3.4   User's Choice: Personal Budgets and Long-term Care Allowances

Needs assessment by (medical) experts is a topic at least as diversely debated as cash benefits for care-dependent persons. While the former, however, has always been a fundamental part of the debate on integrated care, "consumer-directed care appears to be the antithesis of integrated care" (Kodner, 2003: 1). Giving money to persons in need of care, indeed, is a phenomenon that has been spreading over the past 15 years (Evers et al., 1994). It is rooted in claims for independent living – a movement that consists mainly of persons with disabilities at working age but also in traditional cash benefit schemes for disabled persons (invalidity allowances) that have existed in many countries. Furthermore, cash benefits were also to support informal and family carers with some schemes that entitled carers for specific allowances. And, of course, cash benefits are an attractive means for policy-makers to control budgets.

In practice, we can observe quite different approaches, both on the level of financing, and in relation to entitlements that vary between lump sums of 150 Euro up to 1,700 Euro per month depending on assessed needs, kind of services or institutions used. In Germany, entitled persons may choose between cash allowances or vouchers for services-in-kind; a majority of users are opting for cash allowances. In Austria, it is completely up to the recipients to decide whether to use the allowance to buy services or to "pay" informal or family carers. In France, the APA resembles more a voucher system as the allowance has to be used to pay for (informal) care or to co-finance residential care. Also the different forms of the Dutch "individual budget" are more or less earmarked for care – only a small share of this individual budget can be used at the discretion of the recipient, while the main share should be used to buy services, usually with the support of an Insurance Agency. Still, this form of an allowance is intended to increase the user's choice and his/her independence.

With a view on integrated care for older persons, this mechanism might obviously lead to a situation in which the person in need of care (and/or his/her family carer) becomes a kind of case manager, thus shifting the burden. Another consequence might be that the allowance ends up as part of the regular household income so that its specific use for care-related expenditures cannot be retraced and thus generates an alleged "misuse" of public funds, perhaps even by encouraging "black market labour". At the same time, cash allowances could be a first step towards a more general approach towards demand-orientation and greater differentiation, rather than an orientation to allegedly homogeneous target groups such as "older persons". In order to take full advantage of consumer-directed services, a number of preconditions have to be fulfilled (see also Kodner, 2003; Ex et al., in this book):

- Consumers' choice can only be guaranteed if the consumers achieve a considerable overview on supply – knowing that the perfect transparency does not exist, this could be achieved by means of "peer consulting", an independent counselling, initial-contact and brokerage centres (see Germany) or an "omtinker" (see The Netherlands).
- Sufficient competition between providers is another important aspect, in particular guaranteed a sufficient differentiation of services should be fostered.
- Staff have to be trained towards empowering users and service providers will have to develop more user-oriented services.
- Consumer-directed services should be designed by involving the target groups as much as possible, and
- cash allowances should be combined with other tools of integrated care provision (case and care management, joint budgets, joint working etc.).

3.5 Joint Working: Shattering the Cultural Divide

Anybody who has worked with mixed groups consisting of medical, socio-medical and social professionals knows about the cultural cleavages between these groups but also about the fact that structural and hierarchical divisions are often much more significant. Once the various professionals start talking to each other, conflicts and different perspectives often can be resolved. Still, hierarchies remain divisive and may impede development of a common understanding, for instance the definition of "autonomy", or a shared care concept. In particular, the medical orientation towards "healing" often clashes with the needs of persons who depend on long-term care. Also, wrong incentives presented by, for instance, diagnosis-related groups financing (DRG-financing) of hospitals, have contributed to the so-called "cultural" divide between health and social care systems. Furthermore, differences in status and hierarchy that are increasingly challenged by the nursing professions complicate the cooperation between medical, nursing and social care professions (Roth/Reichert, in this book).

A specific group to be addressed in relation to this are medical doctors (general practitioners) who, though having a potentially decisive role in guiding and supporting persons in need of long-term care, also in relation to the LTC insurance, refrain from fulfilling the role as a general reference person ("navigator") for both clients/patients and other service providers due to time constraints, lack of knowledge and missing returns for this task.

The Danish system of care for older persons offers some potential solutions for these aspects. First, the municipalities have to pay for patients at hospitals who have finished their treatment and are waiting for a place in a nursing home. Secondly, some municipalities have concluded cooperation contracts with hospitals stipulating that community care services have to be informed at least 3 days before a patient's discharge, if s/he needs health or social care at home. Thirdly, experiences with "geriatric teams", "mixed meetings before hospital discharge", 24-hours integrated community care and joint training present some first steps towards joint working on an equal footing. In relation to GPs, however, the Danish model rarely has them participating in formalised cooperation with either the hospital or the municipality, unless specific illnesses have to be cured.

Positive outcomes concerning joint working and improved mutual understanding are also reported by almost all model projects trying to combine social and health care services in one or the other way. The mere fact

28

that the different stakeholders are gathered around one table often helps to create an intensive exchange of ideas, trust in each other's capacities and "a new understanding of the other sectors' work (...) both groups of personnel learn from each other and can improve their performance" (Grilz-Wolf et al., in this book). In France, statutory policies have a long-standing history of incentives to support "coordination mechanisms". Based on the experiences of local implementation projects promoting "gerontological coordination", the French report underlines that, unfortunately, the process of improving communication is quite time-consuming and calls for very engaged project leaders. In one project it took about two years to succeed in getting medical doctors and social workers to work together and to gain a fresh look at given situations (Frossard et al., in this book).

Another approach towards joint working on the level of promoting the flow of information and coordination between the different organisations and institutions involved is reported from Germany where coordinating care conferences, round tables and working groups have been installed in several areas. In a broader sense these also concern the planning and structuring of care provision, and agreements on procedures at a regional or local level (Roth/Reichert, in this book).

3.6 Opening the Institutions: Towards an Integration of Housing, Welfare and Care

Future trends in social and health policy have to take into account the notion that the traditional emphasis on target groups and respective solutions will be increasingly confronted with a focus on the solution of social and health problems that regard different target groups with the same type of needs. Furthermore, the increasing migration of family members will trigger the need for new types of support systems within the neighbourhood and the community. Traditional nursing or old-age homes ("total institutions") will hardly survive in this scenario, unless they become pro-active, open and innovative neighbourhood centres providing all kinds of services and facilities to the public, and/or specialising on specific groups, e.g. persons suffering from dementia or other cognitive impairments.

The Dutch government's approach towards demand-oriented care is trying to face this challenge by promoting the concept of "care-friendly districts", i.e. areas in which explicit attention is paid to the improvement of the habitat, the infrastructure, and existing facilities (Ex et al., in this book). Generally, this approach concerns the housing/care interface that has often been neglected within the medical model. Indeed, if care at home is to be supported, then both housing policies and housing organisations become important factors for providing integrated care. In the Dutch reality, respective policies have led to interesting partnerships, e.g. between the Ministry of Housing, Planning and Environment, and Health, Welfare and Sports. The respective "sheltered housing stimulation arrangements" have triggered several initiatives. For instance, housing corporations are, in cooperation with municipalities and institutions for care and welfare, modernising existent residential and nursing homes into new care centres. They are also developing new sheltered care facilities, preferably in cooperation with private funders (op.cit.).

Also the Greek "Open Care Centres for the Elderly" (KAPI) are emphasising the neighbourhood and its social capital to rebuild social solidarity as a part of integrated care provision. KAPIs aim at preventing isolation of the elderly; they should contribute to increase the ability of older citizens to remain active members of society. As mediating centres KAPIs are connecting the elderly to and within their social environment, thus promoting an integrated centre for prevention, health promotion, and social integration (Sissouras et al., in this book).

3.7 Supporting Informal (Family) Care

The role of families and/or informal carers in creating integrated care networks is crucial to their success. This is equally true for prevention and the actual care process as no care system will ever be able to completely cover all long-term care needs by professionalised services. While informal care was, for a long time, taken for granted by service providers, a number of initiatives now exist to ameliorate this situation. These mechanisms range from cash benefits (UK, some regions in Italy) and pension grants (Germany) to training and information, employment (Nordic countries), and respite services such as day-care or short-term care that can be found in almost all countries although availability of these services tends to be very poor.

It is important to notice that, due to the prevailing "family ethics", in those countries where family care is most important (in particular Mediterranean countries) only minor efforts to integrate family carers in providing systems are being observed (Sissouras et al., in this book). Concepts promoted by the EU such as, for instance, social inclusion, subsidiarity and solidarity should help to improve this situation.

The integration of informal care therefore remains a critical area for integrated care delivery, partly due to the fact that family carers often do not even define themselves as carers, and also because professionals in many cases see the family of the person in need of care as an opponent, rather than as a resource.

With the rising number of non-family informal carers, who are often immigrants from outside the EU – and the related problems of "black market employment", "illegal immigration" and consequent poor continuity[4] of care – it becomes more and more urgent to develop strategies of integration and collaboration with the formal health and social care system (see also Motel-Klingebiel et al., 2002; Nesti et al., in this book). To date, no convincing integration strategy has yet been developed, apart from some ambiguous experiences with health professionals (nurses) being "imported" from the Philippines, China, Tunisia or other countries from outside the EU.

31

3.8 Quality Management as an Instrument to create Mutually Agreed Outcomes?

The considerable success of industrial quality certification systems (ISO 9000, EFQM, Total Quality Management, Business Re-engineering) has had a significant impact on the delivery of person-centred and social services during the 1990s, with the consequence that the impetus of case management and coordination issues – one of the most discussed concepts in social policy research during the 1980s – has moved somewhat into the background. With the ongoing market- and managerial orientation it seemed as if public services and social services in particular could catch up in their professional and societal image only by taking on board the "professional approaches" coming from the business-based concepts (for a critical comment see Evers, 1997; Pollitt, 1997). This certainly had a number of positive effects on the changing "culture of care" such as, for instance, an increasing user orientation, a clearer focus on objectives and outcomes, re-organisation processes towards more autonomy of teams and working-groups as against hierarchical decision-making and bureaucratic planning and controlling.

Indeed, quality management can also help to improve inter-organisational coordination if, for instance, indicators and standards concerning structure, process and outcome of different providers or agencies are defined in commonly agreed proceedings, and if the specificities of social and health service provision are recognised during this exercise.

Examples for such an approach can be found in Finland both in terms of a top-down strategy and in bottom-up models. The Finnish Ministry of Social Affairs and Health has addressed the quality issues since the year 2000 by providing a "National Framework for High-quality Care and Services for Older People" and recommendations for quality improvement by involving the municipalities. Single municipalities and projects have used quality management methods in ongoing restructuring and reform processes, e.g. the "Kuopio" project (see for further information Salonen/Haverinen, 2003).

In general, quality management and certification processes have mainly been introduced by single organisations (ISO certification by private non-profit providers in Austria, Germany, Italy and the UK), strategic development processes towards integration by means of quality assurance have been reported to a minor extent (see Alaszewski at al in this book). In Germany, quality management tools have been increasingly applied (Reichert/Roth, in this book; Schubert/Zink, 1997; Reis/Schulze-Böing, 2000) both in the health sector and in connection with the introduction of the long-term care insurance. At the same time, the introduction of a more mixed economy of welfare in Italy triggers the development of regional accreditation systems for social services that are usually based on quality management approaches (Nesti et al., in this book; Bertin, 2002).

3.9 Different Strategies and Instruments to Achieve Integrated Care Systems in Selected EU Member States

Table 3 tries to sketch the situation of key innovations that are underpinning and/or signalling the implementation of integrated care approaches in the participating countries. This assessment is based on the PROCARE national reports and should thus be read as work in progress. However, the overview helps to explain differences and similarities that often run counter to the usual division of welfare state regimes. For instance, the fact that in a "latecomer" country such as Italy quality management and accreditation systems are on the agenda as clearly as in Germany or the UK, is at least as surprising as the fact that Greece, apart from Denmark, is the only country where an explicit approach towards prevention has been developed.

Table 3:   The Status of Different Strategies and Instruments to Achieve Integrated Care Systems in Selected EU Member States

	A	D	DK	EL	F	FIN	I	NL	UK
Case and care management	*	*	***			**	*	**	***
Intermediate care	*	*	**			**	*	**	**
Multiprofessional needs assessment and joint planning			**		**	**	**	**	***
Consumer directed services: personal budget/long-term care insurance	***	***	*		**			***	*
Joint working	*	*	***		*	**	*	**	**
Admission prevention and guidance		*	***	**				**	**
Integrating housing, welfare and care	*	*	***	*	*	**	*	**	*
Integration of family carers (incl. targeted respite schemes, employment)	*	**		*	**	**	*		*
Independent counselling	*	**			*			**	*
Coordinating care conferences		*	**		*				**
Quality management/assurance	*	**	*		**	**	**	*	**

Denotation: ***) broadly perceived and applied as a mainstream method; national standard; **) partly implemented on a local or regional level; *) applied in an experimental stage (model projects).
Source: PROCARE National reports.

33

Again, this overview is intended to show that different combinations of "instruments" or methods can be used to achieve integrated care, depending on national traditions and local conditions. It could nevertheless be suggested that in countries where more methods of integration are being adopted, the political will to achieve development of an integrated service delivery is likely to be stronger.

4 Integrating Health and Social Care Services in Different National Contexts

4.1 The Legal and Structural Framework

The differentiation between health and social care services starts in all countries from the fact that health matters are usually regulated by a specific ministry in the framework of a national health system (UK, Greece, Italy, Nordic countries) or a national social insurance system (Austria, France, Germany, Netherlands), while social care issues are tackled within the social assistance systems that are, depending on respective decentralisation, usually administrated by regional or local entities. In theory, this division of labour is most sensible as social services should be organised as close to the citizen as possible. In the absence of a national framework law, however, this kind of decentralisation in many countries has led to situations where the right to health is defined more broadly than the right to social care – the UK is an example of a system where regulation has become more centralised, while the Netherlands provides an example where national framework legislation and policies are in line with decentralised organisational and provider structures.

Although specific legislation on integrated care is scarce, we can observe an increasing number of policies and respective legislation with respect to long-term care financing and organisation. On the one hand, the number of countries with long-term care schemes has grown remarkably during the last decade (Evers et al., 1994; Pacolet et al., 2000). For a long time only the Netherlands provided for a comprehensive social assurance based funding mechanism for long-term care, whilst countries like Austria, Germany and France started to install specific schemes during the 1990s. In addition, a new scheme was recently introduced in the Netherlands to provide for a "personal budget".

The general trend of these provisions is to allow for cash payments to the person in need of care – not only older persons – and/or their family carers as a way to acknowledge the role of family care and the fact that a complete professionalisation of long-term care will not be feasible. Furthermore, such schemes offer persons in need of care the opportunity to decide more independently on which kinds of services to use. For the integration of services, such schemes are obviously ambiguous as the clients may now

34

choose more independently whether and which kind of service to use. Some of these schemes, in particular the German Long-term Care Insurance and the French "APA", are – at least partly – based on voucher systems.

These trends have nevertheless called for more defined coordination mechanisms between providers or between national and regional levels. In those systems where free market mechanisms have been introduced, accreditation systems and quality control have been developed because the role of public administration was changing from a provider to a "purchaser" of services. Increasingly, public administration authorities seek to increase their steering capacities to guarantee and control services, rather than to produce them directly. While in some countries, this approach can build on a long tradition of third-sector organisations that have always provided an important part of social services (e.g. Germany, Austria, the Netherlands), for both Nordic and Mediterranean countries this development has gained in importance under the title of extended "privatisation" of hitherto public services. This general trend towards "new public management" is producing very exciting results as it is applied in all types of social and health systems in Europe.

Therefore, we can find remarkable legislative initiatives concerning "contracting out", quality control and the promotion of new types of commercial and, in particular, non-profit providers. For instance, in Italy, a national framework law "for an integrated system of interventions and social services" was introduced in the year 2000 in order to regulate, on the one hand, the relationship between public administration and private non-profit providers and, on the other hand, to call for an integrated planning and the coordinated provision of health and social services within so-called "social zones" (districts covering several municipalities within a health district). From 2004/5 onwards regional health and social budgets will be based on respective plans of the social zones so that all actors are given an incentive to participate in round-table discussions and other participative planning procedures.

"Regulating by incentives" can also be observed in other countries. In Germany, where the free market of care services was unleashed with the introduction of the LTCI, providers have to comply with minimum standards and are invited to participate in regional "care conferences" and in ongoing negotiations on quality assurance. In the Netherlands, where the government tries to implement an increasingly demand-driven policy, "care-friendly districts", i.e. areas in which explicit attention is paid to the improvement of the living surroundings, infrastructure, and facilities, are promoted by means of model projects. Those projects that are aiming at improving the interfaces between housing, care, and service are subsidised, thus enhancing interagency-cooperation.

Also in other countries the quest for coordination mechanisms is more based on incentives than on general legislation. The Finnish Ministry of Social Affairs and Health – one of very few examples in Europe where both competences are combined in one ministry – has addressed quality issues by providing a "National Framework for High Quality Care and Services for Older People" as part of the current national "Target and Action Plan". In France, the Ministry for Employment and Social Solidarity promotes local information and coordination centres ("Centres Locaux d'Information et de Coordination"/CLIC) as a means to introduce a more systematic orientation towards joint working (information, assessment, implementation and monitoring) by socio-medical teams. In Greece, and this is partly a first influence of the PROCARE project, a new law on "integrated health and social care services" is currently in the making.

4.2   Legal and Structural Barriers

All these initiatives by central governments show that there is growing awareness towards the need for integrated care provision. However, in general these services are regulated and provided within decentralised structures. Responsibilities are not only divided between "ministries" (health on the one side, and social affairs on the other) but also between central, regional, district and local levels. The lack of federal legislation is therefore only a minor shortcoming, given the enormous regional differences in service provision within the countries. Even in Denmark, a small country with a most developed national care policy for older persons, the responsibilities of implementing health and social policy have been delegated to the counties and municipalities – with resulting inequalities and local differences in budgets and quality.

The Austrian and the German reports provide some illuminating examples of barriers to coordination and integration that stem from decentralised decision-making. In both countries, decentralisation is "doubled" by the fact that social and health insurances are "self-governed" bodies with particular (corporatist) power structures. In Germany, for instance, health insurance companies may now hold contracts directly with selected cross-sector provider networks (physicians in private practice, hospitals, outpatient care and rehabilitation services, etc.) in order to "integrate" outpatient and inpatient care. The primary interest is, of course, to curb cost expansion but nevertheless the *implementation* of the regulation is still not settled as different financial regulations and segmented budgets for outpatient and inpatient provisions continue to exist. In Austria, the division between "cure" and "long-term care" services is particularly strict. For instance, social health insurance funds only a small segment of out-patient services, i.e. those that are prescribed by the general practitioner and defined as preventing hospital care.

Also in France the national incentives to develop CLICs often clashes with the standard organisation of social services on the local/regional level, in particular with the regional implementation of the "autonomy allowance" (APA).

The lack of joint budgets and the differences in financing health and long-term care are generally named as the most significant problems towards integration of service provision in all countries. The concurrent problems in financing health care and the various health reforms to curb cost expansion are hardly ever combined with considerations on long-term care, although "bedblocking", repeated examinations, unnecessary referrals, selective treatment strategies, revolving door effects, technology orientation etc. were identified as the most important cost drivers. Still, long-term care budgets, if reflected in national budgets at all, make up a share of 5 to 20% of general health expenditures in the participating countries. The long-term care sector can then be considered a "latecomer" in social protection systems, and remains relatively poorly developed, partly because resources are usually directed initially towards the predominant problem of financing health care.

The Role of Different Stakeholders

In order to understand the complexity in developing integrated care networks we would like to underline a few features concerning the different stakeholders and the vested interests, concerns, worries and expectations that were mentioned in the national reports.

Given the huge number of boundaries at which the different stakeholders cooperate in funding, contracting, providing and controlling, it becomes difficult to gather them around one table and to arrive at mutually-agreed visions, procedures and objectives. Steering these players by means of market mechanisms – a strategy followed in many countries – does not necessarily lead to positive results for all parties. Obviously, it is more difficult to reach common grounds when more actors are present. In Germany, for example, a long tradition of third-sector organisations has resulted in a further fragmentation of the already shattered responsibilities between social insurance, regions and the state. The added complexity of introducing a free market of care should therefore be approached with caution – in any case, it is essential to develop steering mechanisms (accreditation, quality assurance) that harness providers towards mutually-agreed objectives. Competition is an unhealthy feature that can interfere with integrated service provision, particularly if shared guidelines are missing.

A commonly observed phenomenon of financing is the attempt to shift financial burdens between different funders. The specific mix of private and public funding, together with the different types of user contributions in European health and social care present an interesting policy issue. However, the existing systems lack transparency, and generally fail to provide the clear evidence required to open a fruitful public dialogue. An example is provided by the recently introduced long-term care insurances or benefits in Germany and Austria, which did not generate such a debate – even though both countries have stressed that the provisions from these schemes will only be able to cover a percentage of the costs incurred if the client becomes fully dependent.

The question "who does what" thus remains unresolved both on the structural (political) level and on the "shop-floor" level. On the one hand, for instance, providers or even single professional groups are often forced to acquire contracts and reimbursement from different agencies for the same activity. On the other hand, in most countries, residential and nursing homes have to "compete" for financing from the same budget as community services. Instead of using this kind of contracting for a coordinated or integrated policy in cooperation with the providers, public administrations seem to favour the *"divide et impera"* doctrine. In particular, this doctrine tends to divide the different professional groups, with health care professionals who traditionally have a better regulated educational and job profile, higher pay and higher status than staff in the area of long-term care for the elderly. The respective consequences for the ability and willingness of professional groups in health and long-term care to cooperate and work together can easily be inferred.

Nevertheless, the actual and/or imminent shortage of labour in caring professions might serve to reassure staff about job security, increase the quality of working conditions and improve the image of careers in the social and health sectors. An open question in this respect remains how to integrate informal (and black market) care-giving into the network.

Moving towards user-oriented integrated care delivery necessitates the inclusion of the public, clients and users of services in policy-making, local debates and regional care conferences. Even though it is extremely difficult to gain access to carers and/or care-dependent persons, consultation of this kind is a prerequisite in the formation of a functional equivalent to traditional family-based care. Examples from the Netherlands (one-stop-window and neighbourhood centres), Greece (KAPI) and France (small housing units) show some interesting approaches towards the involvement of the civil society and older persons themselves in developing services and participating in decision-making. Future generations of older persons will certainly be even better informed and they will be prepared to express their needs and expectations as critical and well-informed patients or clients. Thus, the input of "consumer organisations" that act as representatives of clients and client groups will be pivotal to future service development.

4.3   *Current Debates and New Policies*

Given the current context of economic and social policy developments, the debate on integrated provision of health and social care mainly focuses on health care reforms and respective instruments to prevent cost expansion. In a wider context, these kinds of reform discourses have increasingly been based upon market-driven considerations with the aim of reducing supply (for example, of hospital beds by DRG-financing), and to regulate demand (by the introduction or expansion of user fees and other mechanisms to prevent uptake). However, the introduction of quasi-markets in the health realm did not automatically lead to an "integrated" thinking. It rather directed health managers (and politicians) to keep on thinking in health care terms, and to externalise costs towards the long-term care sector without respective shifts in financing and payments. For instance, some reports (see Austria, UK, Germany) made it clear that the reduction of hospital beds and DRG-financing in all countries led to an increased pressure on long-term care services, in particular community care, and that the community sector was further challenged because its client group has increasingly greater

39

medical dependency.[5] Compared to the health care sector, there are only small groups with less political influence that are advocating in favour of social care issues.

What we can observe, therefore, is the development of two separated "quasi-markets", one in the health sector, and the other in the social care sector. As new public management approaches have now also reached social service sectors, competition, cost-efficiency and quality management have contributed to a more competitive management also in social care, thus perhaps creating a basis for a common language to be adopted in integrated care provision.

Are Market Mechanisms Hampering Integrated Care Provision?

At first sight, however, it seems that market mechanisms are preventing integrated care provision. For instance, in the UK the introduction of competitive markets – in the absence of a single health and social care budget – posed a problem to those who were to purchase "continuing care" for patients with long-term support needs. Tensions between acute hospitals and other services, between different providers and with respect to "the lead role" in assessing and implementing care packages have been reported (Lock, 1996; Hudson/Henwood, 2002; see Coxon et al., in this book), thus underlining the social and health care divide, rather than creating incentives for joint working. This experience of market mechanisms without common rules and budgets, for which the UK is the most clear example, should prevent other countries from following a similar path, yet one consequence of this experience has been that a wide debate about joint working now exists in the UK. With its 1999 Health Act the British government has tried to overcome the existing impediments to joint working by allowing for pooled budgets, lead commissioning and integrated providers, thereby initiating a centralised attempt to steer decentralised services. Further policy developments in the UK include the ending of the "quasi market" in health care, and a concerted attempt to promote inter-agency partnership within health and social care.

These developments have contributed to our general impression of a new phase in the debates on integrated care. While most countries related in their national reports that their governments had paid lip service to the prevention of institutional care for a long time, there is now growing evidence of a political change in relation to this issue. Examples include:

- The discourse on "seamless care" (Burda, 1992) that can now be found in many policy documents (e.g. UK, Finland).
- The focus on "intermediate care" (Vaughan/Lathlean, 1999; Department of Health, 2002; see Coxon et al., in this book) and "joint working" (see Ex et al., in this book, for an extended approach of "extramuralisation"; see also Jedeloo et al., 2001).
- The multitude of model projects in the area of coordination and integration might be interpreted as a further milestone towards solutions, even if these projects often lack strategies for follow-up, organisational learning and their translation into mainstream practice.

The Role of Institutional Care

An old feature within the discourse on integration of services is the dichotomy between institutional and community care. The widespread view that "care at home is better than institutional care" has tended to contribute to a situation that impedes rather than facilitates processes of integration. Indeed, a number of scandals and even homicides in nursing homes have highlighted potential negative consequences of institutionalisation and hospitalisation – although incidents of harm and abuse involving family carers may of course be far less frequently reported. Incidents within care institutions have, however, also triggered a number of reforms, innovations and improvements in the residential sector. Still, it is not easy to motivate and sustain staff in institutional care if professionals are constantly confronted with the dreadful image of residential or nursing homes. The discourse on integrated care may contribute to the "either-or" debate by repositioning the role of institutional care in the "chain of care".

From a European perspective, however, we have to be aware that different realities do exist close to each other. While in the Northern countries institutional care makes up to 12% of the provision – and still faces the problem of waiting lists (see Dutch report: Ex et al., in this book) – in the Southern European countries much lower shares of institutional care are on offer (about 3% of older persons are living in institutions in Italy, respectively less than 1% in Greece; see Italian and Greek reports: Nesti et al., in this book; Sissouras et al., in this book). Thus, expansion of institutional care is much more on the agenda in these countries. In Denmark, the construction of residential institutions became prohibited by law and thus has come to a halt; while in the Netherlands major reforms of the institutional sector have been

41

put in place ("extra-muralisation"). In France and other countries "small units" and "assisted living schemes" are being promoted whilst Southern European policy-makers strive, first of all, for a quantitative increase, in particular with respect to the private residential care sector.

In this situation it is high time to develop general standards (also on the European level) concerning accreditation criteria, quality assurance and strategies that promote the inclusion of residential settings in local service networks. The current situation is that some countries are reducing their levels of residential care, whilst others are actively expanding this type of provision, and fundamental issues of quality assurance regularly emerge whenever residential care is proposed. This situation has a knock-on effect on hospital and domiciliary services, both of which have extra boundaries to negotiate when dealing with an additional, privatised resource in the older persons' care sector.

Long-term Care: From "Poor Law" to Citizen's Rights?

42

It is interesting to draw a direct link from improvements in the residential sector to considerations on citizens' rights and integrated service delivery. The strict division between the right to "cure" and the discretionary provisions of social care services has become more and more cynical, in particular in countries with a well-established health system – this remains true whether the health system is based on social insurance (e.g. Austria, Germany and France) or a centralised "national health system" (e.g. Italy, UK). Within all these countries, policies began to shift long-term care from "poor law" provisions towards formal legal systems which have established criteria for quality and financing. In Germany, the LTCI brought long-term care directly in line with health care services, even though different mechanisms of guaranteeing services have been implemented. Also France is moving in that direction, while in Austria the tradition of cash allowances – still based on citizens' rights – was reinforced and financing was guaranteed by the general budget, rather than social insurance. A special case is Finland, where a "National programme for social services to enhance old people's rights to services" is underlining the commitment to improving old-age care (Salonen/Haverinen, in this book).

Still, most of these initiatives are approaching long-term care issues in a distinct cost containment manner, rather than trying to integrate funds and funding mechanisms. This might be due to the fact that most policy-makers try to govern the increasing demand by means of supply-driven policies and mechanisms. Little by little, however, we can observe that first trends towards "demand-driven" policies are beginning to flourish, that is, initiatives that start integration from a user's perspective and from the needs expressed by the users. Examples can be found in Denmark, where prevention is taken seriously by means of "preventative visits of older persons at their homes", but also in Greece, where new programmes with respect to "home care", "Open Care Centres for the Elderly" (KAPI) and new legal initiatives concerning integrated care have been launched. Furthermore, a clear statement towards "demand-driven" policies can be found in the Netherlands, where attempts to identify "hidden care demand" are being made, and a promising step towards integrated services is being taken in the UK, where jointly budgeted health and social care organisations ("care trusts") are on the agenda. The potential difficulty for policy development is that measuring the success of preventative or user-led initiatives is notoriously difficult and this can lead to services that are relatively expensive being curtailed or withdrawn. This means that the opportunity to establish the potential contribution such services make either to disease prevention or to improving an older person's quality of life is frequently lost, and such innovations are regularly re-invented with a short-term lifespan.

43

It follows that many if not most of the initiatives towards integrated care delivery remain in a phase of model projects – and often do not become part of mainstream service provision. Indeed, there is already a long tradition of model projects (with and without evaluation studies) in most of the participating countries. In many cases, these model projects withered away after two or three years, even if results seemed promising. In other cases, and not the least, integration projects failed anyway due to one or the other variable that had been omitted and/or not respected. In both cases, however, experiences faded away with the persons who had been involved and follow-ups were rare. Real organisational learning strategies could not be found but it is no coincidence that many national reports are referring a "new wave" of model projects to be implemented presently.

5 Conclusions: Ambiguities, Necessary Debates and Future Perspectives

What theoretically reads as quite logical and convincing does not necessarily mean that practice is following the allegedly "logical" path. The hypothetical gains of integrated care networks and delivery are difficult to evaluate in terms of scientific research designs. To produce comprehensive evidence of the relative cost-efficiency and cost-effectiveness of services across the countries studied, modelling and evaluating the production functions of social care services would be complex, expensive, and it would require longitudinal studies of large national samples (Davies et al., 2000). On the other hand, even with smaller samples and a fine control-group design it often turns out that (not always) better outcomes cannot be clearly connected to the delivery system (see, for instance, Hultberg et al., 2002). Nevertheless, policy documents in most countries stress the need for integrated services, identifying that "care at home is better than institutional care". However, long-term strategies and solutions building on gained experience and evidence from single model projects are scarce. As an exception, in Denmark, the "Skævinge Project" served as a valid inspiration for the organisation of health and social care in other municipalities with the Ministry of Social Affairs as a promoter and disseminator of good practice. In most other countries, model projects are badly documented, not always evaluated and often stopped without any follow-up activities.

It seems logical, though, to continue linking the development of integrated health and social care policies (joint structures, training, funding) to integrated delivery of services. To date, the allegedly unanimous policies in Europe with respect to long-term care have lacked coherent strategies. Indeed, there is no relevant policy paper that fails to underline that persons in need of care should be supported as long as possible in living at home: residential homes should be reduced, different kinds of providers and services (day-care, short-term care) should be supported, new services are to be developed, social inclusion should be guaranteed, preventative services and person-oriented guidance and assistance are to be extended. Furthermore, family and informal care are to be strengthened, and the whole system of providers should be "coordinated".

However, concrete implementation programmes with priority lists and clear objectives are often missing. In the context of general restrictions to public spending, innovation funds and/or targeted investments remain scarce. Usually, strategies remain restricted to model projects (or even programmes) with a limited time frame, restricted finances and hardly ever any follow-up activities. As a corollary, projects are often under pressure to "produce" results and do not have time for dialogue between persons/organisations involved to develop common grounds and a shared vision.

Dialogues at the front line that involve staff, users and civil society, have not yet been used efficiently to discuss priorities and local needs. However, the almost 50 model ways of working gathered in the nine country reports, also allow for some general lessons to be learned:

- Reforms that intend to integrate health and welfare services must be founded on the integration of financing systems and the overcoming of institutional barriers, especially between outpatient and inpatient care, between health and welfare services, and between professional and informal care.

- Geriatric screening and multidimensional assessment are part of modernising the system in many countries (e.g. Germany, Italy, France, Finland, the Netherlands, the UK and Denmark) – it can be incorporated into practice without too much difficulty, it meets with a high level of acceptance, and it helps to involve different kinds of professions and to improve communication between them.

- Demand-driven, integrated care has to strive to increase clients' control over the care process, e.g. by way of "individual budgets" or other means that increase their purchasing and negotiation power. However, if not combined with other instruments, "cash for care" may also lead to a reduction of public responsibilities and thus a decrease in service provision.

- Innovation programmes promoted by central government can trigger a number of private and local initiatives – a vision of support that goes beyond the traditional notion of care, and integrates care and nursing, adapted housing, local resources, and welfare services (see, for instance, the Finnish national programme). Top-down initiatives should only exist to support bottom-up change processes.

- A central service point for advice, information and help is useful to support clients in clarifying their care needs and to improve cooperation between different organisations that operate according to different logics and have different types of personnel. It is of utmost importance to help staff in developing a new understanding of the other sectors' work.

45

- The success of model projects often depends on the engagement of staff involved and on the structural framework of the projects – clear objectives, competences and guidelines are needed to function successfully. The institutional structure may ease the process of integration, e.g. if institutional care, home help and home nursing are managed by the same agency such as the municipality (Denmark). Also in Greece, it is local authorities that are responsible for the development and implementation of integrated projects (KAPI) as they have first-hand knowledge of the needs of the elderly living in their area.
- Change processes are very time-consuming as it might take years to get a project started and to construct common grounds of working.
- Evaluation has become a common practice. In France, for instance, the evaluation of private and public projects in social and health care has become compulsory. Investment must be accompanied by a programme of reform and modernisation involving the development of greater cooperation and collaboration within and between sectors and joint working practices.
- Collaboration between hospitals and municipalities can be organised in many ways, depending on motivation and existing cooperation. It is not possible though to emphasise the best practice or the best model for cooperation or to expect that a general model can be implemented in all countries.

Perspectives: More Market, Management and IT –
Or More Civil Society?

It is impossible to predict future developments but some trends and their potential impact can nevertheless be outlined. The marketisation track will surely increase with more voucher systems, payments for care and steering mechanisms that try to make use of demand and supply mechanisms. We know, however, that health and care are no more than quasi-markets with their own characteristics and criteria. It will therefore be important to increase regulation (accreditation mechanisms, quality assurance) with respect to providers and, in particular, in relation to employment and human resource development to reduce "black market work" and to increase clients' control over the care process.

In this respect, the importance of management and related tasks will also be enhanced. On the one hand, both social and health staff will have to perform more managerial work in addition to direct care which might also lead to new specialisations and new job profiles, e.g. with respect to case and care management. On the other hand, the necessity of developing steering mechanisms on the national, regional and local level will call for more managerial decision-making with respect to commissioning, contracting, purchasing, planning, evaluating and quality assurance mechanisms.

These developments might be accompanied by a more fervent introduction of information technology, also in the area of social care. Indeed, the "techno track" has already begun with respect to tele-care devices, with the introduction of information technology in the organisation of care processes and the construction of "smart homes".

Even the most advanced technology, though, will not be able to replace human resources and local social inclusion. Therefore, two other evolutionary tracks might be of interest to the development of integrated care. On the one hand, new types of volunteering and new kinds of support networks (intra- and inter-generational) might be interesting resources to build up respectively. On the other hand, shortage of labour in the care professions, illegal immigration and black market work in care will call for new forms of integration and an even extended notion of integrated care networks.

Much will depend on the general development of labour markets and the behaviour of women with respect to family care: Will the Mediterranean countries follow the pattern of the Nordic countries? And if so, to what extent will integrated policies be developed to compensate for the loss of unpaid female labour?

The Role of Research and Development

It has already been suggested that conducting model projects is one of the most frequently applied strategies to develop integrated care networks. Such projects are often accompanied and evaluated by scientific research. Still, many of these projects remain without any documentation or evaluation, and in most cases there is not enough funding for a real evaluation of outcomes and lessons to learn. Compared to medical research, scientific research concerning community care or integrated service delivery is weakly funded and almost not at all published. Denmark, Finland and the UK are countries where targeted R&D programmes can be identified, and have some influence on the practice of organising services. In most other countries, research remains somewhat distinct from practice, and development projects in the area of integrated care organisation depend heavily on single decision-makers and selective project funding. In order to develop evidence-based solutions it will therefore be necessary to improve research and development, in particular with respect to evaluation methods and in relation to the fact that complex change processes need special skills and respective accompanying measures (see, for instance, Broome, 1998).

It is in this context that PROCARE will carry out further investigations, in particular by looking at model ways of working that have been shown to overcome existing barriers and to resolve everyday problems in the cooperation between health and social services. In the end, it will be such examples that will shape the future development of integrated service provision together with public policies that are aware of their responsibility in providing a decent framework for modernisation and reform.

Notes

1   To name but a few examples, we would like to draw the reader's attention to initiatives in the context of the WHO European Office for Integrated Health Care Services (see http://www.euro.who.int/ihb and http://www.ijic.org; Delnoij et al., 2002; van Raak et al., 2003), the Thematic Network in the EU 5th Framework Programme "Managing the integration of services for older people" (CARMEN) but also the activities of the EU Social Protection Committee on "Future strategies on health care and care for the elderly: guaranteeing accessibility, quality and financial viability".

2   Also a current OECD study is investigating into this issue; see Hurst et al., 2003.

3   Not to speak of the additional assessment procedures concerning invalidity pensions/benefits.

4   A relatively widespread practice seems to become that persons from Third World countries are accomplishing full-time care of older persons in EU countries travelling with tourist visa (valid for 3 months). Specialised agencies then cater for a replacement every 3 months (see for instance, Nesti et al., in this book).

5   This phenomenon is also reported for Sweden (see Andersson/Karlberg, 2000), where the "Ädel"-reform succeeded in reducing the number of persons waiting for discharge from the hospital but triggered increasingly heavy burdens on nursing homes and community care.

References

Andersson, G./Karlberg, I. (2000) 'Integrated Care for the Elderly. The Background and Effects of the Reform of Swedish Care of the Elderly', *International Journal of Integrated Care*, Vol. 0/November (http://www.ijic.org).

Audit Commission (2002) *Integrated Services for Older People: Building a Whole System Approach in England*. London: Audit Commission.

Badelt, Ch./Leichsenring, K. (1998) *Analyse und mögliche Neustrukturierung der Sozialausbildungen in Österreich*. Wien: Bundesministerium für Wissenschaft und Verkehr/Bundesministerium für Unterricht und kulturelle Angelegenheiten.

Ballew, J.R./Mink, G. (1991) 'Was ist case management?', pp. 56-83 in: Wendt, W.R. (Hg.) *Unterstützung fallweise: Case management in der Sozialarbeit*. Freiburg im Breisgau: Lambertus.

Barr, O. (1996) 'A Consideration of the Nature of 'Needs-Led Service' Within Care Management in the UK', *Online Journal of Issues in Nursing* (http://www.nursingworld.org/ojin/tpc2/tpc2_1.htm).

Bertin, G. (a cura di) (2002) *Accreditamento e regolazione dei servizi sociali*. Padova: emme&erre libri.

Block, S./Skrobacz, W. (2002) 'In Dialog treten: Dienstleistungen vernetzen. Hilfen effektiver und effizienter anbieten', *Häusliche Pflege*, Nr. 3: 21-24.

Broome, A. (1998, 2nd edition) *Managing Change*. London: MacMillan Press (Essentials of nursing management).

Bundesministerium für Familie, Senioren, Frauen und Jugend (BMFSFJ) (2000) *Case Management – Erfahrungen aus neun Ländern: Materialband und Workshop-Diskussion*. Köln: Kohlhammer.

Burda, D. (1992) '"Seamless" Delivery', *Modern Healthcare*, Vol. 19: 38-42.

Challis, D. et al. (eds) (2002) *Care Management in Social and Primary Health Care: the Gateshead Community Care Scheme*. Aldershot: Ashgate.

Cichon, M./Jesse, A./Pal, K. (1998) 'Preparing for Ageing Societies? An Attempt to Evaluate Pension and Long-term Care Reforms in Europe', pp. 23-58 in: ISSA (ed) *Social Security Documentation. European Series*, No. 26.

Coxon, K./Billings, J./Alaszewski, A. (2003) *Integrated Health and Social Care for Older Persons: Theoretical and Conceptual Issues*. Canterbury/Kent: CHSS (www.euro.centre.org/procare).

Daatland, S.O./Herlofson, K. (eds.) (2001) *Ageing, Intergenerational Relations, Care Systems and Quality of Life – An Introduction to the OASIS Project*. Oslo: NOVA.

Davies, B. (1992) *Care Management, Equity and Efficiency: The International Experience*. Kent: University of Kent at Canterbury/PSSRU.

Davies, B.P./Fernandez, J.L./Nomer, B. (2000) *Equity and Efficiency Policy in Community Care: Needs, Service Productivities, Efficiencies and their Implications*. Aldershot: Ashgate.

Delnoij, D.M.J./Glasgow, I.K./Klazinga, N.S./Custers, T. (2001) *Gezondheid, zorg en stelsel. AMC/UvA-achtergrondstudie bij vraag en aanbod*. Den Haag: Ministerie van Volksgezondheid, Welzijn en Sport.

Delnoij, D./Klazinga, N./Glasgow, I.K. (2002) 'Integrated Care in an International Perspective: EUPHA Proceedings December 2001', *International Journal of Integrated Care*, no. 2 (http://www.ijic.org/cgi-bin/pw.cgi/2002-3/000122/article_content.htm).

Department of Health (2000) *The NHS Plan: A Plan for Investment. A Plan for Reform*. London: Department of Health.

49

Department of Health (2002) *National Service Framework for Older People: Supporting Implementation: Intermediate Care: Moving Forward*. London: Department of Health.

Economic Policy Committee (2001) *Budgetary Challenges Posed by Ageing Population*. Retrieved from http://europa.eu.int/comm/economy_finance/publications/european_economy /reportsandstudies0401_en.htm.

Emke-Poulopoulou, I. (1999) *Greek Old Citizens, Past, Present and Future*. Athens: Ellin.

Esping-Andersen, G. (1990) *The Three Worlds of Welfare Capitalism*. New York: Polity Press.

Evers, A./Wintersberger, H. (1990) *Shifts in the Welfare Mix. Their Impact on Work, Social Services and Welfare Policies. Contributions from Nine European Countries*. Frankfurt/New York: Campus.

Evers, A./Pijl, M./Ungerson, C. (eds) (1994) *Payments for Care. A European Overview*. Aldershot: Ashgate.

Evers, A./Olk, T. (1996) 'Von der pflegerischen Versorgung zu hilfreichen Arrangements. Strategien der Herstellung optimaler Beziehungen zwischen formellem und informellen Hilfesystem im Bereich der Pflege älterer Meschen', pp. 347-372 in: Evers, A./Olk, T. (Hg.) *Wohlfahrtspluralismus*. Opladen: Westdeutscher Verlag.

Evers, A. (1997) 'Quality Development – Part of a Changing Culture of Care in Personal Social Services', pp. 9-24 in: Evers, A./Haverinen, R./Leichsenring, K./Wistow, G. (eds.) *Developing Quality in Personal Social Services. Concepts, Cases and Comments*. Aldershot: Ashgate.

Ewers, M./Schaeffer, D. (Hg.) (2000) *Case Management in Theorie und Praxis*. Bern: Huber.

Flora, P. (ed.) (1986) *Growth to Limits: The Western Welfare States Since World War II*. Berlin, New York: de Gruyter.

Freeman, R. (2000) *The Politics of Health in Europe*. Manchester: Manchester University Press.

Glendinning C./Rummery K./Clarke R. (1998) 'From Collaboration to Commissioning: Developing Relationships between Primary Health and Social Services', *British Medical Journal*, Vol. 317: 122-125.

Gröne, O./Garcia-Barbero, M. (2001) 'Integrated Care: A Position Paper of the WHO European Office for Integrated Health Care Services', *International Journal of Integrated Care*, no. 3 (http://www.ijic.org/cgi-bin/pw.cgi/2001-6/000076/article_print.html).

Grundböck, A. et al. (1997) 'Das Krankenhaus daheim', ProSenectute 3: 13-15.

Haubrock, M./Hagmann, H./Nerlinger, T. (2000) *Managed Care. Integrierte Versorgungsformen*. Bern: Hans Huber.

Hudson, B./Henwood, M. (2002) 'The NHS and Social Care: the Final Countdown?', *Policy and Politics*, Vol. 30, Nr. 2: 153-166.

Hultberg, E.-L./Lönnroth, K./Allebeck, P. (2002) 'Evaluation of the Effect of Co-financing on Collaboration between Health Care, Social Services and Social Insurance in Sweden', *International Journal of Integrated Care*, Vol. 2/October (www.ijic.org).

Huntington, J.A. (1997) 'Health Care in Chaos: Will We Ever See Real Managed Care?', *Online Journal of Issues in Nursing* (http://www.nursingworld.org/ojin/tpc2/tpc2_7.htm).

Hurst, J./Huber, M./Izumi, J./Hennessy, P. (2003) *Trends in Long-term Care in OECD Countries: Evidence from Recent OECD Studies and Preliminary Findings from a Study of 19 Countries*. Paris: OECD.

Jacobzone, S. (1999) *Ageing and Care for Frail Elderly Persons: An Overview of International Perspectives*. Paris: OECD (Labour Market and Social Policy Occasional Papers, No. 38).

Jedeloo, S./De Witte, L.P./Schrijvers, A.J.P. (2001) 'Quality of Regional Individual Assessment Agencies Regulating Access to Long-term Care Services: A Client Perspective', *International Journal of Integrated Care*, Vol. 2/June (www.ijic.org).

Kain, E. (1994) 'New Forms of Health and Social Care in Austria', pp. 12-24 in: Österreichisches Bundesinstitut für Gesundheitswesen (ed.), *New Forms of Health and Social Care: Five National Reports*. Vienna: Österreichisches Bundesinstitut für Gesundheitswesen.

Kanavos, Panos/Mossialos, Elias (1996) *The Methodology in International Comparisons of Health Care Expenditures: Any Lessons for Health Care Policy?* London: LSE Health (Discussion Paper, No. 3).

Kodner. D.L. (2003) 'Long-term Care Integration in Four European Countries: A Review', pp. 91-138 in: Brodsky, J./Habib, J./Hirschfeld, M. (eds.), *Key Policy Issues in Long-term Care*. Geneva: World Health Organization, collection on long-term care.

Kodner, D.L. (2003) 'Consumer-directed Services: Lessons and Implications for Integrated Systems of Care', *International Journal of Integrated Care*, Vol. 3/June (www.ijic.org).

Kodner, D.L./Spreeuwenberg, C. (2002) 'Integrated Care: Meaning, Logic, Applications, and Implications: A Discussion Paper', *International Journal of Integrated Care*, Vol. 2/November (www.ijic.org).

Komp, K./Strümpel, Ch./Grilz-Wolf, M. (2002) *The Understanding of Integrated Care in an International Perspective and in Austria*. Vienna: European Centre (PROCARE Working Paper, nr. 1).

van der Linden, B.A./Spreeuwenberg, C./Schrijvers, A.J.P. (2001) 'Integration of Care in The Netherlands. The Development of Transmural Care since 1994', *Health Policy*, Vol. 55, No. 2: 111-120.

Lock, K. (1996) 'The Changing Organisation of Health care: Setting the Scene', in: Twinn, S./Roberts, B./Andrews, S. (eds.) *Community Health Care Nursing: Principles for Practice* Oxford: Butterworth-Heinemann.

Ludwig Boltzmann-Institut für Medizin- und Gesundheitssoziologie (LBI) (2000) Virtuelles Krankenhaus zu Hause in Österreich (http://www.univie.ac.at/lbimgs/projekte/vh-oenb.html).

Mätzke, N./Wacker, E. (2000) 'Beratung und Fallmanagement: Information und Hilfeplanung für ältere Menschen und ihre Angehörigen', *Blätter der Wohlfahrtspflege*, Nr. 9/10: 220-222.

Motel-Klingebiel, A./Tesch-Roemer, C./von Kondratowitz, H.-J. (2002) 'The Role of Family for Quality of Life in Old Age – A Comparative Perspective', in: Bengtson, V./Lowenstein, A. (eds.) *International Perspectives on Families, Aging, and Social Support*. New York: de Gruyter.

Motel-Klingebiel, A./von Kondratowitz, H.J./Tesch-Römer, C. (2001) 'Unterstützung und Lebensqualität im Alter', pp. 201-227 in: Motel-Klingebiel, A./v. Kondratowitz, H.-J./Tesch-Römer, C. (Hg.) *Lebensqualität im Alter*. Opladen: Leske + Budrich.

Mutschler, R. (1998) 'Kooperation ist eine Aufgabe Sozialer Arbeit: Zusammenarbeit und Vernetzung als professionelle Verpflichtung – Regionale Arbeitsgruppen als Standard beruflicher Sozialarbeit', *Blätter der Wohlfahrtspflege*, Nr. 3/4: 49-52.

Niskanen, J. (2002) 'Finnish Care Integrated?', *International Journal of Integrated Care*, Vol. 2/June (www.ijic.org).

Pacolet, J./Bouten, R./Lanoye/, H./Versieck, K. (1999) *Social Protection for Dependency in Old Age in the 15 EU Member States and Norway*. Leuven: HIVA.

Pacolet, J./Bouten, R./Lanoye, H./Versieck, K. (2000) *Social Protection for Dependency in Old Age. A Study of the 15 EU Member States and Norway*. Aldershot: Ashgate.

Pollitt, C. (1997) 'Business and Professional Approaches to Quality Improvement: A Comparison of their Suitability for the Personal Social Services', pp. 25-48 in: Evers, A./Haverinen, R./Leichsenring, K./Wistow, G. (eds.) *Developing Quality in Personal Social Services. Concepts, Cases and Comments*. Aldershot: Ashgate.

van Raak, A./Mur, I./Hardy, B./Steenbergen, M. and A. Paulus (eds) (2003) *Integrated Care in Europe – Description and Comparison of Integrated Care in Six EU Countries*. Maarssen: Elsevier Gezondheidszorg.

Ranta, H. (ed) (2001) *Sosiaali- ja terveydenhuoltolainsäädäntö 2001* (Statutory social welfare and health care services 2001). Helsinki: Kauppakaari; Talentum Media Oy.

Reis, C./Schulze-Böing, M. (Hg.) (2000) *Planung und Produktion sozialer Dienstleistungen. Die Herausforderung neuer Steuerungsmodelle*. Berlin: ed. Sigma.

Schnetzler, R. (2000) 'Die Case-Managerin/der Case-Manager: ein neuer Beruf', *Managed Care* 8: 20-23.

Schubert, H.-J./Zink, K. J. (1997) *Qualitätsmanagement in sozialen Dienstleistungsunternehmen*. Neuwied usw.: Luchterhand

Seng, T. (1997) 'Managed Care – Instrumente und institutionelle Grundlagen', *Sozialer Fortschritt* 12: 289-293.

Sissouras, A./Ketsetzopoulou, M./Bouzas, N. (1998) *The Elderly in Greece: Analysis and Proposals for a National Programme*. Athens: Institute of Social Policy, National Centre for Social Research.

Steiner, A. (1997) *Intermediate Care: A Conceptual Framework and Review of the Literature*. London: King's Fund.

Steiner-Hummel, I. (1991) 'Case Management in der Altenhilfe', pp. 162-180 in: Wendt, W.R. (Hg.) *Unterstützung fallweise: Case Management in der Sozialarbeit*. Freiburg i.B.: Lambertus.

Tester, S. (1999) *The Quality Challenge: Caring for People with Dementia in Residential Institutions in Europe, A Transnational Study*. Edinburgh: Alzheimer Scotland – Action on Dementia (with Alzheimer Stichting Nederland, NZi Institute for Health Care Management, Federazione Alzheimer Italia and Fundacion Alzheimer España).

Vaughan, B./Lathlean, J. (1999) *Intermediate Care: Models in Practice*. London: King's Fund Publishing.

Wendt, W.R. (1991) 'Die Handhabung der sozialen Unterstützung. Eine Einführung in das Case Management', pp. 11-55 in: Wendt, W.R. (Hg.) *Unterstützung fallweise: Case Management in der Sozialarbeit*. Freiburg i.B.: Lambertus.

Wendt, W.R. (2001) *Case Management im Sozial- und Gesundheitswesen*. Freiburg i.B.: Lambertus.

Wendt, W.R. (2002) 'Case Management – Stand und Positionen in der Bundesrepublik', pp. 13-36 in: Löcherbach, P. et al. (Hg.) *Case Management: Fall- und Unterstützungssysteme in Theorie und Praxis*. Neuwied: Luchterhand.

Wistow, G./Waddington, E./Lai Fong Chiu (2002) *Intermediate Care: Balancing the System*. Leeds: Nuffield Institute for Health.

Zawadski, R.T. (1983) 'The Long-term Care Demonstration Projects: What They Are and Why They Came into Being', *Home Health Care Services Quarterly*, Vol. 3, No. 4: 3-19.

CHAPTER 2

Integrated Health and Social Care for Older Persons: Theoretical and Conceptual Issues

Andy Alaszewski, Jenny Billings, Kirstie Coxon

1 Introduction

This paper provides the theoretical and conceptual framework to the field-work component of the PROCARE programme. The first section explores the need for and impediments to providing integrated care for older people in Europe. The second section is a discussion of the alternative approaches and definitions of integrated care, which emphasises the importance of a person-centred approach. The third section examines the alternative ways in which the impediments to integrated care can be overcome. The last section considers ways in which integrated care can be evaluated.

1.1 Identifying the Need for and the Impediments to Integrated Care

In this section we consider the factors that make integrated support of older people particularly important and then consider the particular impediments to the provision of integrated care that often result in services for older people being more fragmented than those for younger people with similar health and social difficulties.

1.1.1 The Importance of Integrated Care for Older People

While all users of health and social care should be able to access and experience seamless or integrated care, for older service users integration is especially important. Older service users tend to suffer from a combination of health problems, and may at the same time experience increasing isolation, declining social support and increased personal vulnerability.

1.1.2 Impact of Ill Health on Older People

Ageing is associated with increasingly complex and often inter-related problems encompassing physical, psychological and social health. Older people tend to experience higher rates of chronic illness such as diabetes, heart disease or disability associated with strokes. When older people experience an acute episode of illness resulting from, for example flu or a fracture following a fall, not only is treatment more complex and based on a wider range of expertise and skills but recovery and recuperation are often slower and longer. Grimley Evans (2001: 408) has identified the following characteristics of illness in later life:

- Rapid deterioration if untreated
- High frequency of multiple disease
- Cryptic or non-specific presentation
- High incidence of secondary complications
- Frequent need for active rehabilitation
- Frequent need for help in resettling in the community

The complexity of treating older people is reflected in their length of hospital stay. In most European countries the development of a more active approach to treatment, especially surgery, has meant the average length of hospital stay has been progressively cut. For example, across PROCARE participating countries, the mean length of acute care stay in days has dropped from 10.3 in 1980 to 6.7 in 1999 (OECD data, 2002).

However, the reduction of the length of stay of older people has fallen more slowly than that for younger people with the result that in all European countries older people stay on average three times as long in hospital. For Example, in the UK the mean acute care length of stay was 6.2 days in 2000 (OECD, 2003), but the average length of stay for a person admitted to the specialty of geriatric medicine was 23.4 days (compared with 8.2 days for "general medicine", that is, medical admissions of patients younger than 60). Perhaps not surprisingly, patients admitted for "rehabilitation" had longer mean stays of 49 days (Department of Health/DoH, 2002a), and this is likely to reflect the fact that, at least in the UK, length of stay for the older person is related in part to the problems of arranging a safe discharge back to the person's own home.

This trend is also evident in surgery. Generally the majority of people being admitted for surgery are younger. UK admission figures for 2001-2002 show that only 18% of surgical patients are aged 75 or above, and only 14% of cardio-thoracic surgery patients are over 75 (DoH, 2002a). Whilst this is in some ways unsurprising given that combinations of heart and respiratory problems, arthritis, diabetes, cognitive difficulties and sensory impairments may mean that surgical and anaesthetic procedures are particularly diffi-cult for older people, there remains evidence that surgery which benefits younger persons attracts numerous performance targets, whilst waiting lists for operations such as hip replacements and cataract surgery remain long. For example, according to central government statistics, which may them-selves mask wide variations between regions, the mean waiting time for general surgery in England is 63 days, for orthopaedic surgery 170 days and for ophthalmology 144 days (DoH, 2002a).

The complexity of providing health care for older people requires col-laboration between and integration of a range of different health and social care professionals. This can be seen in relation to medication. Many older people are routinely prescribed a range of medication to manage their chronic health problems. These medications are usually prescribed and reviewed by their community physician and where necessary a community nurse will help the older person manage their medication. If an older person is admit-ted to hospital and professionals do not collaborate then there can be con-siderable problems with medication:

- New medication may be prescribed which interacts negatively with existing medication;
- Routine medication may be cut or changed without due regard to ongoing health problems;
- Ward nurses may take over the administration of all medication, deskilling the older person.
- These difficulties may be exacerbated if on discharge professionals do not collaborate and community health and social care workers are unaware of or choose to disregard the decisions made in hospital (DoH, 2001b).

When older people are acutely ill, it is often in the context of enduring long-term illness. As a result not only is their treatment complex, lengthy and expensive, it also requires the coordination of a range of skills and expertise contributed by different agencies. If these skills are not effectively integrated, there is at best inefficiency with one agency duplicating or undoing the work of another and at worst there may be serious harm for the older person because treatments interact negatively or because they fall through the welfare net.

CHALLENGES OF MAINTAINING OLDER PEOPLE'S HEALTH

While the health of older people has undoubtedly improved with people managing to remain healthier for longer, it is still the case that ageing is associated with increased risk of physical and mental disability. Such disability increases the vulnerability of older people to harm. While some risks are well recognised and documented, for example the increased risk that older people have of falling (Cryer/Patel, 2001), other risks have been recognised more recently. In the UK there is a growing awareness of and literature on elder abuse and the risks of financial exploitation, emotional harm and violence from carers and others (Stanley et al., 1999). Protecting older people from harm requires effective collaboration between emergency services such as police, fire and ambulance as well as from the more routine services.

56   There is also a subjective dimension to vulnerability. Mental well-being can be linked to a personal sense of security (Wilkinson, 2001). In modern society it is possible to identify the phenomenon of anxious or timid prosperity in which increased levels of collective safety and welfare are paradoxically associated with increased levels of anxiety about personal security (Taylor-Gooby, 2000). Increases in objective levels of "safety" do not necessarily lead to increases in perceptions of individual well-being, as demonstrated, for example, in studies of fear of crime, which consistently show that the least "at-risk" group, namely elderly females, are the most fearful (Jefferson/Holloway, 1997). The literature also indicates a relationship between physical disability and low self-esteem (Taleporos/McCabe, 2002) and a reduced perception of self-efficacy (Schieman/Campbell, 2001), which are also likely to contribute to psychological vulnerability and perception of risk. Thus if health and welfare agencies are to maximise the well-being of older people they not only need to objectively enhance safety, they need to develop means of empowering older and functionally disabled people that challenge such perceptions of risk or vulnerability.

These issues indicate a number of existing challenges to the ideal of a holistic and proactive (or preventative) approach towards helping older people stay healthy and socially integrated. In some European countries, there is evidence of policies that aspire to ever wider cross-departmental collaboration. For example, recent policy documents from the Dutch government demonstrate the growing interest in housing and welfare issues, and recognise that these issues have been neglected (Ex et al., in this book). This approach is based on the premise that the needs of older people go beyond the basic provision of care. Frail elderly people also want suitable housing, and to be able to participate in society, social contacts and recreation. There is evidence that the "person centred" approach to care which this requires is being addressed by organisations in the Netherlands. For example, a policy document of "Arcares" (the Dutch professional association of homes for the elderly) shows a person-centred approach, stating that the service providers should look at care problems within the broader perspective of the client's well-being, and that clients' unique life styles and preferences should be identified and taken into account (Arcares, 2002). Because the older person's need for care and services is integral in nature, it follows that supply should include an integral package of care, welfare and housing-services. This integral approach has led to the insight that communication between separate departments who are supplying care could lead to an overall reduction in demand. For instance, participation in activities may prevent loneliness and depression, and consequently may reduce the demand for social care.

One consequence of providing specialist accommodation (such as sheltered or warden housing) is that older people may move away from their immediate family or neighbourhood, and therefore may be both living alone and socially isolated. Even where this is a result of personal choice, there is a danger that such individuals will fall through the welfare net if there is weak integration between different parts of the health and social care systems. Although some European countries appear to have successfully addressed this problem, the PROCARE National Reports in this book suggest that integration frequently breaks down at the point of discharge from hospital.

Cultural Diversity in Europe – The Role of Families and "Informal Care"
The risks to older people with long-term care needs are being exacerbated by the decline of social support in industrial societies. Social trends in such societies are now well established and recognised. At the same time as the population is ageing through increased longevity, the "informal" support from families is reduced by increased economic migration together with the trend for women to remain longer in paid employment (Kavanos/McKee, 1998). Furthermore, changing social norms and expectations mean that even

57

where such family is available they are less likely to accept an obligation to provide care and support. In some Northern European countries such as Denmark, family care is not even factored into care provision (Colmorten et al., 2003), the consensus being that the state will provide support to older people. In the UK, services "top up" the level of family care available, although family support is not a legal obligation. In fact, "informal" or family carers provide the majority of long-term social care in the UK (Twigg/Atkin, 1994). By contrast, in Germany there is both a legal obligation and social expectation that families will provide and finance continuing health and social care (Roth/Reichert, in this book). However even in this system actual enforcement of such obligations is limited and there is evidence of shifting social norms and expectations.

AGEING AND GENDER

A wealth of research has been carried out on both older people and on the social situation of women. However, research on ageing from a gender perspective is still scarce, despite the fact that women are overrepresented in the ageing population. In many cases, differences in the standard life courses of men and women become more pronounced in later life. Also, women are more affected by care than men in two ways: as those cared for and as those who care. Specifically, 18% of the population (that is, almost every fifth person in Europe) are women aged 50 or more (European Commission, 2002-2004). Yet women and men do not receive the same (or similar) care, even for the same conditions. American studies show women are less likely to receive high-tech services, and tend to receive less aggressive care for conditions such as heart disease and cancer (McKinlay, 1996). Men are taken more seriously than women in health care, and women's health problems may be attributed to psychological or emotional factors rather than to physiological disease processes (Macintyre et al., 1999).

In terms of women's higher life expectancy and the ageing of the population as a major trend in European countries, women are a specific target group of integrated health and social care. They are often the carers of the person in need of care – as professionals or as immediate family – but may also be in receipt of care. Older women are very often dependent on community or institutional care. While older women often care for their husbands or other male relatives until their death, due to their own longer life expectancy, they may not be able to rely on this kind of help. One main difference in the life situation of older men and women is that women can be seen as the "covert resources of the social policy" with respect to their roles as informal carers (family care and volunteers). Also, the social and financial situation of older women is usually more tenuous than that of older men. Older women have less income and fewer benefits than men, and in general have worse living conditions than men of their age do (Bundesarbeitsgemeinschaft der Senioren-Organisationen et al., 2001).

Thus, it should be kept in mind that most people working in integrated care close to the users are women, that most service users – meaning those in need of help and care as well as informal carers – are also women, whereas those in the higher management positions of integrated health and care services (or making policy decisions) are likely to be men. It is therefore important to consider which aspects of the PROCARE study findings reflect gender issues, and which can be generalised between women and men.

COMMENT

In modern society, health and social care agencies have to deal with a major paradox. Major social changes such as the decline of infectious disease and improvements in nutrition have enabled an increasing number of people to live longer. Other social changes such as reduced family size, increased personal mobility and rising divorce rates mean that the level of social support for older people is falling. In these circumstances, improved integration is not an option – it is an imperative. One advantage of the advances in home care and rehabilitation which have taken place is that there is greater understanding of how to care for people at home in a cost-efficient way, and an argument for integration is that it both epitomises best practice and correlates well with the expressed preferences of both users and carers.

1.2 Ageism and Age Discrimination

"Ageism" refers to cultural and social processes that discriminate against older people because they are old (Tinker, 1996), excluding them from the mainstream of society and depriving them of their full rights as citizens. This discrimination is based on the stereotyping of older people as intrinsically incompetent and dependent and less likely to benefit from treatment (Bytheway, 1995).

Ageism may be evident in the decisions individual professionals make about treatment as well as in institutional decision-making especially in terms of access to services and allocation of resources. Both forms of ageism act as impediments to integrated care:

> Ageism is a process of systematic stereotyping of people on the basis of age. Wade suggests that such stereotyping allows younger people to see older people as different; "thus they subtly cease to identify with their elders as human beings (Brooker et al., 1997: 8).

PROFESSIONAL DECISION-MAKING AND AGEISM

In publicly-funded services, clinicians should ground their decisions in clinically relevant data. However analysis of clinical decision-making indicates that non-clinical factors, such as age, gender and ethnicity influence clinical decisions. For example in the treatment of heart disease in the UK older women are less likely than other groups to receive active treatment (Dudley et al., 2002; Bowling et al., 2001):

> Older people, and older women in particular, are less likely to receive appropriate cardiological investigation – from echo-cardiography to measuring cholesterol concentrations. Older people are more likely to have more severe disease and to be treated medically rather than surgically (Bowling et al., 2001: 286).

The net effect of such ageism is that many older people with heart disease do not experience an integrated service. They will tend to experience clinical delays and inappropriate referrals, i.e. to specialists in geriatric medicine rather than cardiologists. This increases the likelihood that they will enter the hospital system for emergency treatment of a heart attack or stroke rather than for routine investigation and preventative therapy. This leads to more complex treatment and rehabilitation, and a consequent increase in the need for sophisticated service coordination.

INSTITUTIONAL AGEISM

This term relates to a potentially ageist agenda which may exist within the collective decision-making of health and social care agencies. As Bowling et al. (2001: 286) note, institutional ageism is rarely explicit. It is not politic to admit that older people are being deprived of access to services because of their age, and it is often concealed within arguments about clinical effectiveness or value for money, i.e. that older people will not benefit from certain services or procedures. In the UK, the Government's "National Service Framework for Older People" has identified the existence of age discrimination in the provision of health and social care:

> Some evidence suggests there has been age discrimination in certain areas of health care. In 1991, 20% of cardiac units operated upper age limits and 40%

had an age-related policy for thrombolysis... Many older people and their carers have also found that palliative services have not been available to them... For social care, there is some evidence that councils can discriminate against older people where they apply commissioning strategies that are not sufficiently flexible to take account of individual needs... There is also considerable variation across the country in the range of services available to older people and their families or carers. Older people from black and minority ethnic groups can be particularly disadvantaged and are likely to suffer more discrimination in accessing services (DoH, 2001a: 16-17).

Institutional ageism can affect integration directly and indirectly. Health and welfare agencies often provide services to a range of users. If low priority is given to older users then less time and resources within the agency may be given to ensuring that services for older people are effectively integrated both within the agency and with other agencies. For example in social services departments in England high priority is given to child protection and to the lead role that social services departments play in coordinating overall child protection services. There are serious consequences for senior managers if they fail to protect a child. Yet failure to protect an older person appears to go unnoticed, or may be attributed to their age and condition rather than being considered a weakness or shortcoming of the care system. Also, there is less pressure to coordinate services for older people. While there is pressure on social services to speed up assessment to reduce hospital bed blocking, individual failures tend not to attract media and ministerial concern, so there is less interest in and incentive for collaboration.

COMMENT

It is generally acknowledged that both individual practitioners and health and welfare agencies discriminate against older people. Such ageism is extremely difficult to combat as it is based on perceptions that have been internalised. Individuals and agencies are likely to be unaware and even deny that they are discriminating.

Ageism creates a major impediment to effective integration of services. If older people are denied early access to health and social care then they are more likely to access services in an emergency, which reduces the time and scope for integration. Agencies themselves may recognise the benefits of effective collaboration but given limited time and resource may concentrate on collaboration for other service users who are perceived to be more vulnerable, e.g. children, or more dangerous, e.g. individuals with mental health problems.

1.3 Organisational Complexity

The main impediment to the provision of integrated care for older people comes from the fragmentation and lack of coherence of the health and social care system. The structure of health and social care systems in Europe tends to be divided horizontally between levels of government and vertically between agencies with different functions. Such structural divisions tend to reinforce conflicts between professions and with boundary and demarcation disputes in which professions often use their control of information and knowledge to maintain or increase autonomy and control. These tensions are heightened by competition between professions and agencies over the allocation of scare resources.

STRUCTURAL COMPLEXITY

While the social care system should be a unified entity which responds in a coherent and integrated fashion to users, in reality it is highly fragmented and competitive with different parts ready to blame each other when things go wrong.

62

In most of the PROCARE countries it is possible to identify a vertical division of functions. Central government is normally responsible for policy-making, setting the framework of resource allocation and establishing the legal framework of the health and social care system. The actual delivery of services is delegated to the sub-national level. At this level there tends to be a further split between regional/county level and municipal/district level. This split is particularly important for health and social care because the responsibility for the provision of health care often resides with the larger regional/county government while the smaller municipal/district government takes responsibility for the provision of social care. For example, in Denmark, the regions (counties), of which there are 16, are responsible for health care. Social care is the responsibility of the 275 municipalities, and this leads to widespread variations in service provision (Colmorten et al., in this book). Similarly, in Austria, health care is regulated mainly by federal government, whereas social care is the responsibility of the nine provincial governments (Grilz-Wolf et al., in this book). A recurring feature of the UK system has been attempts to create geographical co-terminosity for health and social care agencies (Alaszewski et al., in this book), so that health and social care are provided for the same distinct population albeit by different organisations, as this seems likely to reduce barriers to integrated working, however this has not been achieved successfully to date.

Horizontal functional division reinforces these vertical divisions. At central government level responsibility for the range of policies affecting older people is frequently divided between and within ministries. At local levels similar divisions exist between agencies responsible for the delivery of health and social care. A common finding at least in the Northern European countries featured in the PROCARE study is that whilst local authorities are responsible for personal care, housing and transport provision, these services are each provided by organisationally distinct sections of the responsible authority and that planning and strategic approaches tend to happen individually and in isolation of other departments (e.g. UK, Finland, Netherlands). These organisational divisions tend to impede the provision of integrated care, as the following excerpt from the Finnish national report illustrates:

> A large-scale development between social and health sectors was begun in the year 1991, when the Ministry set up a working group to make a proposal for an action programme to help improve the service structure. The programme recommended, for instance, the improvement of cooperation between social and health care services by uniting the municipal health and social service committees and respective agendas (Seiskari, 1997: 149).

> However, until 2000 only 38% of Finland's municipalities (N=448) had followed this recommendation and even in that case health care and social welfare services continue to be separately arranged on the practical level (Salonen/Haverinen, in this book).

Such structural fragmentation of services creates integration problems that are now well documented and are a product of contradictions within contemporary systems of government. Policy contradictions may also be described as resulting from the diversity within national systems, for example differences between sources of funding for health and social care between countries, and the diversity that may result from a mixed market of private, public, lay and voluntary care providers.

While governments are committed to integrated services they are also preoccupied with the problems of funding the welfare system and therefore of obtaining maximum value for money from the public funds allocated. To achieve best value, governments are developing performance assessment structures based on performance indicators. When resource allocation and incomes of senior personnel in welfare agencies are linked to performance then there is an incentive to maximise performance. This can result in "creaming" (McKinlay, 1975: 365), eliminating or rendering "invisible" cases that jeopardise the achievement of performance targets. Older people are par-

63

ticularly vulnerable to creaming, as they are likely to need more resources than other users over a longer period of time. They can effectively "clog up" the system. McKinlay identifies four techniques for eliminating unwanted cases:

> *Firstly* the eligibility requirements for the agency's service can be constructed in such a way that the official can exclude the client on first encounter... *Secondly* after accepting a client, an official can prematurely terminate contact while at the same time giving token recognition to some problem... *Thirdly* an official may only recognise a highly segmentalised area of the client's social life as relevant to his agency, and disregard other spheres of activity or problems... Fourthly, and probably the most effective and frequently employed technique of invisibility is for some official to recognise related problems, yet abdicate responsibility by referring the client to another agency (1975: 365).

At a system level such behaviour is irrational as it harms the very users who have the greatest need for care and support and ensures that the most vulnerable users do not receive an appropriate and integrated service. However at unit level it is highly rational. It enables individual units to manage a potentially overwhelming level of demand and achieve their performance targets.

RESOURCES

Much of the systemic irrationality of the current system can be related to the current mechanisms of resource allocation both in systems funded from general taxation such as the UK's NHS and those funded through social insurance such as the German and Austrian systems. In both cases, resources are separately allocated for health and social care with health care receiving the largest share. Little resource is specifically used to provide incentives for the provision of integrated care. Roth and Reichert note in their review of integrated care in Germany:

> Regulations for financing are a basic prerequisite for improving the coordination or integration of health and social services for older people. Connected with this are essential incentives for participant activities (Roth/Reichert, in this book).

The separate funding of health and social care for older people in Germany is a serious impediment to integration, which as Roth and Reichert (in this book) note can only be achieved through additional and targeted funding:

> To this extent, reforms to integrate health and welfare services must be founded on the integration of financing systems and the overcoming of institutional barriers, especially between outpatient and inpatient care, between health and welfare services, and between professional and lay care...Such approaches have

> not yet been developed in Germany, as already explained, and it seems that their
> way is still blocked by many insuperable obstacles and unsolved problems.
> (Roth/Reichert, in this book)

It appears then that while central governments exhort agencies providing health and welfare services to integrate their services, they may actually provide few financial incentives to encourage collaboration, and this factor represents a further impediment to achieving integrated health and social care.

PROFESSIONAL EXPERTISE

Professional expertise is one of the major assets of modern health and social care systems. Indeed systems are shaped by and based on areas of professional expertise. However reliance on such expertise can create impediments to integration especially when professional boundaries are aligned with and reinforce organisational boundaries.

While professionals may justify their status and control of resources in terms of their altruistic interests in providing services, the reality is rather different. In the welfare sector, it has been suggested that professionals have developed a dominant position through monopolisation of specific skills and knowledge, and by excluding competitors who can undermine their dominant position (Freidson, 1970; Johnson, 1972). Thus professionals establish and police boundaries that maintain their status and rewards. As McKinlay (1975) notes, one way of creating and maintaining status is to associate with high-status clients. Thus while a profession is ideologically committed to serving all clients:

> In the competition for increased prestige, it may be that one way to advance
> one's claims is to seek a "higher" class clientele, rather than being identified as
> a lower status servant of the poor (1975, p. 364).

Such professional considerations may reinforce organisational tendencies to cream and to avoid or to pass older service users on to other agencies.

DYSFUNCTIONAL CONFIDENTIALITY

One tactic used by professionals to protect their status is to emphasise the privileged status of the relationship that they have with their clients or users, especially the confidentiality of this relationship. Confidentiality can be used to restrict the flow of information between professionals and agencies. This professional justification for the restriction in the flow of information can be reinforced by data protection legislation, which specifies that data obtained for one purpose and stored electronically should not be reused for another purpose. This is designed to protect the privacy of the individual but paradoxically in health and social care may increase intrusion into users' privacy as each agency and professional deprived of the information collected by other agencies needs to duplicate information collection and assessments.

Such restrictions on the free and easy movement in information are increasingly seen as a major impediment to integration. For example in England, the Department of Health has identified such problems in the following way:

> Assessments are often duplicated with no coherent approach across health and social care services. This problem is exacerbated by the fragmentation of information systems, which unnecessarily duplicate information held about individuals. Failure to share such information can result in failure to deliver the best package of care. Care provided on the basis of assessment may not be well coordinated or follow the complex pathway that an older person might follow (DoH, 2001a: 24).

ORGANISATIONAL BOUNDARIES – CONCLUSION

While professionals provide the key skills and expertise for the care and support of older people, they may also act as an impediment to the development of an integrated service. Professional groups seeking to enhance their status may seek to avoid low-status clients who are considered to be professionally unrewarding. It is no accident that in the medical profession, geriatric medicine is a low-status specialty that is continually under threat, while in social work, child care and protection is considered to be the area in which social work can use the full range of its professional skills, whereas when providing social care of older people many social workers consider they are being de-professionalised and their role is restricted to that of bureaucratic care managers who fill in forms. Furthermore competition between professions tends to reinforce boundaries between care agencies as professions strive to create and maintain professional empires. This tendency reinforces the tensions between agencies and in particular restricts the flow of information as each profession claims ownership of the information it has collected and uses.

COMMENT

Given the organisational complexity of health and social care systems for older people in all European countries and the incentives to and opportunities for organisations to cream to maximise their performance, it is perhaps hardly surprising that older service users do not receive seamless care and experience the system as highly fragmented. The inferior service which many older service users receive when compared to younger service users is a product of ageism, the assumption that older people are less valuable as citizens and will benefit less from the resources allocate to their care and support. It might be anticipated that professionals with their commitment to the interests and well-being of their clients would actively counter ageism. While there is some evidence that some professionals do, there is little evidence that the majority of health and social care professionals have actively engaged in anti-discriminative practice. Older people are still often regarded as low-status clients who do not enable professionals to use the full range of their skills and should be avoided or passed on as quickly as possible.

1.4   Summary and Comment: Impediments to Integrated Care

Tudor-Hart (1971) coined the phrase "inverse care law" to describe one of the paradoxes that lies at the core of the health and welfare systems in contemporary late modern societies. This "law" infers that, the greater the need a person or population has (for a service), the lower the delivery of service will be for that person/population. Integration of health and social care for older people presents an exemplar of the inverse care law. Older service users need more integrated services, their ill health is rooted in complex and interacting causes, if these causes are not identified and treated then change can be rapid and treatment urgent and expensive, recovery may be slow and partially necessitating long-term health and social care. There is little evidence that the health and social care system has adjusted to or prioritised the needs and interests of older people. Instead, the increased pressure on resources combined with an increased emphasis of value for money provides agencies with strong incentives to avoid or pass on as quickly as possible older people. There is little evidence that the professionals employed by these agencies have sought to counteract these tendencies through anti-discriminatory practice. It is difficult not to conclude that the fragmentation and lack of integration of the health and social care system is the product of deep-rooted ageism which has to date permeated the whole health and welfare system.

2   Approaches to Integrated Health and Social Care

The diversity of definitions of "Integrated Care" found across the PROCARE national reports reflects the way that integrated care tends to be treated, especially in policy documents, as a self-evident concept that does not need definition or analysis. Such a taken-for-granted approach may be functional in policy statements that are aiming to construct a broad consensus and gloss over potential tensions but are not helpful to local service providers who are seeking to develop integrated services, or to researchers who are seeking to identify and evaluate integrated services. This section is designed to provide an overview of different approaches to integration and to identify the approach that will be the most productive of future research.

Since our interest in integrated care is grounded in concerns about the quality of services, a starting point for our analysis is a consideration of quality in health and social care. Donabedian (1980) has provided a framework for analysing quality that identifies three approaches: structure, process and outcome. "Structure" focuses on the resources available to organisations and care providers. The "process" of care involves the relationship between staff and users, and the approach taken to care delivery. "Outcome" is more difficult to define, but relates to a change in the client's health status *"which can be attributed to antecedent health care" (p. 83)*. Donabedian (1980) proposes a utilitarian definition of "quality of care", suggesting that interventions which can be judged as effective and beneficial to the population and are affordable in broad terms demonstrate quality within care provision. He also argues that:

> ... the attributes that are part of the quality of life – for example the maintenance of autonomy and self-respect – are also attributes of a desirable client-practitioner relationship and, in this way, become part of the definition of quality (Donabedian, 1980: 30).

Since integration of services can be seen as a dimension of service quality, Donabedian's (1980) framework can be used to classify approaches to integrated care. We will first examine whether it is possible to identify structural approaches to integration before exploring process and outcome approaches.

2.1   *Structural Integration*

ORGANISATIONAL STRUCTURE

The structural approach to integration involves bringing together staff and resources in one single organisation under a single unified hierarchical structure. Since such integrated organisations are usually located within the public sector and funded from public resources their creation, structure and functions require legal sanction. While such an organisation may be internally divided into functional departments, externally it presents as a unified service. Thus a key characteristic of an integrated organisation is a single point or portal of entry for potential users at which all their requirements can be assessed and an appropriate provision of services agreed.

In the United Kingdom the development of "Care Trusts" provides one model of structural integration (Alaszewski et al., in this book). Such Trusts are intended to be single organisations that provide community-based health and social care to a given population, and this may be a targeted group (such as older people) within a given geographical area. However, to date, the model is tending to develop in the specialty of mental health rather than in older people's health care.

STRUCTURE AND TECHNOLOGY

Modern technology, especially information technology, can be used to create virtual organisations, that is, organisations which are formally separate but because they have full and rapid exchange of information, function as a single entity. In the Netherlands the "One-Window Model" (Ex et al., in this book) has features of the integrated organisation model especially with its emphasis on a single point of contact or portal of entry for older people who wish to access services.

> The *Vraagwijzer*-window (query-guide window) ... is a central point where people may go and address their questions to an adviser in the area of care and well-being. People are served immediately, or are brought into contact with those that can help them on their way. This may concern application of rent subsidy, or the arrangement of an intake-interview at the RIO [Regional Assessment Board]. Sometimes these windows function as a gateway to the RIO's: clients may apply for an assessment concerning home care or admission to a nursing home (Ex et al., in this book).

While the One-Window model focuses primarily on the point of access, it is clear from the account given in the Netherlands Report (Ex et al., in this book) that it is intended to facilitate the development of a virtual integrated organisation for older people:

69

> The central issue is whether the query guide window, as a so-called "front-of-fice", manages to make effective contacts with various provisions and functions in the "back-office": (in fact) the local service providers. The better the mutual cooperation between these providers, the better the chance that the query-guide window facility will succeed. And that is what finally constitutes both the field of tension and challenge (*Congreskrant* OL2000, 2002). (Ex et al., in this book)

COMMENT

The structural approach to integration centres on the creation of integrated organisations that bring together a range of services, resources and staff. While such organisations may function through distinctive departments, a key integrating feature is the provision of a single point of entry at which the range of an individual's requirements is assessed and arrangements made for the provision of these services.

2.2 Joint Working: Process-centred Collaboration

Process-centred integration focuses on caring activities rather than on the organisational context within which such activities take place and can be defined as:

> ... collaborative actions or activity, undertaken between health and social service organisations and practitioners ... with the ultimate aim of providing an improved service to the client or patient (Hiscock/Pearson, 1999: 151).

As Wildavsky noted in 1979, there is universal support amongst service providers that they should "contribute to a common purpose at the appropriate time and in the right amount to achieve coordination" (p. 132) but that organisational and professional boundaries create major impediments. Similarly, Donabedian (1980: 18) noted that:

> ....with several providers of care, failures in continuity and coordination are more likely; these attributes thereby become more important as determinants of the quality of care.

The process-centred approach to integration focuses on ways of overcoming impediments through the use of incentives or closer working between professionals, and there is evidence of this approach across Europe, and specifically in France and Greece where a model of "gerontological teams" can be identified.

In France, the use of the term "coordination" is derived from the French government's promotion of this form of cooperation between professionals since 1982. Since the 1980s, a lot of coordination structures have employed a coordinator, or "case manager". Coordination is a central aim of French gerontological policy – for example, there is a 5-year programme for the creation of 1,000 "Local Information and Gerontological Coordination Centres" (2001-2005).

The coordination model aims to achieve integration in all three stages of Donabedian's (1980) model. Structural integration is managed by the development of a single access point (or office) that handles all initial enquiries from older people and their carers. Process integration is achieved through fostering joint working, and the intention is that person-centred and "seamless" services will be the outcome of the "coordination" approach. In France, the word "coordination" means a more flexible and horizontal arrangement than the term "integrated care" suggests. The coordination is a voluntary organisation of professional people who pool their means and resources to develop information, social or health care, and prevention services designed to resolve complex or urgent problems that have been identified as priorities over a given geographical area, according to criteria decided in advance on a consultation basis. So the number of organisations involved in coordination can vary over time (see Frossard et al., in this book).

INCENTIVES FOR INTEGRATION

There is a major body of literature that explores the use of incentives to facilitate interagency collaboration. Benson (1975) has argued that health and social agencies form parts of local networks and these networks are held together by mutual dependencies, because individual agencies hold resources that other agencies need to accomplish their tasks. This insight provides the basis of interventions designed to increase dependency and integration through the manipulation of resource allocation.

In insurance-based systems with their strong emphasis on resource allocation and economic incentives, such approaches are essential. In Austria, progress towards integration has been made through the development of a specialist fund, the "long-term care allowance", which provides one incentive for the development of more integrated care:

> As a first step, the formerly scattered and unequal cash benefit schemes for frail persons in need of care were comprehensively regulated within the "Bundespflegegeldgesetz" (Federal Long-Term Care Allowance Act), which

came into force on July 1, 1993. According to this law, all people with disabilities and/or chronic illness who are in need of at least 50 hours of attendance and care per month are entitled to a long-term care allowance (Grilz-Wolf et al., in this book).

2.3 Interdisciplinary Working and Teams

An alternative approach to process integration is closer working between the professionals engaged in providing support for older people. A common theme running through the PROCARE reports is integrated care as interdisciplinary working or team working. In most countries in the PROCARE study there is pressure for and evidence of inter-professional working and the development of inter-professional teams. For example, the Danish Report identifies the formation of multi-professional geriatric teams. The hospitals have led the way in the formation of these teams and professionals employed by the hospital form the core team, which usually has a doctor, a nurse, and secretary. In addition some teams include therapist, occupational and physiotherapists and social workers. The most developed teams include local authority social care staff as well as hospital staff. The aims of the teams are:

> To ensure a coherent treatment and follow-up after discharge from hospital... to treat the elderly as close as possible on own surroundings and prevent admission to hospital or re-admission. The team is supposed to ensure a coordination of the effort for the elderly between the [hospital and local authority] sectors. The target group for the geriatric teams is elderly with complex health problems and/or loss of function (Colmorten et al., in this book).

In the United Kingdom there has been consistent pressure on individual professions to work collaboratively or to participate in team working. It is therefore hardly surprising to find that in the UK, joint and team-working form a prominent part of current initiatives in integrated health and social care, especially in the development of intermediate care. For example, the central feature of Community Assessment and Rehabilitation Teams (CART) is multi-professional working.

This service model was one of the earliest developments in intermediate care, with many schemes set up during the mid-1990s, prior to the "winter pressures" funding (Vaughan/Lathlean, 1999). With respect to joint working, the important difference is that a multi-professional team is central to the service design and is housed in one location, usually in a health service setting. CARTs take referrals both from hospital and community settings, both pre-admission and post-discharge. The intention is that the intervention be available before a point of crisis requiring hospital admission is reached. The teams are usually made up of nurses, occupational therapists and physiotherapists, and should conduct an integrated assessment of the individual. One professional will take the lead role, depending on which therapy is most needed – for example, if the person has had a number of falls, and the assessment suggests that physiotherapy would be the most appropriate intervention, the physiotherapist will take on the lead role of assessment and evaluation (see also Alaszewski et al., in this book).

COMMENT

Process-centred approaches focus on the ways in which care activities are integrated. They are less concerned with the agencies or organisations that form the basis of the structural approach. They by-pass the organisational level by focusing either on the overall ways in which resources in the system can be used to create incentives for the integration of care activities, or more directly on the development of inter-professional teams bringing together the skills and expertise from different agencies into one integrated team.

73

2.4   Person-centred, Seamless Care

As Donabedian (1980) notes, approaches that discuss quality in terms of either structure or process are limited as they are describing the means not the end. The "ends" of health and social care systems are their outputs, the care and support which older people receive. It is self-evident that health and social care systems for older people are designed to improve the lives of the people that use them. Traditionally, health services have focussed on creating functional improvements in health of service users. It is possible to apply this type of approach to services for older people using measurement instruments such as the Minimum Data Set (MDS) (InterRAI, 2001) which assess individual functioning. However, because these instruments are designed to assist professionals in complex assessment, rather than to identify the clients' experience of receiving care, there is a risk that the key features of integrated care may be missed if a quantitative or standardised approach to evaluating integrated care is applied. A central theme found across the PROCARE participating countries is that integrated care may be defined by the way in which users experience it. They should experience it as continuous or seamless care that does not have gaps, waiting or overlap conflict between different components. While such care should help older people live a more effective life, improvements in functional ability may not necessarily be the most important outcome. For example, older people suffering from dementia or dying may benefit most from services that are flexible and adjust to changing circumstances.

Seamless Care

Thus integrated services should be those that provide continuity of care from both subjective and objective perspectives. A recent review defined aspects of integrated care delivery as follows (Freeman, 2000: 23):

*   "Experienced continuity: The experience of a coordinated and smooth progression between services"
*   "Flexible continuity: To be flexible and adjust to the needs of the individual over time"

In some of the PROCARE reports it is possible to identify this approach to integrated care with an emphasis on either seamless care or responsiveness to the needs of individual service users. For example, the Finnish Report emphasises "seamless" care:

> Seamless service chains are defined as an operating model, where the services received by a client... within social and welfare and health care services... are integrated into a flexible entity which will satisfy the client's needs regardless of which operating unit provides or implements the service (Ranta, 2001, from Salonen/Haverinen, in this book).

While the Dutch Report focuses on responsiveness to user demands:

> Demand-driven care ... simultaneously means *integrated care* for, when the requests and needs which the client may experience in various areas are met, integrated care is provided (Ex et al., in this book).

Models of Seamless Care

While most of the models identified in the PROCARE reports are "structure" or "process" oriented, it is also possible to identify models whose design appears driven by the pursuit of "seamless care" as an outcome. The Danish report provides one exemplar of this model, which is the service provided by the municipality of Skaevinge. The starting point for the integrated service was the existing specialised services provided by five separate departments within the municipality including one for residential care managing a large nursing home, one for home nursing, one for home help, one for health care and one for social work support (Wagner, 1994). These health and social care components were integrated into a single service providing integrated health and social care up to 24 hours a day to older people in a given geographical area. Within this service there are autonomous multi-professional groups. These groups share a common value system and goals, i.e. facilitating user self-care, and can respond rapidly to changes in user requirements. This may mean that an older person can be nursed through an acute illness at home, thereby avoiding the upheaval of hospital admission. All citizens are eligible and might have equal access to provided health and social care, irrespective of living at home or on institution.

The Skaevinge scheme is based around a former nursing home, which was converted into individual apartments without having to change the original layout. At the same time a health centre was established, putting together home nursing, public health nursing and day centre under one roof. Here, the various professional and technical groups work closely together for the first time. The centre directs its attention not only to the 63 older people who live in the new apartments but also equally toward other older people in the municipality (see Colmorten et al., in this book).

2.5   Summary and Comment – Approaches to Integrated Care

While "integration" forms an important part of the policy rhetoric in all European countries that form part of the PROCARE programme, it remains possible to identify a number of different approaches. Since the fragmentation of the delivery into competing health and social care organisations is one characteristic of all the countries, it seems self-evident that structural change, that is, the creation of single agencies providing both health and social care is one possible solution. Indeed in the UK some commentators see the creation of integrated "Care Trusts" as the way forward. However, given the time and energy absorbed by such reforms and the institutional inertia evident in some countries (e.g. Germany), an alternative approach is to focus on the activities of caring either by providing incentives for integrated working (as in the Austrian long-term fund) or through encouraging the development of inter-professional care teams (such as the UK's Community Assessment and Rehabilitation Schemes). Both organisational restructuring and the integration of care activities through interdisciplinary teams are a means to an end, namely the development of integrated care. It is possible to recognise a third approach, which focuses directly on the provision of seamless or continuous care. Such a person-centred approach is typified in the "Skaevinge" 24-hour health and care scheme in Denmark.

3 Assessing Integration: Organisational and Person-centred Outcomes

Since integration of services for older people is likely to be beneficial, all governments in the PROCARE study had policy statements that endorsed it, and most supported this with legislation and in some cases there were also resources specifically allocated to supporting integration. In such a context it is important to assess the extent to which reality of service provision matches the policy rhetoric.

To do this it is important to identify tools that assess the nature and degree of integration. Since we have identified different approaches to integration it should follow that we are also able to identify different approaches to its evaluation. In this section we will examine three approaches starting with those that seek to measure integration in terms of service outputs (3.1). We will then consider those that focus on the objective and subjective experience of users (3.2) before finally considering approaches that take a broader societal perspective considering issues such as social integration (3.3).

3.1 Care Pathways and Need: The Systems Approach

The "service output" research or audit approach to evaluation is likely to be predominant during the process of managing effective service integration, although it does assume that integration can be assessed in terms of measurable outputs. It is possible to consider outputs in terms of process, i.e. the continuity of care, and in terms of direct impact of users, i.e. changes in users' levels of functioning and health.

"CONTINUITY OF CARE" AND "CARE PATHWAYS"
It is likely that an expected outcome of integration might be improved continuity of care, but in practice, measurement of "continuity" can prove extremely difficult. Freeman (2000) acknowledges that continuity is an ambiguous and contested concept, and identifies two contrasting dimensions of

continuity. One dimension concerns the stability of the caring relationship with the minimisation of disruption to this relationship. This type of continuity takes several forms:

- *Longitudinal continuity:* Care from as few professionals as possible consistent with other needs.
- *Relational or personal continuity:* Providing one or more named individual professionals with whom the patient can establish and maintain a therapeutic relationship.
- *Geographic continuity:* Care is given/received on one site.

The second dimension addresses mechanisms that provide continuity by counteracting disruption of care especially across organisational boundaries and include:

- *Continuity of information:* Excellent information transfer following the patient.
- *Cross-boundary and team continuity:* Effective communication between professionals and services and with patients.

One way of overcoming such ambiguities is to focus on the health and social care provision within a locality as a single system and then examine the pathways that individual users take through this system. Soft systems technologies developed in "Operational Research" (the use of mathematical or computer models to analyse an organisation's operations) have been used to simulate such pathways. If the system is integrated then individual users' path through the system should be smooth and direct without blockages and delays, and individuals being cared for in each service should meet the criteria for that service.

This approach is clearly articulated in the UK's Department of Health review of discharge from hospital to community services. The review stresses the importance of a systems approach built around the needs of users:

> Whole system working does not have restrictive service boundaries – it puts the individual at the centre of service provision and responds to their needs… The whole system is not simply a collection of organisations that need to work together, but a mixture of different people, professions, services and buildings which have individuals as their unifying concern and deliver a range of services in a variety of settings to provide the right care in the right place at the right time (DoH, 2003: 15)

If health and social care agencies do function together as a system then individual users should have smooth pathways or journeys through the care system following "agreed and explicit routes" (DoH, 2003: xi) in which the services provided are appropriately adjusted as their needs change. In particular there should be no delays or backlogs that prevent a person moving on when they are ready. The PROCARE national reports suggest that there are waiting lists for social care across many northern European countries, including the UK, the Netherlands and Denmark. The Department of Health summarises the UK position in the following way:

> The research literature on hospital discharge goes back at least thirty years and there is remarkable consistency in the research findings, which continue to report on the breakdowns in routine discharge arrangements. In particular, older people make up a disproportionate number of those whose discharge from hospital is delayed and who are waiting for other services (DoH, 2003: 1)

In Denmark, the "Skaevinge" project has contributed to the development of older people's care across the country (see section 2.3). A ten-year local evaluation of the project produced the following observations:

- Older persons believed that their health status had improved. They were asked in 1985 and again in 1997.
- Even though the number of persons with 75 years or more had increased by 30%, the operational expenditures have decreased.
- There is the same amount of staff in 1996 as there was in 1986.
- The preventive care efforts have entailed a surplus of capacity, which among other things has been used to establish acute beds and rehabilitation places in the community to prevent unnecessary admissions to hospitals.
- The use of bed days at hospitals has been reduced by 30-40% for all citizens in the community.
- The municipality has not had waiting days at hospitals during 10 years for older people whose hospital treatment is completed.
- There is no waiting time for (supported housing) apartments in the health centre or for home help.

The use of and expenditure to sick insurance is less than in the rest of the county. These findings are believed to result from the emphasis placed by the municipality on preventative care, flexibility and individualised health and social care (Wagner, 2000).

ASSESSING NEED AND MEASURING THE IMPACT OF SERVICES

Given the centrality of need to the operation of health and social care agencies, there are a plethora of different approaches available for the assessment of individual need. Indeed in the UK the government has sought to reduce the confusion by supporting the development of a single integrated assessment though as yet has not commended a single model (DoH, 2002b). Most of these assessments focus on the individuals' functional abilities, i.e. their ability to perform activities of every day living such as walking or maintaining bowel or bladder control, and identify deficits. These deficits can be used as an indicator of a person's need and an overall assessment can indicate their level of functioning and need. One example of such an assessment is the Minimum Data Set (MDS). This set of instruments has been developed to enable comprehensive assessments of older people to be undertaken (and repeated as indicated) in a number of settings. It is now used in a variety of countries including Canada, Japan, the UK and Italy (InterRAI, 2001).

Instruments that aim to assess need such as the MDS could potentially be used to support the integration of health and welfare systems. Different components of the system should have different functions and therefore should be designed to meet different needs. One approach to evaluation is to examine the extent to which the needs of the service users actually match the needs criteria specified by each service. A study of intermediate care in East Kent (UK) found a mismatch between the needs criteria of services and characteristics of older people actually being treated within the service:

> This section shows that each of the intermediate care services were providing for people who did not meet al.l their criteria. CART [Community Assessment and Rehabilitation Teams] admitted people not meeting the Rehabilitation Potential criteria, Recuperative Care admitted people not meeting the Mobility criterion and Day Hospital admitted people not meeting the Rehabilitation and Cognition criteria... some people admitted to [hospital rehabilitation] wards may have been potential candidates for ICS [Intermediate Care Services] (Carpenter et al., 2002: 57)

COMMENT

The effective assessment of need opens up the possibility of assessing the health and social care agencies as systems in terms of their outputs, in particular the impact they have on the functional ability of older people. For example the MDS is currently being used to evaluate home care for older people in a number of European countries, and also in North America and Canada. However such an approach assumes that the main purpose of services is to improve the functional ability of people using them. For some services and for some users there may be other more important purposes, for example the purpose of palliative care may be to help individuals die with dignity and for older people with dementia minimising the impact of mental changes may be crucial. The needs approach tends to emphasise individual deficits, and it is also an approach in which the individuality of service users tends to get lost in the aggregation, for example when there are delays in discharge, individual older people are classified as "bed blockers". The individual experience subsequently tends to be lost and the overall assessment of integration tends to be in utilitarian terms, i.e. aggregation of the benefits of the defined population. In the next sections we consider approaches that focus more on the individual and his/her experience of integration, and it is this aspect of integrated care that is to be explored during the empirical phase of the PROCARE study.

3.2   Risk and Integration

An alternative way to thinking about the nature of the relationship between service users and health and social care agencies is in terms of risk rather than need. As Kemshall notes in a recent study:

> **Risk, particularly an individualised and responsibilised risk, is replacing need as the core principle of social policy formation and welfare delivery (Kemshall, 2002: 1).**

While the needs approach focuses primarily on functional deficits, a risk approach focuses on the change that an individual is likely to experience. In its narrowest form the risk approach is concerned with identifying and protecting individuals from harm but in its broader form it is concerned with individuals' own aims and experiences. We will deal with the narrower harm minimisation approach first.

HARM MINIMISATION AND THE SAFETY CULTURE
The "harm minimisation" approach was initially developed as a pragmatic response to serious problems that did not seem amenable to the more traditional "needs approach" (Alaszewski et al., 1998: 142-143). The most obvious example is drug use. The recognition of HIV/AIDS resulted in a shift from identifying drug use as a behaviour that needed to be eradicated through police and other action to developing strategies to minimise the harmful consequences of drug use through needle exchanges and other schemes (Strang/Stimson, 1990: 330). The overall success of this approach is judged in terms of the reduction of harm.

Integrated care can be assessed in terms of harm minimisation. It is possible to examine the ways in which health and welfare agencies contribute to the safety of the older service users by reducing the overall incidence of harm. For example, in Denmark, all municipalities are obliged to conduct two preventive home visits a year to citizens aged 75+ in order to identify and reduce risk factors in the home of the elderly person, and 85% of the municipalities fulfil that obligation. The presence of a proactive preventative system of this nature is unique to Denmark, although similar projects are present, albeit less widespread, in other countries. While the harm minimisation approach provides a more dynamic and more focussed way of assessing the impact of integration on individual users, it is still essentially utilitarian, assessing and aggregating collective benefit in terms of the harm prevented. The individual experience still remains elusive.

Some commentators are critical of the risk approach as it tends to emphasise the vulnerability of service users to harm and can be seen as fostering a protective paternalist approach to service delivery that undermines the autonomy and independence of older people. For example Alaszewski and Manthorpe note the tendency of risk management to create restrictive services which "... exaggerate the vulnerability of older people, restricting them unnecessarily and resulting in over protection" (2000: 197).

Such restrictions tend to occur when risk is equated with danger. Such a narrow restricted approach treats risk assessment and management as a technical activity of identifying and counteracting hazards such as the various factors that may result in falls. Little attention is payed to the broader and far more complex issue of values. Implicit within the approach is a set of values, for example that the main priority of services should be to protect individuals from physical harm especially death. These values are deeply embedded within professional practice and ethics and in the United Kingdom, following high profile scandals in which services have failed to protect vulnerable individuals, have been given formal government recognition as the basis of clinical governance. It seems self-evident that harm minimisation is socially beneficial. However, if we adopt a broader definition of risk as:

> The possibility that a given course of action will not achieve its desired and intended outcome but instead some undesired and undesirable situation will develop (adapted from Alaszewski/Manthorpe, 1991: 277),

then we can consider what is desired and factor in personal values, especially those of users and carers, which allows a richer picture to develop.

81

Studies of users and carers indicate that they are undoubtedly aware and concerned about the possibility of harm but may not give it the same over-riding priority as professionals and agencies (Heyman, 1998; Alaszewski et al., 2000: 47-70). They may wish to balance harm minimisation against other personal priorities, such as independence or privacy.

If this approach is taken seriously then it is only possible to assess the full extent of integration by considering how and in what ways agencies assist (or hinder) users and carers achieve their desired goals. Thus the start-ing point has to be users' and carers' desired and intended outcomes, and evaluation must include their experience of services and the ways in which they perceive their interaction with services assists or hinders achievement of their goals. Any study that addresses these issues will need to have a strong qualitative component using naturalistic methods such as in-depth inter-view and observation (Ong, 1993: 57-63; Murphy, 2001). It is difficult to see how standardised assessment instruments that seek to identify need, or structured patient satisfaction questionnaires, can capture the complex and dynamic nature of user and carer interaction with services.

COMMENT

The assessment of integration in older people's services still tends to be very much within the traditional "need" paradigm, in which the emphasis is on the functional deficits of individual users and the ways in which services respond to such deficits. The development of risk-based approaches facili-tates a broader, more dynamic approach. Harm minimisation identifies the factors that make older people vulnerable, (e.g. falls), and can be used to evaluate integration in terms of the overall minimisation of harm. The harm minimisation approach still tends to aggregate individuals into "at-risk" groups and gives precedence to agency and professional values. It needs to be expanded to take account of the values of older people and their carers if it is to form the basis of a fully person-centred approach. There is consider-able policy rhetoric about developing person-centred care but it takes the form of providing information to users, rather than adjusting the service to the wishes of the user. For example, in the UK's National Service Frame-work discussion of person-centred care, communication is a way process:

> Information should be provided at key points in the pathway, or stages of treat-ment. Many older people live with long-term illness, frailty or disability; if they have appropriate information, they will be better able to participate in manag-ing their own condition and lives (DoH, 2001a: 27)

Although elsewhere in Europe there is evidence of programmes to encourage more active consumerism in older people, including the provision of internet technology in older people's homes or facilities (e.g. Ex et al., 2003: 17), this remains a one-way process where older people are the recipients of care, rather than empowered to take part in care provision processes. A recent UK study identified that older people feel disadvantaged by the lack of information about services, and noted that "the concept of advocacy was rarely recognised amongst older service users" (Joseph Rowntree Foundation, 2003).

The UK "single assessment process" guidance does specify that user's perspectives and expectations must be recorded (DoH, 2001a). But as yet it is not clear that tools currently being used actually include these perspectives and if they do there is little evidence that the information is being used to shape care or evaluate services. The questions that lie at the heart of the person-centred approach are relatively easy to articulate, for example: "What do older people and their carers want, and do they get this?" To answer such questions one needs to access the perceptions and experiences of older people and their carers. This requires the use of relatively costly and labour intensive research methodologies and at present there is little evidence of substantial investment of research time into these methodologies. There is also an issue of the scope of the questions: Should the assessment be restricted to the relationship between users, cares and services or should it take into account the whole of their life experience? It is to this issue we turn in the next section.

3.3 Collective or Community Perspectives: Social Inclusion

While health and social care agencies focus on their own specific tasks, it is possible within some countries to identify a broader policy agenda that addresses the ways in which vulnerable and deprived individuals and groups relate to the wider society. This policy agenda is driven by concerns that certain groups do not engage with civil society and that this disengagement represents both wastage of resources and also a threat to the society. For example if grievances are not expressed through the normal political system they may be articulated as destructive behaviour directed either at the self (e.g. suicide or self-harm), or others (e.g. vandalism and civil disorder). These anxieties are long-standing and can be traced back to work of

19th century sociologists. For example, Durkheim (1933) identified the growth of "anomie", the declining moral and social integration of individuals in society. In current terminology this process is referred to as "social exclusion".

SOCIAL INCLUSION AND OLDER PEOPLE

The measures to counteract social exclusion focus on individual engagement in social networks, to encourage participation in society as a full citizen. In the UK government, there is a social exclusion unit (SEU) located within the Cabinet Office whose function is to ensure that there is an integrated government response to exclusion or in the Prime Minister's terminology, a "joined-up solution to joined-up problems". The prime focus of the SEU is on the exclusion of younger people as they appear to be seen both as the most vulnerable and also the most dangerous. However since older people are also citizens, the general measures designed to improve social integration through community building such as neighbourhood renewal include them.

It is clear that neighbourhood renewal is based on integration of all services provided within a neighbourhood and that it is not only designed to improve service but also to increase engagement. In the first issue of the Social Exclusion Unit's (SEU) review, there is an interview with Joe Montgomery, Director of the SEU's main programmes. He describes the function of the SEU strategy in the following way:

> Our work is about tackling the root causes of deprivation through improvements to mainstream public services, and the involvement of people in their own communities. By driving up standards in areas such as education and health, we are focussing efforts on changing the prospects of people who live in deprived neighbourhoods...We also support communities by putting them at the heart of the neighbourhood renewal process... Local people and organisations can easily identify the problems they face and propose solutions. Our approach is about removing barriers so that local people can also ensure these solutions are implemented. In many ways, the Government's success will be judged by the success of neighbourhood renewal. The proof will be that in communities and in families we see real improvements across health, education, employment and quality of life (Inclusion News, 2003).

It is perhaps another example of institutional ageism in the UK that the Social Exclusion Unit does not have any programme that explicitly addresses the social exclusion of older people. Social inclusion is addressed in the National Service Framework but in a rather weak form as "The promotion of health and active life in older age" (DoH, 2001a: 107). The main focus is on health promotion designed to minimise decline. Wider participation is briefly considered but only in terms of safety and risk and the main responsibility for social inclusion is given to other local government agencies:

> A neighbourhood that is perceived to be safe will enable older people to feel safe in their own home, and able to go out at will. The NHS and social care agencies should collaborate with local community safety partnership and other community-based activities…Access to wider community facilities, libraries, education, and leisure for example, will enable older people to participate in and contribute to society (DoH, 2001a: 112).

ASSESSING SOCIAL INCLUSION

Given the relative invisibility of older people in the social inclusion debate, it is difficult to identify and develop approaches that assess the extent to which service integration actually contributes to inclusion of older people within society. Therefore at this stage we are speculating on the type of information that might be required. One approach might be to focus specifically on the older person/community relationship and the other to take a more holistic approach.

85

An approach which focuses on the older persons community relations would seek to explore the extent to which services support older people in accessing the wider community physically and socially. For example, does domiciliary care provided by health and social service agencies merely "warehouse" older people at home keeping them clean, fed and safe – or does it enable them to maintain and develop their social inclusion by helping them to physically move outside their home using local facilities, thereby maintaining their social networks?

Part of the problem with any framework that is used to assess the effect of services on older people is the variety of contexts in which it has to be used. For example the situation of an older person who has just been discharged from hospital following a bout of pneumonia is very different from an older person who is developing dementia and this in turn is different again from the needs of an older person dying of cancer. Both the needs and risk approach deal with this difference through assessing need or risk and then assessing how far services address either the need or risk. It is not clear how a social inclusion approach would take into account such variations. One possible solution is to by-pass the issue by focussing directly on a more holistic assessment of the individual, especially whether individuals are thriving or flourishing.

This approach has been applied successfully at the other end of the life course, to young babies. In child care services social workers and other professionals have a legal duty to integrate their services to ensure children are protected from harm and to intervene when they judge there is a significant risk of harm. While some evidence such as physical bruising or fractured bones is a strong indicator of harm, in many cases it is absent or forms part of an overall picture. The holistic assessment of a harmful relationship identifies:

> Significant impairment of the child's health or development, including non-organic failure to thrive (Lyon/de Cruz, 1993: 6)

Thriving is contextually defined. In the case of young babies it can be defined in terms of physical development:

> Babies have an expected normal level of growth (weight and length), which is based upon their weight and size. Those that fall well below this expectation, with no apparent physical explanation, are considered to be causes for concern, and neglect (both physical and emotional) is thought to be a likely cause of this (Corby, 1993: 46-47).

While this approach to assessment developed as a technical and pragmatic response to a socially sensitive situation, it can also be seen as an example of an ethical approach to assessment that has a long and complex history (Alaszewski et al., 2000: 171-175). Aristotle, the Greek philosopher, argued that ethics is concerned with judging what is "good" and that one way of defining goodness is in terms of the purpose or end of an action or thing. Almond, a contemporary philosopher interested in medical ethics, defines ethics in the following way:

> The notion of flourishing... derives from the idea that every kind of object has its own essential end or function... a musical instrument is for making music. The Greek word for excellence, *arete* is the word we translate as "virtue". So the excellence of a chair, a knife, a musical instrument, consists in it's being able to fulfil its essential function (*ergon*) well. We might speak of an ideal chair, or an ideal knife, with approval. The idea that this generates, then, is that for an object or a creature to flourish, is for it to be in a state or situation that allows it to fulfil its essential function well. As far as human beings are concerned, this may well be a matter of displaying the traditional virtues (emphasis in the original: Almond, 2000: 100).

If this approach were applied to assessing integrated services then it would need to start from the specific context. For example in terms of dying it may be possible to define a "good" death as one in which an individual dies with dignity. Part of this process may be related to the dying person's preference for where death should take place, part would relate to the effective management of physiological processes such as pain and part to the social context that is culturally appropriate for the dying person, the family and friends s/he wishes to have involved and his/her involvement in social processes after death such as funeral arrangements. Thus a holistic assessment of dying would assess the extent to which integrated services had contributed to or hindered a good death. Similarly this approach could be applied to assessing the effectiveness of rehabilitation after a stroke. Part of rehabilitation relates to the improving physical functioning, however a crucial element is the way in which an individual normalises their life and recreates their personal identity through social integration. Again, holistic assessment would measure the overall contribution of services to the process of rehabilitation.

3.4 Summary and Comment: Assessing Integration

There appear to be no good reasons why older people should not be included within policy development designed to increase the engagement of vulnerable individuals within mainstream society, yet barriers to the inclusion of this group clearly remain. If person-centred policies are taken seriously then they imply integration of coordination of *all* locally delivered public services: health, social care, police and housing to name just a few. The services will be increasingly judged not just in their own functional terms but how they contribute to the broader social goal of social inclusion. As yet there are few measures to assess the ways in which services contribute to social integration. We would suggest that the virtue approach provides the conceptual basis for a holistic person-centred approach to such assessments.

While it is important to analyse and describe integrated care, it is also important to assess the effectiveness of different models. There are a number of different approaches each with its own strengths and weaknesses. Just as the process of defining and understanding "Integrated health and social care" is in its early stage, so too are methods for evaluating ways of collaborative working. These methods of evaluation can be summarised as follows:

CONTINUITY OF CARE
This approach concentrates on the care system and examines whether the components work together to provide a smooth pathway or whether there

are delays especially at common boundaries, for example between acute hospitals and community services. A systems approach can be used to examine whether individuals are appropriately being cared for in specific parts of the service by comparing the admission criteria for a service with the specified patient needs. This approach is being developed using well-established operational research methodologies and does facilitate modelling of care systems. However it does also aggregate individuals into groups so it is not clear how individuals experience and are affected by the system.

MEETING NEEDS

Since it can be argued that health and social care systems exist to meet the needs of the individuals that use their service, it seems self-evident that integration should be assessed in terms of whether collaboration between services leads to a situation where health and social care agencies can meet these needs more effectively. A standardised approach to this is now well established and several European governments have invested considerable resources in developing tools and data systems. However, there remain a number of challenges to this approach. Not only does this tend to aggregate individuals into groups, it also tends to focus on their negative aspects, things they cannot do without help, and information tends to be decontextualised. Furthermore it is difficult using this approach to disaggregate the effect of integration from that of individual services.

HARM MINIMISATION

This builds on current interest in risk assessment and management and focuses on identifying and counteracting causes of harm and measuring the impact of interventions in terms of reduced harm. Since such interventions rely on integrated action by health and social care agencies, harm minimisation could be used as an indicator of integration. At the moment this approach has only been applied in the UK in specific areas such as falls, an area highly relevant for older people. In Denmark, there is evidence that a proactive visiting service is being supported by government and implemented across the country, so that all individuals aged over 75 receive two home visits a year, specifically to identify and reduce risk factors, and this includes social, emotional and physiological risk factors which may indicate falls, depression or social exclusion (Colmorten et al. 2003). The problem associated with this type of service is that with the emphasis on overall levels of harm, the approach is built on the professional's value system, which may privilege harm minimisation over the older person's own goals and values.

PERSON-CENTRED RISK EVALUATION

The "risk" approach can be used as the basis of a person-centred evaluation if the values and goals of users and carers are acknowledged and a serious effort is made to examine whether services are recognising individual difference in values and enabling individuals to achieve their personal goals. While there is considerable government rhetoric about person-centred services, there is less evidence of a developing technology for person-centred assessment of integrated care. There are intrinsic difficulties to developing person-centred assessments. They will need to be grounded in naturalistic research methodologies that are expensive to apply universally. Furthermore such methodologies are not familiar or well understood within the biomedical establishment that currently dominates the funding of health and social care research.

89

SOCIAL INCLUSION AND ACCESS TO THE COMMUNITY

If older people are to have full rights as citizens it is important that they are able to access all community facilities and to establish and maintain social networks. Thus integration can be assessed in terms of how it enables older people to overcome the physical and social impediments to maintaining social networks. While the research tools to examine the ways in which older people participate already exist, it is not clear that they have yet been used to address this specific issue.

HOLISTIC ASSESSMENT BASED ON VIRTUE ETHICS

Social inclusion can be seen as a means to an end, as a mechanism for ensuring older people have flourishing lives. It is possible to use virtue ethics to develop a context-sensitive person-centred methodology for assessing the contribution of integrated services. In some areas such as palliative care or stroke rehabilitation the outlines of this approach can be sketched in, however substantial work is needed if this approach is to be more generally used.

4   Conclusion

As welfare systems mature in the European Union it is possible to identify a new post-Fordist approach. The initial Fordist stages of the welfare state were characterised by a standardised approach and fragmented service delivery in which each agency sought to deliver standardised services at the lowest possible cost. This provides incentives for agencies to reduce their costs by passing on difficult and costly cases, which usually includes older people. In such systems individuals, especially vulnerable individuals with complex needs are not likely to receive an integrated service that provides continuity of care. The post-Fordist system is intended to radically change individual experience of services so that users experience a seamless service that adjusts flexibly and quickly to their changing needs and wants.

Given the importance of integration and partnership to current welfare reforms, it is hardly surprising that there are a variety of initiatives designed to enhance integration. An obvious starting point is the creation of new agencies combining both health and social care functions, yet the costs of such structural reform, both in terms of finance and of wide-ranging organisational change, are often judged to be prohibitive. A further alternative is to use information technology to effectively create a virtual agency whose components share information and decision-making. Structures are of course a means to an end, and therefore some models by-pass structural reform, concentrating instead on integrating processes either by providing incentives and additional resources or by encouraging teamwork that brings together information, expertise and decision-making. Finally some models concentrate directly on seamless care by either providing a single access point through which users can access all services or guaranteeing comprehensive 24-hours care.

Since all countries in the PROCARE study are committed to some form of integration of health and social care, it is important to assess the extent to which the different models being used actually achieve integration. However just as there are different models of integration so there are also different ways of assessing integration. Three of these approaches fall within a utilitarian framework assessing the overall system or aggregated benefits or gains from integration:

- "Continuity of care" identifies the delays, blockages and losses which result from lack of integration,
- The "needs approach" examines the ways in which integration contributes to meeting need, and
- The "harm minimisation" approach examines the ways in which integration can ensure safety and reduce harm.

The other three approaches are:

- The "person-centred" approach, which explores the individual experiences and benefits of integration. A "person-centred risk evaluation" model can also be identified, and this examines the individual's personal attributes and risk factors, and the extent to which integration enables individuals to remain safe and avoid harm.
- The "social inclusion" approach, which examines the way in which integration enables individuals to fully participate in society, and finally
- The "virtue ethics" approach, which considers the ways in which integration contributes to thriving old age.

91

References

Arcares (2002) *Zorg en huisvesting*. Utrecht: Arcares.

Alaszewski, A./Alaszewski, H./Ayer, S./Manthorpe, J. (2000) *Managing Risk in Community Practice*. Edinburgh: Balliere Tindall.

Alaszewski, H./Manthorpe, J. (2000) 'Older People, Nurses and Risk', *Education and Ageing* 15: 195-209.

Alaszewski, A./Harrison, L./Manthorpe, J. (1998) *Risk, Health and Welfare*. Buckingham: Open University Press.

Alaszewski, A./Manthorpe, J. (1991) 'Measuring and Managing Risk in Social Welfare – A Literature Review', *British Journal of Social Work* 21: 277-290.

Almond, B. (2000) 'Commodifying Animals: Ethical Issues in Genetic Engineering of Animals', *Health, Risk and Society* 2: 95-105.

Benson, J. K. (1975) 'The Inter-Organisational Network as a Political Economy', *Administrative Science Quarterly*, 20: 229-249.

Bowling, A./Bond, M./McKee, D. et al. (2001) 'Equity in Access to Exercise Tolerance Testing, Coronary Angiography, and Coronary Artery Bypass Grafting by Age, Sex and Clinical Indicators, *Heart*, 85: 680-686.

Brooker, C./Davies, S./Ellis, L. et al. (1997) *Promoting Autonomy and Independence among Older People: An Evaluation of Educational Programmes in Nursing*. London: English National Board for Nursing, Midwifery and Health Visiting.

Bytheway, B. (1995) *Ageism*. Buckingham: Open University Press.

Bundesarbeitsgemeinschaft der Senioren-Organisationen (Bonn)/Europäisches Zentrum für Wohlfahrtspolitik und Sozialforschung (Wien)/de senectute (Paris)/Institut für Soziale Infrastruktur (Frankfurt) (2001) *Chancengleichheit für ältere Frauen in Politik und Gesellschaft. Dokumentation einer europäischen Konferenz am 1./2. Februar 2001 in Brüssel*. Stuttgart, Marburg, Erfurt: Verlag Peter Wiehl.

Carpenter, I./Challiner, Y./Coxon, K. et al. (2002) *An Evaluation of Intermediate Care Services for Older People*. Canterbury: CHSS, University of Kent.

Corby, B. (1993) *Child Abuse: Towards a Knowledge Base*. Buckingham: Open University Press.

Congreskrant OL2000 (2002) *Denken en werken vanuit de burger*. Den Haag: OL2000.

Cryer, C./Patel, S. (2001) Falls, Fragility and Fratures (Paper). Proctor and Gamble Pharmaceuticals, UK.

Department of Health (2001a) *Older People: National Service Framework for Older People*. London: Department of Health.

Department of Health (2001b) *Medicines and Older People: Implementing Medicines-related Aspects of the NSF for Older People*. London: Department of Health.

Department of Health (2002a) *Hospital Episode Statistics* December 2002 http://www.doh.gov.uk/hes/tables/tb00701a.pdf.

Department of Health (2002b) *The Single Assessment Process – Guidance for Local Implementation*. London: Department of Health.

Department of Health (2003) *Discharge from Hospital: Pathway, Process and Practice*. London: Department of Health.

Donabedian, A., (1980) *The Definition of Quality and Approaches to its Assessment*. Michigan: Health Administration Press.

Dudley, N. J./Bowling, A./Bond, M. et al. (2002) 'Age- and Sex-related Bias in the Management of Heart Disease in a District General Hospital', *Age and Ageing*, 31: 3-4.

Durkheim, E. (1933) *The Division of Labour in Society.* Free Press.

European Commission (2002-2004) *MERI: Mapping Existing Research and Identifying Knowledge Gaps Concerning the Situation of Older Women in Europe.* Frankfurt: Institut fur Soziale Infrastruktur.

Freeman, R. (2000) *The Politics of Health in Europe.* Manchester: Manchester University Press.

Freidson, E. (1970) *The Profession of Medicine.* New York: Dodd, Mead and Co.

Grimley Evans, J. (2001) 'Ageing and Medicine', in: Davey, B./Grey, A./Seale, C. (Eds.), *Health and Disease: A Reader,* 3rd Edition. Buckingham: Open University Press.

Heyman, B. (1998) (Ed) *Risk, Health and Health Care: A Qualitative Approach.* London: Arnold.

Hiscock, J./Pearson, M. (1999) 'Looking Inwards, Looking Outwards: Dismantling the "Berlin Wall" between Health and Social Services?', *Social Policy and Administration,* 33: 150-163.

Inclusion News (2003) 'Hot Seat: Joe Montgomery', http://www.socialexclusionunit.gov.uk/inclusion_news/issue_1/articles?hs_j_montgomery.doc (accessed 4th March 2003).

InterRAI (2001) Interrai Home page – Minimum Data Set (MDS) links: http://nt8380.hrca.harvard.edu/Default.htm

Jefferson, T./Holloway, W. (1997) 'The Risk Society in an Age of Anxiety: Situating Fear of Crime', *British Journal of Sociology,* 48: 255-266.

Johnson, T. (1972) *Professions and Power.* London: Macmillan.

Joseph Rowntree Foundation (2003) 'Older People's Views on Information, Advice and Advocacy' (Findings) http://www.jrf.org.uk

Kavanos, P./McKee, M (1998) 'Macroeconomic Constraints and Health Challenges Facing European Health Systems', in: Saltman, R. B./Figueras, J./Sakellarides, C. (Eds.), (1998) *Critical Challenges for Health Care Reform in Europe.* Buckingham (UK): Open University Press.

Kemshall, H. (2002) *Risk, Social Policy and Welfare.* Buckingham: Open University Press.

Lyon, C. M./de Cruz, P. (1993) *Child Abuse,* 2nd Edition: Family Law. Bristol.

Macintyre, S./Ford, G./Hunt, K. (1999) 'Do Women Over-report? Men's and Women's Responses to Structured Prompting on a Standard Question on Long-standing Illness', *Social Science & Medicine* 48: 89-98.

McKinlay, J.B. (1975) *Processing People: Cases in Organisational Behaviour.* Surrey (UK): Holt, Rinehart and Winston.

McKinlay, J.B. (1996) 'Some Contributions from the Social System to Gender Inequalities in Heart Disease', *Journal of Health and Social Behaviour* 37: 1-26.

Murphy, E. (2001) 'Micro-level Qualitative Research', in: Fulop, N./Allen, P./Clarke, A./Black, N. (Eds.), *Studying the Organisation and Delivery of Health Services: Research Methods.* London: Routledge.

OECD (2003) *OECD Health Data* http://www.oecd.org (Frequently Asked Data).

Ong, B. N. (1993) *The Practice of Health Services Research.* London: Chapman and Hall.

Schieman, S./Campbell, J. E. (2001) 'Age Variations in Personal Agency and Self-Esteem: The Context of Physical Disability', *Journal of Aging and Health* 13 (2): 155-185.

Stanley, N./Manthorpe, J./Penhale, B. (Eds.) (1999) *Institutional Abuse: Perspectives across the Life Course.* London: Routledge.

Strang, J./Stimson, G.V. (Eds) (1990) *AIDS and Drug Misuse: The Challenge for Policy and Practice in the1990's.* London: Routledge.

Taleporos, G./McCabe, M. P. (2002) 'The Impact of Self-esteem, Body Esteem, and Sexual Satisfaction on Psychological Well-being in People with Physical Disability', *Sexuality and Disability* 20 (3): 177-183

Taylor-Gooby, P. (2000) 'Risk and Welfare', pp. 1-18 in: Taylor-Gooby, P. (Ed.), *Risk, Trust and Welfare*. Macmillan: Basingstoke.

Tinker, A. (1996) *Older People in Modern Society*, 4th Ed. London: Addison Wesley Longman.

Tudor-Hart, J (1971) 'The Inverse Care Law', *Lancet* v.1: 405-412.

Twigg, J./Atkin, K. (1994) *Carers Perceived: Policy and Practice in Informal Care*. Buckingham: Open University Press.

Wagner, L. (1994) *Innovation in Primary Health Care for Elderly People in Denmark*. Gothenburg: The Nordic School of Public Health.

Wagner, L. (2000) 'Ti år efter – aktionsforskning anvendt i udvikling af ældres pleje og omsorg (Ten Years After – Action Research used in Development of Health and Care for Elderly)', in: Gress, N./Graugaard, K. (Eds.), *Klinisk Sygepleje 1, 2 og 3 – Praksis & Udvikling (Clinical Nursing 1, 2 and 3 – Practice & Development)*. Viborg: Akademisk Forlag.

Wildavsky, A. (1979) *The Art and Craft of Policy Analysis*. Basingstoke: Macmillan.

Wilkinson, I. (2001) *Anxiety in a Risk Society*. London: Routledge.

National Reports

CHAPTER 3

Providing Integrated Health and Social Care for Older Persons in Austria

Margit Grilz-Wolf, Charlotte Strümpel, Kai Leichsenring, Kathrin Komp

1   Introduction

Traditionally, there has been a distinct division of "cure" and "care" in Austria, leading to enormous differences between the areas of health care and social care provision: Health care has been regulated mainly by federal government (exception: hospital system) whereas social care has been the responsibility of the nine provincial governments. Health care was and is financed by contributions of the social health insurance, by taxes and by patients' co-payments. Social care was financed through a variety of individual measures in the context of social assistance schemes, many of them different from province to province. Also, health care has always been legally well regulated, whereas many areas of social care still are not subject to specific legislation (Barta/Ganner, 1998; Rubisch et al., 2001: 8).

The Austrian Constitution stipulates that, unless competencies are covered by the social insurance system, all matters concerning social care, e.g. services and institutions for frail older persons, for people with disabilities or children, are a matter to be dealt with by the regional governments (provinces/Länder). As a federal framework law on social assistance has never been agreed upon, there are nine different Social Welfare Acts with various differences concerning the extent of benefits, eligibility criteria and means-testing (Leichsenring, 1999: 1).

Thus it can be stated that, for a long time, with respect to policies for persons in need of care – i.e. all matters concerning institutional housing – the regional governments have shaped community care and related financial benefits, exclusively. These policies were characterised by an extension of institutional housing and care in nursing homes until the beginning of the 1980s. Since that time, policies were developed to increase the extension of community care services and to look for additional and/or alternative ways of financing measures to cope with social problems related to long-term care (Leichsenring, 1999: 2). Also, there has always been a large proportion of informal, family care provision in Austria (estimation: 80% of all care is informal, family care, mainly by women).

During the past ten years, political debates on necessary reforms but also concrete measures to improve social care in Austria have been quite in line with general reform trends in Europe (Leichsenring/Pruckner, 1993):

- Firstly, persons with help and care needs are increasingly considered as self-confident clients of social services and persons who – depending on their individual potential – are able to decide on their care arrangements (see 3.3.1). Especially younger persons with physical impairments acted as forerunners with respect to equal rights legislation and claims for "personal assistance". Issues of user satisfaction, users' choice of services and users'/clients' rights have become increasingly important in the last few years.

- Secondly, the broad consensus is that care in the community is preferable to institutional care. The slogan "care should be provided at home as long as possible, rather than in an institution" can be found in most policy documents concerning social care. In the last few years care in the community has been developed, which reacts to but also poses new challenges for the interface between health and social care.

- Thirdly, it has become clear that services have to be developed to support informal or family carers to ensure that care at home is more adequate, and less expensive than institutional care. Support services and provisions for family carers are being developed increasingly, but there is still a lot to be done in this area.

An important step in social care provision was taken in 1993 when the Federal Long-Term Care Allowance Act ("Bundespflegegeldgesetz") was put into effect. The above-mentioned issues were debated during the preparation of the Federal Long-Term Care Allowance Act, which allots a cash benefit to individuals according to their levels of help and care needs, for the whole of Austria. This is one of the first laws regulating social care on the federal level (see below).

Another development to harmonise the area of social care that went together with the implementation of the Long-Term Care Allowance Scheme was the state treaty between the federal state and the federal provinces concerning the development plans for social care facilities. Such development plans were compiled in each region, in order to set objectives in relation to a minimum standard of community care services, institutional care facilities and intermediary structures in terms of quantity, quality, working conditions and coordination (Rubisch, 1998).

In the same way as progress was made towards improved coordination within the sector of social services, policies in the health care field have also been focusing on coordinating and harmonising health provision during the last few years. A health care reform has been implemented since 1997, with the aims of improving transparency regarding costs and services and of supporting hospitals with regard to optimal resource allocation in order to provide a basis for performance-oriented budget flows from the federal state. Also in this case an agreement between the federal and provincial governments was necessary (Hofmarcher/Rack, 2001: 107-116).

A further agreement on health care reforms has come into effect for the time span 2001-2004 with a focus on uniform planning of the Austrian health care system, including the primary, secondary and tertiary sector with the aim of regionally coordinated planning. Another focus is on improving the management of the interface between different levels and types of health provision.

This paper will give an overview on the legal and structural framework of the varied and fragmented health and social care provision and the ensuing issues on financing health and long-term care. After a short description of the process of care provision with respect to institutional care, community, family and health care there will be a short section on the stakeholders involved in these processes as well as suggestions for the improvement of the integration of health and social care. In order to introduce the model ways of working in Austria, we will provide a comparison between the understanding of integrated care in an international perspective and in Austria. Furthermore, a theoretical model of integrated care provision will introduce the presentation of practical examples. Finally, conclusions will be made concerning lessons learned from the existing situation and from model projects that have been carried out.

99

2 Legal and Structural Framework – The General Discourse on (Integrated) Care Provision

2.1 Legal Framework on Health Care and Social Welfare Services

The legal framework of health and social care services is characterised by the fact that health and social services are strictly divided concerning legislation and competencies. Whereas health care and its financing is subject to the logic of social insurance, social care functions according to the logic of social assistance. A large variety of provincial laws lead to differing regulations in health care and especially in social care between the provinces. For example, old persons' homes as well as education for staff in these homes are part of the social services and thus legislated by the provinces. Hospitals and the education of nurses are subject to basic regulation by federal laws.

This same rationale is true for the division between health insurance and social assistance: Only strictly medical services are the responsibility of the health insurance, long-term care is partly regulated by the Long-Term Care Allowance Act as well as by provincial laws (in particular provincial social assistance laws).[1] In Europe, this distinction between health provision and long-term care provision is particularly strict in Austria and Germany (Barta/Ganner, 1998: 6-7).

A sound legal framework has a long tradition in health care in Austria but not so in social care. Whereas some provinces have had social care provisions legislation since the late 1970s others did not have such legislation until as late as 1990 (Barta/Ganner, 1999: 7-8). There has been an especially poor legal framework for training and education of staff in long-term care services for the elderly. The first law in Austria regulating the professional framework and education of staff working in help and care for the elderly and people with a disability was passed in 1992 in Upper Austria. Since then other provinces have followed this example. However, there is hardly any standardised provision in Austria, as the provincial laws differ quite substantially (Badelt/Leichsenring, 2000; Wild, 2002).

On federal level the Ministry for Women and Health is responsible for health care and the Ministry for Social Security and Generations has the social care agenda. Many of the responsibilities for the provision of health and social care lie with different departments of the provincial governments. Also, 26 Social Insurance Agencies[2] are responsible for the provision of social insurance (health insurance, pension insurance, unemployment insurance). The Ministry for Education, Science and Culture is responsible for academic education and thus – as there is neither an academic education for Social Work nor for Nursing Sciences – only for medical doctors (Hofmarcher/ Rack, 2001).

Concerning the legal framework, social insurance (including health insurance) is regulated by the *General Social Insurance Law* (Allgemeines Sozialversicherungsgesetz).

The basic legal framework for hospitals is set in Article 12 of the Austrian Constitution and in the *Federal Hospital Law* (Bundeskrankenanstaltengesetz). Details on hospital provision in the individual provinces can be found in the *Provincial Hospital Laws* (Landeskrankenanstaltengesetze).

On federal level since 1967 there has been a law dealing with the education and professional profile of staff in nursing which was revised in 1997 as the *Health and Nursing Law 1997* (Gesundheits- und Krankenpflegegesetz 1997). This regulates the education of registered nurses and nurses' aids ("PflegehelferInnen"). However, it does not include provisions for other staff involved in the care of older people, e.g. in old persons' homes. For this group of professionals, the laws of the provincial governments apply. This leads to quite varied educational and professional standards between the different Austrian provinces (Barta/Ganner, 1998; Kalousek/Scholta, 1999: 13 ff).

The provision of long-term care is regulated in provincial laws, among others in the provincial Social Assistance Laws.

Since 1993 a federal law was passed to standardise provision for long-term care allowances throughout the country. Since then the *Federal Long-Term Care Allowance Act* (Bundespflegegeldgesetz) has been the main instrument to regulate and finance long-term care on federal level (see section 2.3 for details).

Another development to harmonise and improve the area of social care that went hand in hand with the implementation of the Long-Term Care Allowance Scheme was *the state treaty between the federal state and the federal provinces*[3] concerning "Needs and development plans for social care facilities". Such plans had to be compiled in each province, in order to set objectives in relation to a minimum standard of community care services, institutional care facilities and intermediary structures in terms of quantity, quality, working conditions and coordination (Rubisch, 1998). These needs and development plans had to include the legal framework in each province, a structural analysis of demographic and sociological data, personnel

needs in the social care sector, minimum standards for provision, development aims with cost assessment as well as an implementation plan
(Eiersebner, 2000: 46).[4] In addition, provincial governments committed
themselves to implement these plans until the year 2011.

In summary, it should be underlined that not only a legal framework
for integrated care in Austria is missing, but that the existing legal framework leads to a lack of coordination within the individual fields (especially
long-term care), which results in fundamental barriers to integrating health
and social care. Nevertheless, there have been some improvements over the
last few years such as the implementation of the Long-Term Care Allowance Scheme as well as the "Needs and development plans for social care
facilities".

2.2 Financing Health Care and Social Welfare Services

The main pillars of financing health care and social welfare services stem
from the above-mentioned legal regulations.

2.2.1 Financing Health Care

Approximately one half of total health care expenditure in Austria is financed
by means of health insurance contributions, a fifth is financed from public
budgets and a fourth of health care expenditure is financed by private households, i.e. non-prescription medicine and patients' co-payments
(Hofmarcher/Rack, 2001: 33). Thus, actors in financing are the federal and
provincial governments, regional and local governments, social health insurance, private insurance as well as the patients themselves (BMSG, 2001).
147 out of Austria's 321 hospitals – i.e. 72% of all hospital beds – are financed
through public funds.

From 1990 to 2000 the costs of these publicly-funded hospitals have
doubled (BMSG, 2001: 101). This created a necessity to change the method
of funding, in particular with a view to the fact that the type of health provision has changed, patients are more intensively cared for and different,
more expensive, methods of treatment have emerged. Thus, in 1997 the
Austrian Procedure and Diagnosis-oriented Hospital Financing System was
introduced, which is similar to Diagnosis Related Groups (DRG) Funding.
Rather than financing lump sums according to the number of days spent in

hospital, in this system the hospital is reimbursed by the provincial funds according to a flat rate per case to abolish the undesirable incentive of extending a patient's length of stay. The provincial funds are financed by the so-called structural funds that distribute budgets between the provinces according to predefined indicators (BMSG, 2001:102-103).

2.2.2 Financing Long-Term Care: The Long-Term Care Allowance

During the 1980s, the social welfare expenditures for institutional housing had risen from 2.9 billion to 6.4 billion ATS (from about 200 million Euro to about 500 million Euro) per year, while expenditures on other welfare benefits had just doubled (Pratscher, 1992: 77). Thus, regional governments were eager to receive additional funding from the federal state. Another pressure group that was interested in additional payments for long-term care were persons with disabilities who demanded equal treatment with war veterans. Since the 1950s, war veterans had been entitled to a special long-term care allowance in seven levels up to more than 20,000 ATS (about 1,450 €) per month. Similar cash benefits had also existed since the 1960s within the pension insurance and within the Social Welfare Acts, however, at much lower levels than the war veterans allowance, with different eligibility criteria and with inadequate coverage. The ensuing debate on a long-term care reform was thus focused on the introduction of a comprehensive system of long-term care allowances. The following measures were taken since the beginning of the 1990s:

- As a first step, the formerly scattered and unequal cash benefit schemes for frail persons in need of care were comprehensively regulated within the "Bundespflegegeldgesetz" (Federal Long-Term Care Allowance Act), which came into force on July 1, 1993. According to this law, all people with physical, mental or psychological disabilities who are in need of at least over 50 hours of attendance and care per month are entitled to a long-term care allowance. This benefit, which is not means-tested, is paid in seven levels, ranging from 145 Euro to 1,532 Euro per month (12 times a year), depending on a medical assessment of the entitled person's monthly care needs (see Table 1). If residents of old-age and nursing homes are entitled to a long-term care allowance, 80% of the entitlement is paid directly to the provider (usually the provincial government). The person entitled to the long-term care allowance receives a lump sum of 10% of level 3, i.e. 41 Euro per month (Pfeil, 1994; Barta/Ganner, 1998) as a personal allowance.

- At the same time, in the already mentioned state treaty between the federal state and the provinces the former guaranteed to cover the additional means that are needed to finance this new scheme – from general tax revenues – whereas the latter ensured to amend their old long-term care allowance regulations according to the new standards (see also Leichsenring, 1999; Rubisch, 1998).

The comprehensive long-term care allowance scheme is a benefit that is neither part of the social insurance system nor an element of social welfare or social assistance schemes. However, it follows rationales of both these systems. This scheme increased public expenses (federal state and provinces) on cash benefits compensating for care needs from about 1 billion Euro (in the first year) to about 1.8 billion Euro (in 2002) per year. When policies to reduce public spending became stricter in 1995, some legal amendments also concerned the comprehensive long-term care allowance. For instance, the benefits have not been automatically adjusted according to the inflation rate since 1996. In another amendment in 1998, however, definitions concerning the assessment in levels 4, 6 and 7 were improved so that the number of persons in these higher levels increased.

Table 1: The Austrian Comprehensive Long-Term Care Allowance (2002)

Level	Care needs per month	Amount per month in Euro	Share of beneficiaries per level[1]
I	> 50 hours	145	18%
II	> 75 hours	268	37%
III	> 120 hours	414	18%
IV	> 180 hours	620	14%
V	> 180 hours of heavy care	842	8%
VI	> 180 hours of constant attendance	1.149	3%
VII	> 180 hours of care in combination with complete immobility	1.532	2%
Total number of beneficiaries			354,500

Note: 1) As different entities are administering the long-term care allowance on the federal and provincial levels, comprehensive data are scarce.

Source: Petzl, 2003: 244.

Altogether about 350,000 persons, more than 4% of the population, receive the allowance together with their pension (federal level) or a social assistance benefit (provinces). The average age of recipients is about 78 years, i.e. almost 90% of them are above the age of 60 (Petzl, 2003: 250).

SUBSIDIARITY IN PRACTICE: CONTRIBUTIONS OF PERSONS USING SOCIAL WELFARE SERVICES AND INSTITUTIONS

All in all, it is important to mention that long-term care allowances can cover only part of the real costs of home help and care as well as care in nursing homes. In Austria, services and institutions for older persons are generally provided in the framework of the provincial Social Welfare Acts and therefore financed by public subsidies and means-tested contributions of users. On average, the allowance amounts to about 385 Euro per month per recipient. Only about 5% are assessed in levels six and seven, and even in institutions this share is not extremely different. With, for instance, monthly costs between about 1,100 Euro and 3,600 Euro per bed in a nursing home, it is obvious that other sources are needed, i.e. the resident's pension (except 20% pocket money), contributions of family members (only in some regions, spouses and/or children are charged; see Barta/Ganner, 1998: 12-14) and, finally, social assistance schemes. In 2001 expenditures for persons in institutional care that were covered by the provinces' social assistance budgets were about 832 million Euro (Statistik Austria, 2004), about 50% (estimate) of which were covered by income from residents' pensions and long-term care allowances or their families' contributions.

Similar procedures apply to community care services that charge, according to the client's income, between 3 and 18 Euro – on average about 5 Euro – per service hour.[5] Since the beginning of the 1990s, community care services have increased considerably. On average, an increase of at least 60% of service hours provided could be observed during the second half of the 1990s (BMSG, 2001). Provincial governments currently spend about 300 million Euro (Statistik Austria, 2004) on social services, of which about 25% are covered by user contributions.

The complicated situation in financing long-term care in Austria may be illustrated using the example of home care services. Generally, home help and care services are financed from different sources (Wild, 2002: 25-26):

- Social assistance budgets of the provinces
- Social assistance budgets of the municipalities
- Provincial funds
- Health insurance agencies
- Clients' private funds (including long-term care allowances)

In some provinces, the provincial funds contribute to home care payments, in others they do not. Also, the type of financing through the health insurance agencies is different from province to province. In general, health insurance agencies reimburse providers for so-called "medical nursing care", i.e. specific tasks provided by home nurses and supervised (prescribed) by the General Practitioner. This, however, does not mean that each activity provided by a home nurse is included in the list of these specific tasks. As reimbursement thus obviously becomes quite complicated and GPs are hesitant to get involved in such arrangements, some regional health agencies simply transfer a (small) lump-sum to the regional governments to integrate their budget on community care services.

Figure 1 provides a rough overview of the various (potential) cash-flows between the stakeholders involved. Variations depend on the type of service a client uses, the province in which s/he lives, his/her GP and, of course, the supply and the organisation of services that exist in his/her vicinity.

Figure 1: Overview of Financial Flows in Long-Term Care Provision

106

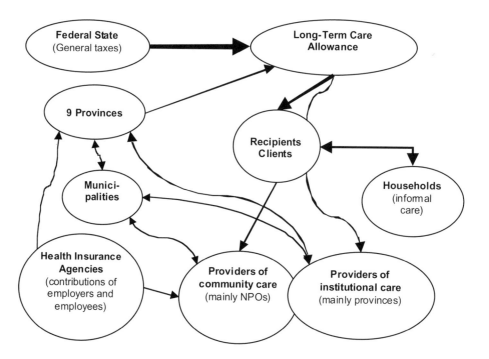

Source: Adapted according to Wild, 2002: 26.

It has become clear until now that this kind of financing is quite far from a "joint budget" and an integrated provision of health and social care services. However, while transferring money still is relatively easy to manage and to coordinate, this becomes much more difficult if we turn to the process of coordination and integration of various services which will be outlined in the following section.

2.3   Process of Care Provision

2.3.1 Institutional Care

Both in institutional housing/care and in community care there is a strong tradition of voluntary non-profit providers in Austria. According to Badelt (1999: 81), about 26% of institutions for older persons (45% of total places in residential housing and 25% of total places in nursing homes)[6] are provided by non-profit organisations, 53% by public providers (46% of total places in residential housing, 67% of total places in nursing homes), and about 21% by smaller commercial providers (10% of total places in residential housing and 8% of total places in nursing homes). There are remarkable regional differences in terms of quantity, quality and coverage.

Table 2:   Capacities of Institutional Care in Austria (2002)

Province	Population 2002	of these 65 years and older	of these 75 years and older	Total no. of places	of these in Residential Care	of these in Nursing Care	of these in Short-term Care	No. of institutions
Burgenland	278,600	50,136	22,257	1,487	0	1,487	0	26
Kärnten	561,126	91,137	42,378	3,195	982	2,213	0	45
Niederösterreich	1,549,658	248,656	113,169	10,499	2,548	7,851	100	99
Oberösterreich	1,381,933	204,620	93,005	11,961	0	11,630	331	110
Salzburg	518,587	69,901	32,369	5,201	1,698	3,454	49	82
Steiermark	1,186,379	196,252	91,241	8,315	0	8,315	0	163
Tirol	675,070	90,307	40,842	4,786	1,221	3,522	43	74
Vorarlberg	351,570	43,588	18,752	2,131	889	1,156	86	60
Wien	1,620,170	250,121	129,389	20,936	10,666	10,141	129	81
Austria	*8,123,093*	*1,244,718*	*583,402*	*68,511*	*18,004*	*49,769*	*738*	*740*

Source: Departments for Social Affairs of the Provincial Governments, compiled by the Salzburg Provincial Government (Spring 2002).

In general one can say that, today, older persons move to institutions only when being in need of help and/or care. Thus, the average age of residents has risen to above 80 and the general health status of residents has declined. Confronted with this "ageing" of their residents, residential homes tend to convert apartments for residents in good health into departments or beds for persons in need of care. Similar to other European countries, almost all of the traditional old-age homes – most of which had been built during the 1960 and 1970s – now dispose of "nursing beds" or "long-term care wards". Altogether there are 68,511 places in senior and nursing homes for Austrians above the age of 60 in 740 institutions (see Table 2). And there are about 49,800 "nursing" beds in old-age and nursing homes and 18,004 places in residential care for less frail elderly.

2.3.2 Community Care

In the area of community care, services are almost exclusively offered by private non-profit providers. Although the general objective of both federal and regional governments has been to extend the number of community care services and to increase their efficiency, e.g. by improved coordination mechanisms, it can be noticed that additional efforts in terms of investments have remained limited until today. Notwithstanding some positive developments in terms of professionalisation, regional differences remain huge. For instance, while in Vorarlberg more than 80% of long-term care allowance recipients use one or the other service, this is only about one third in Carinthia and the Burgenland. All in all 56,5% of persons receiving long-term care allowance use social services (Badelt et al., 1997: 79). Only in Vienna where services had already been relatively well developed, the number of service hours did not increase after the introduction of the long-term care allowance. While other provinces are increasingly catching up, services in Vienna seem to have already entered another phase of community care development: Similar to many other European countries services are targeted towards a smaller number of clients. However, it is the relative amount of user contributions that seems to regulate access, rather than professional assessment procedures.

Concerning coordination of services and institutions in health and social care, some provinces have installed so-called health and social districts but even the designation of these (in some regions: virtual) entities varies (Bahr/Leichsenring, 1996). A general framework for such integrated health and social districts was developed in the beginning of the 1990s by the Federal Institute for Health but neither the provincial governments nor regional branches of the health insurance (sickness funds) have implemented this coordination model (see Section 3: Model Ways of Working).

2.3.3 Personnel in Old-Age Care

Although some improvements towards better training and professional working conditions have been realised (Leichsenring, 1999), Austria is still lacking in nation-wide regulations for social service professions. Home-helpers, geriatric helpers and family helpers are still trained on the basis of regional regulations[7] (sometimes even specific providers' curricula) so that a minimum standard remains to be developed. Given this background, wages are very low and working conditions rather strenuous. For instance, the average hourly wage of a home-helper is about 7.5 Euro, and working times often depend on short-term demand.

The analysis of the provinces' needs and development plans shows that quite a large amount of additional personnel is needed in community care as well as in institutional care for the elderly in the next 10 years. However, shortage of staff in the area of care for the elderly is on the agenda already today. This is also why the necessity of better training and further education for staff in this field is being stressed (Schaffenberger et al., 1999).

As a specific Austrian feature it is worth mentioning that, due to the curricula of social worker's education, social workers only play a marginal role in the provision and organisation of care services for older persons.

2.3.4 Family Care

Traditionally, family care plays an important role in care provision in Austria, as it is undoubtedly the main source of care. According to the evaluation of the long-term care allowance scheme (Badelt et al., 1997) currently about 90% of the recipients are mainly cared for by a family member. This finding is underlined in a more recent study on "Quality Assurance in Social Care" (Nemeth/Pochobradsky, 2002). About 23% of these carers combine work and family care (more than one third of all family carers below the age of 60). Altogether about 1.5% of all employed persons are carers of older kin. Generally, however, it is daughters and daughters-in-law who carry the main burden of care: about 59% of all family carers are between 40 and 60, one third above 60 and about 15% are younger than 40. About 25% of all family carers who care for persons receiving long-term care allowance have reduced or abandoned their employment according to the care needs of their dependent family member (Badelt et al., 1997: 175). Family carers are confronted with multiple burdens, such as back aches, too much responsibility as well as time or financial problems (Nemeth/Pochobradsky, 2002).

Services to support family carers, such as counselling, respite care, etc. have developed over the past few years (Farkas/Leichsenring, 1994). However, there are still very few day centres, opportunities for short-term care and day care for older persons. Also, family carers are confronted with a lack of information on all aspects of the care situation (Nemeth/Pochobradsky, 2002). Austrian experts in this area suggest that it would be very important to expand such provisions as well as information on family care in order to improve the situation of family carers (Kalousek/Scholta, 1999: 8-12; Schaffenberger et al., 1999; Nemeth/Pochobradsky, 2002).

The amendment of the comprehensive long-term care allowance act in 1998 facilitated the inclusion of family carers into the social security system. Family carers who care for a dependent person with substantial care needs (long-term care allowance levels 4-7) may contribute to the pension insurance (using part of the long-term care allowance), while the state takes over the employer's contribution (Rubisch, 1998).

To sum up, the status of informal carers in Austria remains precarious as specific and systematic measures to acknowledge and support family care are still lacking. The importance of family ethics is the main factor why it remains the most preferred and accepted way of long-term care for frail (older) persons (Bahr/Leichsenring, 1996; Rosenmayr/Majce, 1998).

2.3.5 Managing Pluralism in Vienna

As the organisation of services – as well as their mode of financing and their degree of development, quality and professionalisation – differs from region to region, in the following some more information is provided with respect to Vienna.

In Vienna, the municipality, which is at the same time a provincial government, hardly plays any role as a supplier of community care services for older persons except for home nursing ("Mobile Schwestern"). In particular, home help services (and some home nursing) are provided exclusively by private voluntary organisations, which are reimbursed by the municipality. Currently about 20 voluntary organisations offer their services, but five big suppliers dominate the market (Wiener Volkshilfe, Wiener

Hilfswerk, Sozial Global, Rotes Kreuz, Wiener Sozialdienst). These providers are offering a wide range of services while others concentrate on one or two services. Altogether, these services generally remain limited to the "classical" ones such as home help – the most important –, home nursing, "meals on wheels", cleaning services, or repair services and alarm systems. On average, not more than 5% of Viennese citizens above 60 use one or the other of these services (Table 3). While the supply of social services for the elderly is officially still subdivided in the single segments mentioned above (e.g. home help, home nursing), some providers consider this situation inadequate and increasingly try to offer integrated community care services such as, for instance, in Lower Austria and other provinces.

Table 3:   Number of Users of Community Care Services in Vienna (1997)

Type of service (1)	No. of users/ year (2)	Share of users in total population above 60
Home help	17,709	5.0%
Cleaning services	9,043	2.6%
Meals-on-wheels	11,155	3.2%
Hospice	353	0.1%
Befriending	3,304	0.9%
Repair services	622	0.2%
Laundry services	1,557	0.4%

Notes: (1) except community nursing care; (2) There are about 330,000 Viennese above the age of 60 out of which about 125,000 are above the age of 75.

Source: Amt der Wiener Landesregierung (MA 47), 1997.

The Department "Soziale Dienste" acts as a purchaser, coordinator and controller of these services on the municipal level, i.e. general contracts, planning and budgeting are regulated between this Department and single providers. Local supply is coordinated by organisational branches of that department, so-called "Soziale Stützpunkte" (social coordination and support centres – see also below). Altogether there are 10 "Soziale Stützpunkte", each covering a specified area of the city. Their staff mainly consists of district nurses who are responsible for the first contact with the client, i.e. the assessment of the client's needs in his or her home. On that basis an individual care plan is drawn up which serves as a guideline for the kind of care that is subsequently supplied by the single providers. It is up to the individual coordination nurse to contact the local providers, unless the client expresses certain preferences. In the recent past some of the "social coordination and support centres" have been integrated into "Gesundheits- und Sozial-zentren" (health and social centres). There, information is offered not only about home care and home help, but also about residential homes, social work etc. In addition, they organise day care and other social services on a local level (Leichsenring/Stadler, 1998). Currently, there are five centres of this kind in Vienna.

2.3.6 Health Care Provision

In Austria there are 16,600 independent physicians (5,800 general practition-ers and 7,400 specialists). Three-quarters of them have a contract with one or more health insurance agencies as 99% of the Austrian population is cov-ered by health insurance. There are also 750 outpatient clinics and 1,600 outpatient hospital departments that offer health care services.

In Austria there are 321 hospitals with 70,300 beds (1 December, 2000). This means 8.7 beds per 1,000 inhabitants. More than 2 million patients were treated in Austrian hospitals in 2000. The Austrian hospital law distinguishes between general hospitals (118 hospitals with 62% of all beds), 98 special hospitals (21% of all beds) with specific aims, such as accident hospitals, or for specific groups such as geriatric or children's hospitals as well as 105 other hospitals (nursing homes for chronically-ill patients, convalescence homes, etc.) with 17% of all beds. The third group are institutions like nurs-ing homes for the chronically ill, rehabilitation homes, birth clinics etc. (105 hospitals with 17% of all beds). As mentioned above, 70% of the beds in 147 hospitals are public; 38 hospitals with 8% of beds are private, non-profit. The third group of hospitals belongs to the provinces (51% of beds) and to municipal governments, religious organisations, private persons, etc. Apart from some huge hospitals in Vienna and the provincial capitals, most of these institutions are quite small (BMSG, 2001: 51-52).

The Austrian Hospitals and Major Equipment Plan (Österreichischer Krankenanstalten- und Großgeräteplan – ÖKAP/GGP) is an important pil-lar of the Austrian Health Reform that was started in 1997. Its aims are to ensure structural quality and to optimise the allocation pattern of health care and the interactions with the (public) health system and between its sectors. The ÖKAP/GGP regulates numbers of beds, key areas and geographical position of the public hospitals. Detailed regulations are fixed in provincial hospital plans (Landeskrankenanstaltenpläne) (BMSG, 2001: 52).

Looking at the development of hospital provision over the last 20 years, one can say that the amount of hospitals per 100,000 inhabitants has stayed relatively constant. The number of beds per 1,000 inhabitants has decreased from 11.2 in 1980 to 8.6 in 2000 and the average stay has decreased significantly from 7.2 days in 1995 to 6.3 in 2000. The admissions per 100 inhabitants have increased from 19.5 to 29.3 a year from 1980 to 2000. These developments are in line with those in other EU countries. They show that medical treatment is becoming more efficient. At the same time the consequences for home help and care are self-evident (Hofmarcher/Rack 2001: 75-80).

Table 4:   Characteristics of Hospital Provision in Austria (1991-2000)

	1991	1992	1993	1994	1995	1996	1997	1998	1999	2000
Number of beds in a hospital per 100,000 inhabitants	9,8	9,6	9,4	9,4	9,3	9,2	9,1	8,9	8,8	8,6
Admissions per 100 inhabitants	23,7	24,0	24,1	24,5	24,8	25,2	26,7	27,9	28,9	29,3
Average length of stay in days					7,2	7,1	6,7	6,6	6,5	6,3

Source: "Krankenanstalten in Zahlen": www.kaz.bmsg.gv.at

2.4   Stakeholders

There are a great variety of actors involved in the different processes of health and long-term care in Austria: the federal and provincial governments are responsible for funding and provision, controlling/inspection as well as for developing and planning provision. In addition, local governments have provision as well as planning functions. The social insurance agencies have an important role in financing and administrating health care and long-term care provision. Non-profit organisations as well as informal family carers provide most help and care services for older people.

From this follows a large number of interfaces where the different stakeholders cooperate in funding, contracting, providing and controlling. However, it seems difficult to steer the different systems towards one mutually agreed objective.

A common phenomenon concerning the financing of these different systems (like "medical home nursing" and home help) is to try pushing certain types of provision or financing to other actors. The void or ambiguities which result from this behaviour are often negatively felt by clients/patients and/or their informal carers. Also, it is unusual that stakeholders reflect on potential consequences for the other systems that might stem from reforms in one sector. For example, the DRG-based financing system for hospitals that was introduced in 1997, among others, aimed at and succeeded in reducing the average length of stays in hospitals but, at the same time, put pressure on community care provision. Another example is when the provincial governments profited quite substantially from the implementation of the Long-Term Care Allowance Scheme – however, rather than using the money that was economised on lower bills for institutions to invest in further community care services or innovation, it was mainly used to rebalance regional social assistance budgets.

Another pertinent conflict line dividing the stakeholders can be identified between the different professional groups. Health care professionals have a better regulated educational and job profile, higher pay and higher status than staff in the area of long-term care for the elderly. This has a variety of consequences for the ability and willingness of professional groups in health and long-term care to cooperate and work together.

Important stakeholders in long-term care provision in Austria are the non-profit organisations such as the Austrian Red Cross, Caritas, Diakonie, Volkshilfe and Hilfswerk. With a few exceptions (Austrian Red Cross) they either have religious (Caritas, Diakonie) or political party (Volkshilfe and Hilfswerk) affiliations. Whereas non-profit organisations' links to religion are quite common in many countries, links to political parties are an Austrian specificity: the Austrian political culture is characterised by a long tradition of pillarisation, where all areas of society have been linked to the main political parties (schools, seniors' organisations, sports clubs etc. etc.). As a result, in Austria, choice – in terms of being able to choose between different providers linked to different political parties – has been considered an important feature, in particular for the older generation and in rural areas. To date, an important sign for the diminishing influence of ideological cleavages between the providers can be seen in the fact that the most important ones have formed a working group ("Bundesarbeits-gemeinschaft Soziale Wohlfahrt") with the aim of harmonising their interests towards federal government policies and e.g. to develop quality criteria for social services.

Concerning patients'/users' interests, the interest organisations of people with disabilities of working age were most engaged in influencing care policies, in particular the introduction of the long-term care allowance. The large seniors' organisations (also affiliated to the political parties) also play a role when it comes to representing older people's interests in health and long-term care. However, until now they have focused more on issues of pensions than on health and social care issues. Family carers are not organised on the national level, but there are smaller – self-help type – organisations for caring family members (e.g. carers of persons with Alzheimer's Disease or with psychiatric diseases). As mentioned above the clients/patients and their carers are usually the last link in the chain of provision and have to compensate for ambiguities and gaps in the responsibilities of the other actors.

2.5   *Demands and Plans for Improvement*

The important points in the discourse on long-term care and health provision for the elderly in Austria can be identified from several documents that express demands or plans for the improvement of these provisions. During 1999, the UN-Year of the Elderly, the Austrian Federal Government convened several working groups, consisting of experts – providers, interest groups, representatives of political parties and local, regional and federal government, researchers and older people themselves – in the field (20-40 experts each). One working group was on help and care of the elderly in home care and institutions. A variety of recommendations to improve the provision of long-term care for the elderly were elicited (Kalousek/Scholta, 1999), for instance:

- *More support for family carers:* better and more information for caring relatives, educating general practitioners to play a role in networking and giving information, better coordination between providers and more training and support services for family caregivers.
- *Better interface between institutional and home care:* implementation of care and case management and improving quality assurance. In its brochure on developing quality, the "Bundesarbeitgemeinschaft Freie Wohlfahrt" (2002: 2) states case management as an important quality criterion.
- *More choice* for clients in provisions.
- *Transparent financing systems:* Harmonising financing, e.g. for home care, is demanded from different sides (Wild, 2002).

- *Standardised federal legal regulations* concerning education and professional profile of all staff in the field of elderly care.
- *Standardised federal training system for staff*, with different modules and scope for mobility between different professions.
- *Improvement of care provisions* on the weekends, nights also short-term and day care.

The conclusion of the needs and development plans for long-term care of the provincial governments also include some of these points, they are (Schaffenberger et al., 1999):

- expanding services for care of the elderly (especially day care and day centres),
- improving provision to meet the needs of the old and people with dementia,
- improving structures to enable integration of different provisions,
- improving and securing quality and economic outcomes of provisions.

Finally, some reform steps in the health reform also concern older people, like (Hofmarcher/Rack, 2001):

- creating 57 new geriatric wards until 2005,
- improving hospice and palliative care provision,
- improving home health services and day clinics.

3   Model Ways of Working

3.1   *The Understanding of Integrated Care in Austria*

The term integrated care has experienced growing popularity over the last few years. The increase of attention towards Integrated Care and its variants is accompanied by a growing number of meanings attributed to these terms. As a basis for future discussion and research projects it is essential to clarify the use of these terms. Therefore, this section shall reflect the understanding of Integrated Care in Austria.

3.1.1 The Terminology Used in Austria

When talking about integrated care in Austria, one usually refers to case management. Both in theory and in practice this concept has been predominant since the issue has gained public interest. Other concepts of integrated care and the idea of integrated care itself are of subordinate interest and use in Austria. They only exist in connection with case management, often lacking explicit definitions. Accordingly, there is a variety of literature on case management in Austria but hardly any publication on care management or on integrated care as a self-contained idea. Even coordination, the second popular idea in the field of integrated care in Austria, is being used in a rather imprecise way. In the following the use of the terms integrated care, care management and cooperation will be shortly described and the term case management will be considered in detail.

There is no explicit definition of the term "integrated care", but from its use and concepts one might draw a few conclusions. Firstly, the idea of integration refers to the horizontal as well as to the vertical level. Secondly, the aims of the process are to guarantee demand-orientation, a continuity of service provision and a high standard of quality (Grundböck et al., 1997: 13; Kain, 1994: 13ff.; LBI, 2000). It is impossible to concisely compare the use of this term on the international and the Austrian level on the basis of this scarce information. Statements concerning the nature of care management are just as fragmentary as the ones about integrated care. In Austria, care management stands for the design of the cooperation between care providers (Grundböck et al., 1997: 14; Grundböck et al., 1998: 101).

The question whether this design refers to a particular case or cooperation in general thus remains open. However, as a basic definition we may conclude that care management is a contract between different service organisations on the management level. Another kind of vagueness can be found when talking about coordination, cooperation and networking: there is no distinct separation between these terms, usually though, the term cooperation is applied. In contrast to this vagueness the internal structure of the conglomerate at stake is very elaborated. There is a multitude of suggestions on how to subdivide and therewith characterise the different ways of networking, cooperating or coordinating. The characteristics used for this task are closeness (from formal agreements to agreements concerning working procedures), type of involved institutions (from service providers to decision-making bodies) and number of partners (from intra- to inter-institutional arrangements) (Bahr/Leichsenring, 1996: 25; Grundböck et al., 1998: 191; Grundböck et al., 2000: 221; Hofer, 1999: 26; ÖBIG, 1993: 225). Thus the vague definitions are met by a complex content, which stands out because of the attention it pays to decision-makers, e.g. on the political level.

117

The concept of integrated care preferably talked about and mainly used in Austria is case management. This term, as it is used in Austria, stresses the individual case with its specific needs and its long-term aspect. The basic idea is that all cooperative and organisational tasks are taken over by a single person, preferably a qualified nurse. In this function s/he should represent the contact person for the patient, his or her relatives and the internal as well as external service providers. Even though it is her/him who collects information about the market for care services and the development of the patient's needs, it is still the patient him- or herself who makes the decisions (DWPS, 1998: 5ff.; Grundböck et al., 1997: 14; Grundböck et al., 1998: 101; ÖBIG, 1993: 228; RKW, 2001: 3). There is the – not undisputed – suggestion to distinguish between an internal and an external variation of case management on the organisational and personnel level. The external variation refers to the relationship between the case manager and her/his client and works on the level of the "market" for care services. The internal variation refers to the client-orientation within the individual. All in all the use of the term case management in Austria resembles its international use. The Austrian specificity is that a specific profession, namely nurses are defined as the ideal case managers. Unfortunately, the question whether the term case refers to the person or the situation the person is in remains unanswered.

In summary the idea of integration within the process of care delivery is being realised in a multitude of concepts, which can still be expected to grow in number and evolve in quality. Examples for the diversity of possibilities of realisation are the concepts of case management, which is need-driven, care management, which also pays attention to the financial perspective, and networking, which describes a certain quality of cooperation. The Austrian discussion about integrated care concentrates on the matter itself, thus neglecting definitions. The – often rudimentary – definitions partly resemble, partly contradict their international equivalents. The concept of case management is in the centre of attention as well as the variant prevalently realised. In the practical model ways of working in Austria, case management is very often reduced to discharge management (see 3.3).

3.2 Approaching Model Ways of Working in Austria

As becomes clear from the description of the current system of help and care for the elderly in Austria, there is a need for better care systems, which is much discussed at present. In the late 1980s and early 1990s several research as well as practical projects were initiated which have multiplied since then.

Looking at models for integrated care systems, there are three types, which can be seen as a basis for description and analysis:

- The theoretical models, which describe the model ways of working and demonstrate the (positive) aspects of an integrated care system.
- The practical models (projects) that try to implement the theoretical concepts.
- The speculative models that can support the analysis of problems of integrated care systems and the systems development (Lindell/Olsson, 1999: 39).

Currently, the main focus should not be put on finding new theoretical model ways of working for integrated care, as the already existing theoretical models give us sufficient background for practical model ways of working. At this stage, it is more important to adapt the theoretical models to the practical situation in our societies (Grimm, 2002: 53-59).

This chapter is focused on two theoretical models in Austria, on prac- **119** tical models that illustrate these as well as on the connection between theory and practice. The two theoretical models are the *Integrated Health and Social Care Districts* (Integrierte Gesundheits- und Sozialsprengel) and *The Virtual Hospital at Home* (Das virtuelle Krankenhaus zu Hause).

3.3   *Theoretical Model Concepts of Working*

3.3.1 Integrated Health and Social Care Districts

In 1990 the government defined the introduction of *Integrated Health and Social Care Districts* ("Integrierte Gesundheits- und Sozialsprengel", in the following: IGSS) in Austria as a major aim of future health policy. The Austrian Federal Institute of Health (Österreichisches Bundesinstitut für Gesundheitswesen/ÖBIG) developed the respective theoretical concept (ÖBIG, 1993 with the idea that *IGSS* should be regional organisations for coordination and cooperation of health and social care organisations within a defined geographical area. The concrete work of an *IGSS* should be guided by the regional situation. Also, they were to analyse the existing provisions, to guarantee the existence of health and social care organisations and to act as partners for the patients and their families by helping them find the organisations to meet their specific needs.

An *IGSS* was to be comprised of a part of a city or several local governments with a number of inhabitants between 10,000 and 20,000 persons in all.[8] The health and social care districts have to cooperate with public services for financing, controlling and strategical arrangements.

The objectives of the concept are:

- to improve and guarantee the provision of health and social care in a district,
- to coordinate and harmonise the services of health and social care organisations,
- to optimise the cooperation and exchange between the health and social care organisations,
- to increase the effective output of the health and social care organisations in a district by catering to the special requirements of the patients,
- to help patients and their families to find the correct organisation for their needs,
- to initiate and develop health programmes.

The *IGSS* concept improves and extends the health and social care systems in a region. This also improves the situation for the elderly in need of care at home as it will be possible to find the best organisation(s) to meet their special needs and requirements. Also they help to improve the quality of care by securing its continuity and avoiding over-provision or the doubling of services.

They should develop preventive and rehabilitative health programmes to prevent and/or delay the development of diseases or disabilities responsible for an augmented need of care.

The conceptual guidelines for an *IGSS* mainly outline them as information centres about health and social care organisations in a particular district but do not include advice and counseling of the elderly in need of care, e.g. concerning which kind of health or welfare organisation they should select for their special needs.

In Austria there are different practical ways of working which are supposedly developed along this theoretical concept of *IGSS* (see A1).

3.3.2 The Virtual Hospital at Home

In 1998 the "Ludwig Boltzmann-Institut für Medizin- und Gesundheitssoziologie" in Vienna – a research centre for health and medical sociology – developed a theoretical concept for integrated care in Austria (LBI, 1999). The concept is based on international experience of "hospitals at home", empirical fieldwork and practical models for integrated care in Austria (Pelikan et al., 1998: 14).

In the concept *Virtual Hospital at Home* social care providers offer a "hospital at home" for patients. In practice, this means that social care providers have to organise an individual network of providers for every patient to manage his/her illness at home. The starting point is the cooperation between health and social care systems and, especially relevant with regard to the structure in Austria, the construction of a network between health and social care systems and different social care providers (see 2.4; Pelikan et al., 1998: 16-17).

This means integrating health and social care systems without establishing a new organisation, i.e. virtual integration. So, *The Virtual Hospital at Home* offers care following hospital characteristics, in case of a patient's need, at the time of the patient's need and in the patient's own home, provided by a combination of adequate providers (LBI, 1999: 14). The theoretical model "Virtual Hospital at Home" was developed by a study of the LBI where existing model ways of working were collected and analysed. Also, the project "Ganzheitliche Hauskrankenpflege" ("Holistic Home Nursing") was carried out in Vienna from 1996-1998 in cooperation with the Viennese Red Cross to implement the model in practice.

121

To summarise one can say that the focus of the theoretical models and the model ways of working in Austria is to improve cooperation between the different health and social care systems (see 2.4. and 2.5), not the integration of health and social care systems into one system.

3.4   *The Practical Model Ways of Working*

The starting point of all practical model ways of working in Austria is a holistic approach. This means that the older person in need for care is seen in relation to his/her biography and environment and not as an isolated entity (Österreichisches Hilfswerk, 2001: 29). All practical model ways of working in Austria try to see the person in need of help and care not as a helpless object of care but as a self-determined user with his/her own needs and wishes.

In the concrete, practical work, networking and cooperation between patient, hospital and social care system(s), the main prerequisite is to provide better care for the elderly. The target is to overcome the division of provision of health and long-term care for the elderly. The model ways of working try to find optimal ways of cooperation between established health and social care systems. They do not establish new organisations (Schmidt, 2002: 12-13).

The different model ways of working in Austria can be divided into four types (LBI, 1999: 36-39):

a) *Extramurally organised model ways of working:* The starting points of these model ways of working are the providers of social care, in general private non-profit organisations offering home help, meals-on-wheels etc. – and (in most provinces except Vienna) home nursing. These social care providers exist in all of the provinces and cooperate with the medical field, represented by a general practitioner (see Annex A1).

b) *Vertically integrated extramurally organised model ways of working:* Within the nursing and the care sectors pre-conditions for cooperation and substitution are created; the social care sector is the point of departure. The scope of action is the region of the hospital and the social care organisation (see Annex A3).

c) *Vertically integrated intramurally organised model ways of working:* These model ways of working have the same background as the vertically integrated extramurally organised models; the only difference is that in this case the point of departure is the hospital (see Annex A4).

d) *Intramurally organised model ways of working:* In this model, the professionals working in a hospital are responsible for the mobile care of patients at home. For example, teams of nurses offer medical care for the patients at home under supervision of the hospital staff (for example the integrated community care of patients with cystic fibrosis in the "Lainz hospital" in Vienna).

This categorisation represents ideal-type models. There has been some criticism of this as in reality the models partly overlap and cannot always be put clearly into one of these categories. In Austrian reality a number of variations of these ideal-type models can be found in every province, most of them defined as model projects, others as large-scale mainstream practices. Still, for the target group "older persons" we did not find an example for an *intramurally organised model way of working*. Most of the model projects considered in the analysis are situated in Vienna (14 out of 27), four in the province of Upper Austria, three in the province of Salzburg, two in Styria and one in each of the provinces of Burgenland, Niederösterreich, the Tyrol and Vorarlberg.

The reason for this situation might be that networking and cooperation is easier – but also more important – in a city than in rural areas. And/

or that in rural areas the informal care of the elderly in need of help and care, such as family care and neighbourhood help is more common, and institutional as well as home care provision is less available.

The different spheres of competence between the government and the provinces (see 2.1-2.5) have, on the one hand, resulted in various cooperation agreements between local governments and hospital systems of a province. On the other hand, local level model ways of working have developed in which one specific hospital cooperates with one specific social care organisation.

For example in August 1996 the hospital system of Vienna (Wiener Krankenanstaltenverbund) and the local government department of Vienna for care at home (Magistratsabteilung 47, Betreuung zu Hause) made a cooperation agreement concerning patients in need of long-term care. The target of this cooperation agreement between seven hospitals and different social care organisations in Vienna was to improve the cooperation and coordination between health and social care organisations focused on discharge management. For the realisation of these cooperation agreements, working groups in some districts of Vienna were established.

In 1999 the hospital system of Vienna (Wiener Krankenanstalten-verbund), a municipal health department of the City of Vienna (Magistrats-abteilung für Angelegenheiten der Landessanitätsdirektion) and the Austrian Umbrella Association for Social Security Agencies (Hauptverband der Österreichischen Sozialversicherungsträger) have commissioned the Ludwig Boltzmann-Institut for Medical and Health Sociology to carry out a feasibility study on patient-oriented integrated care in Vienna (LBI, 2000b). The result was an action plan and a federal recommendation for a best practice model of integrated care in Austria (see 3.1.2).

The important points of this action plan are:

- to optimise the process between the allocation of care and discharge management,
- to advance case management and to support professionals in social care services,
- to construct a network between intramural and extramural services,
- to construct a regional information pool for the patients.

Also, in July 2002 the practical model "Patient oriented integrated care" was started in Vienna (Districts 14-17) (see A4) (www.univie.ac.at).

The latest model in Austria officially started in October 2002. The project is called "MedTogether" (www.medtogether.at) and aims to improve the

123

management of the interfaces between health provision and social care organisations throughout Austria[9] (see 2.1 and A5).

Although the different health and social care systems on different levels try to find new model ways of working and although similar in structure (discharge management, cooperation), there is no exchange between the different model ways of working. The reasons for this situation are that there is no specific government programme for integrated care, that the different spheres of responsibilities of the state and the provinces complicate the cooperation of health and social care organisations, and that the social organisations compete with one another (see 2.1-2.5).

Thus, the government and the particular health and social care organisations are looking for solutions to work together, but they do not try to integrate the different health and social care systems into one system.

So the common targets of the model ways of working are (only) to give elderly in need of care the possibility to live at home. Therefore health and social care organisations try to improve cooperation between each other. The background of all model ways of working is discharge management (see 3.1).

4   Conclusions: Lessons to Learn

What becomes clear in this report on the Austrian situation is that *different types of financing of health and social care* and the fact that health is subject to federal regulation and social care is subject to provincial regulation makes the coordination of these two areas very difficult. Because of this legal distinction between health and social services there has been no integration of these fields on the federal level until now.

The involved actors in these fields – federal government, provinces, health and social service organisations, communities, health insurances – have been aware of this dilemma for quite a long time and a number of efforts have been made to improve the situation (see 3). A feasibility study (LBI, 2000b) has shown that there are different model projects of integrated health and social care. While looking at these different models in Austria it became clear that theoretical models available on an international level have to be tailored to fit the individual situation in the country, and to be able to develop new paths.

In Austria, it has been realised that it is not possible to radically change structures that have grown over the past 30 years, and that are very closely related to the political structure ("pillarisation"). It seems as if it was hardly possible to *integrate* the health and social service systems in Austria into one system. However, there are extensive efforts to improve the *coordination* of health and social services and it is considered as being important to build up an infrastructure for care and case management (Wild, 2002: 24).

One of the latest efforts to improve the management of the interface between health and social care is the government-initiated project *"MedTogether"* (see 3). This is a project operating on the federal level with the aim of initiating regional networks. An important aspect of this project will be to involve all stakeholders in health care and social networks in the project. This project is a reaction to suggestions from different sides concerning the need for improvements in this area (see 2.4). Another important improvement from earlier projects will be using better project management structures and to once more implement the method of benchmarking between the involved projects. These improvements cannot be reached on a federal level but are mainly relevant on a local level. Efforts in this direction are made, for example, in the patient-oriented integrated care projects in Vienna, that are being implemented currently.

A specific issue of *coordination within social services* in Austria concerns the coordination between different providers and between provinces in the provision of social services. This is due, on the one hand, to the varied legal frameworks in the provinces and, on the other hand, to issues of competition between different providers (especially those linked to different political parties). One lesson to be learned from the models aimed at improving health and social care is that social service providers have learned to work together better. Due to the number of social service providers and the fact that there are several in one region, they have been under pressure to participate in the model projects and thus to work together and keep the logic of competition in the background.

One of the main issues in all these models is the effort to combine a *reduction of cost increases with improved quality of life* for the clients and other people involved. It is still open whether these aims can be combined. Especially, if social services are given more responsibilities and have more clients due to shorter length of stay in hospitals and improving opportunities for home care services, there is a need to improve social services' infrastructure as well as staff's education, working conditions etc. These improvements would then also involve further spending.

A main lesson that has been learned from the models that have been implemented in Austria so far concerns the cooperation and working together between different organisations that operate according to different logics and have different types of personnel. It was shown that after overcoming first doubts, people cooperating in these projects develop a *new understanding of the other sectors'* work and both groups of personnel learn from each other and can improve their performance.

The success of model projects depends on the *engagement of those involved* in them and in the structural framework of the organisations at hand. We have seen that, in successful projects, the staff members have to take up the ideas of a project within the organisation to be able to take it outside and to cooperate with staff from other areas.

It has also become clear that projects need clear competencies and guidelines to function successfully. The *split competencies and regulations* in the area of health and social services that these projects strive to overcome are at the same time the *barriers* for successful work of these projects.

Another issue is criticism on the *Integrated Health and Social Districts* (IGSS) that can be found especially in Tyrol and Vorarlberg. Some experts argue that they are only a group of providers that integrate social service provision and nothing more. From our point of view some of the envisaged aims in coordinating regional social service provision have been reached (see 3). The IGSS have shown professional ways of working. Also, the IGSS have always been oriented towards the needs of the clients. They are existing regional networks in which providers from different political backgrounds and with a long tradition of competition have learned to mutually work together. However, working together with regional hospitals and other health providers has been missing until now.

With respect to the new project *"MedTogether"* which aims at building up new regional networks in the area of health and social care, it will be interesting to see, whether they will connect to *existing networks* like the IGSS, whether the existing networks will be flexible enough to adjust to new networks or whether new networks, in the worst case, lead to a disintegration of the existing ones. *"Medtogether" does endeavour both to use existing networks and to support new ones.* Another issue to be noticed is that while there have been studies that looked at different model projects and thus the model projects could learn from each other, there are no *apparent links and networks* connecting the different projects and enabling ongoing exchange. This is, for instance, noticeable in the respective projects' websites.

Last but not least, there is a discussion in Austria on the issue whether *the increased coordination and integration of social services* – as e.g. in IGSS – might lead to *less choice of services* for the service users. However, with respect to the lack of staff and services, which is to be expected, these worries will certainly vanish, in particular if the only distintion in providers' qualities remains to be their political or religious affiliation.

All in all one can say that the fragmented situation of health and social service provision in Austria has been recognised and that there have been several efforts made to improve this situation. However, there is still a lot to be done in order to be able to speak of integrated health and social service provision in Austria.

Notes

1   A specific problem with regard to split competencies in health and social care concerns the hospitals for the chronically ill (Chronische Krankenanstalten). They belong to the area of social care but partly offer the same medical provisions as hospitals. This leads to the phenomenon that persons receiving a certain medical provision in a chronic hospital have to pay for this themselves, while another person receiving the same provision in a regular hospital will have this covered by the health insurance.

2   The social insurance agencies are autonomous bodies. However, in this area federal legislation regulates their functions and governmental agencies are represented on their boards.

3   Article 15a of the Austrian Constitution allows for special coordination agreements between the federal state and the provincial governments in a specific field (such as health care) that both territorial authorities have competencies in. The aim of these agreements is to harmonise provisions throughout the country and to improve policy efficiency (BMSG, 2001).

4   As the general framework provided for these plans was quite vague and different institutes or consultants compiled them for each single provincial government, they are hardly comparable as they lack in comparative data sets and common criteria (Schaffenberger et al., 1999).

5   Although there are different types of charging mechanisms, it should be noted that billing is usually accomplished by the local or regional administration that reimburses the providers and charges the clients about 1% of their income (e.g. pensions plus long-term care allowance minus housing costs).

6   As most institutions, i.e. also former old-age homes, have at least some nursing beds, a distinction between old age and nursing homes has become more or less impossible.

7   Since September 1997, in Vienna special training is needed for home-helpers according to the new "Wiener Heimhilfegesetz" (Viennese Home Help Act). This act determines that home-helpers have to attend a course to the extent of 400 hours (200 theory and 200 practice). Those courses are carried out by the private non-profit organisations them-

selves. Sozial Global, Wiener Sozialdienste, Wiener Volkshilfe and the Wiener Rotes Kreuz are the main providers of this service.

8   Austrian municipalities/communes comprise entities with some 300 inhabitants as well as, for instance, Vienna with its more than 1.8 million inhabitants. Thus, in general, an IGSS would comprise about 5 smaller municipalities/communes.

9   Thus, once more it will be necessary to formulate agreements between the federal and the provincial governments according to Art. 15a B-VG (Art. 5 and 6) of the Austrian Constitution.

References

Amt der Tiroler Landesregierung (2002) *Ich brauche Hilfe. Pflege, Betreuung und Behindertenhilfe in Tirol*. Innsbruck: Amt der Tiroler Landesregierung.

Badelt, Christoph (1999) 'Der Nonprofit Sektor in Österreich', S. 61-83 in: Badelt, Christoph (Hg.), *Handbuch der Nonprofit Organisation*. Stuttgart: Schäffer-Poeschel.

Badelt, C./Holzmann, A./Matul, C./Österle, A. (1997) *Analyse der Auswirkungen des Pflegevorsorgesystems*. Wien: BM für Arbeit, Gesundheit und Soziales.

Badelt, Ch./Leichsenring, K. (1998) *Analyse und mögliche Neustrukturierung der Ausbildungen im Sozialbereich*. Wien: Bundesministerium für Unterricht und kulturelle Angelegenheiten und Bundesministerium für Wissenschaft und Verkehr.

Badelt, Ch./Leichsenring, K. (2000) 'Versorgung, Betreuung, Pflege', S. 408-453 in: Bundesministerium für Soziale Sicherheit und Generationen (Hg.), *Ältere Menschen – Neue Perspektiven: Seniorenbericht 2000*. Wien: BMSSG.

Bahr, C./Leichsenring, K. (1996) *"leben und pflegen" – Beratung und Koordination im Sozialsprengel*. Evaluationsstudie. Wien: European Centre.

Barta, H./Ganner, M. (1998) *Alter, Recht und Gesellschaft. Rechtliche Rahmenbedingungen der Alten- und Pflegebetreuung*. Wien: WUV-Universitätsverlag.

Bundesarbeitsgemeinschaft Freie Wohlfahrt (2002) *Qualitätsmerkmale der mobilen Pflege und Betreuung*. Wien: BAG Freie Wohlfahrt.

Bundesministerium für Arbeit, Gesundheit und Soziales (BMAGS) (1999) *Soziale Sicherheit ein Leben lang. Ein Wegweiser durch die Leistungen des Bundesministeriums*. Wien: BMAGS.

Bundesministerium für Soziale Sicherheit und Generationen (BMSG) (2001) *Bericht des Arbeitskreises für Pflegevorsorge*. Wien: BMSG.

Bundesministerium für Soziale Sicherheit und Generationen (BMSG) (2001) *Das Gesundheitswesen in Österreich*. Wien: BMSG.

Dachverband der Wiener Pflege- und Sozialdienste (DWPS) (1998) *Case Management in den sozialen Stützpunkten der MA 47* (http://bildung.dachverband.at/DOWNLOADS/hyperpdfs/case. pdf).

Dachverband der Wiener Pflege- und Sozialdienste (2001) *Entlassungsmanagement durch ambulante Anbieterorganisationen im Hanusch-Krankenhaus der Wiener Gebietskrankenkassen. Case Management an der Schnittstelle Krankenhaus und extramurale Betreuung*. Wien: Dachverband der Wiener Pflege- und Sozialdienste.

Eiersebner, E. (2000) 'Bedarfsplanung am Beispiel der Bedarfs- und Entwicklungspläne in Österreich', S. 43-63 in: Manfred Lallinger (Hg.), *Altenpflege zwischen Makrosteuerung und Marktwirtschaft*. Stuttgart: Akademie der Diözese Rottenburg-Stuttgart.

Evers, A./Leichsenring, K./Pruckner, B. (1994) 'Payments for Care: The Case of Austria', S. 191-214 in: Evers, A./Pijl, M./Ungerson, C. (Eds.), *Payments for Care. A Comparative Overview*. Aldershot: Avebury.

Farkas, U./Leichsenring, K. (1994) 'Eine gemeinsame Sprache finden – Beratung und Koordination zur Entlastung von Angehörigen in Niederösterreich', S. 157-169 in: Evers, A./Pruckner, B. (Hg.), *Pflege in der Familie? Politik, die hilft.* Tagungsbericht. Wien: Europäisches Zentrum/BMJuF.

Grimm, K. H. (2002) 'Die strukturelle Planung zwischen Pflegender und Patient als Basis pflegerischen Denkens und Handelns', *PflegeForschung,* 06/2002: 53-59 (http://www.pr-internet.com)

Grundböck, A. et al. (1997) 'Das Krankenhaus daheim', *ProSenectute* 3: 13-15.

Grundböck, A. et al. (1998) 'Ganzheitliche Hauskrankenpflege – ein Modellprojekt des Wiener Roten Kreuzes', S. 91-112 in: Pelikan, J.M. et al. (Hg.), *Virtuelles Krankenhaus zu Hause – Entwicklung von Qualität und Ganzheitlicher Hauskrankenpflege.* Wien: Facultas.

Grundböck, A. et al. (2000) 'Case Management in einem Wiener Modellprojekt zur ambulanten Versorgung von Patienten mit komplexen Betreuungsbedarf', S. 217-250 in: Ewers, M./Schaeffer, D. (Hg.), *Case Management in Theorie und Praxis.* Bern u.a.: Hans Huber.

Hofer, E.M. (1999) 'Wer ist nun der ideale Case Manager?', *Lazarus* 1/2: 26f.

Hofmarcher, M./Rack, H. (2001) *Health Care Systems in Transition. Austria.* Copenhagen: The European Observatory on Health Care Systems.

Kain, E. (1994) 'New Forms of Health and Social Care in Austria', pp. 12-24 in: Österreichisches Bundesinstitut für Gesundheitswesen (Ed.), *New Forms of Health and Social Care: Five National Reports.* Vienna: Österreichisches Bundesinstitut für Gesundheitswesen.

Kalousek, M./Scholta, M. (1999) *Arbeitskreis 5: Pflege und Betreuung im häuslichen und institutionellen Bereich.* Endbericht. Bundesministerium für Soziale Sicherheit und Generationen.

Leichsenring, K. (1995) 'La prestation dépendance en Autriche', *Années Documents Cleirppa,* No. 231 (mars): 9-16.

Leichsenring, K. (1999) 'The Austrian System of Social Protection for Persons in Need of Care', pp. 119-146 in: Observatorio de Personas Mayores (Ed.), *Vejez y protección social a la dependencia en Europa.* Madrid: Ministerio der Trabajo y Asuntos Sociales/IMSERSO.

Leichsenring, K./Pruckner, B. (1993) 'Zwischen privater Pflicht und öffentlicher Verantwortung – europäische Trends und sozialpolitische Perspektiven der Pflegevorsorge', *Österreichische Zeitschrift für Politikwissenschaft,* 22 (3): 291-311.

Leichsenring, K./Stadler, M. (1998) *Purchaser-Provider Relationships and Quality Assurance in the Area of Personal Social Services in Vienna.* Vienna: European Centre (Austrian National Report in the framework of the EU project 'Qualification for Development' coordinated by SMAER, Bologna).

Leichsenring, K./Pleschberger, S. (1999) *Needs Assessment and Allocation of Long-term Care Services for Care-dependent Persons in Austria.* Vienna: European Centre.

Lindell, M./Olsson, H. (1999) *Grundlegende Modelle in der Pflege. Theoretische Aspekte und praktische Beispiele.* Heidelberg: Altera.

Ludwig Boltzmann-Institut für Medizin- und Gesundheitssoziologie (LBI) (1999) *Virtuelles Krankenhaus zu Hause in Österreich. Bestandsaufnahme und Analyse von Modellen der Qualitätsverbesserung der Spitalsentlassungen bzw. der integrierten ambulanten Versorgung akut kranker Menschen.* Wien: LBI.

Ludwig Boltzmann-Institut für Medizin- und Gesundheitssoziologie (LBI) (2000) *Virtuelles Krankenhaus zu Hause in Österreich* (http://www.univie.ac.at/lbimgs/projekte/vh-oenb.html).

Ludwig Boltzmann-Institut für Medizin- und Gesundheitssoziologie (LBI) (2000a) *Integrierte Versorgung /12. Organisation der Patientenbetreuung zwischen dem Donauspital und der Betreuung zu Hause – Abschlussevaluation.* Wien: LBI.

Ludwig Boltzmann-Institut für Medizin- und Gesundheitssoziologie (LBI) (2000b) *Integrierte Versorgung /13. Machbarkeitsstudie für ein Modellprojekt „Patientenorientierte, integrierte Krankenbetreuung (in Wien) – Enbericht*. Wien: LBI.

MA 47 – Betreuung zu Hause/Dachverband Wiener Pflege- und Sozialdienste (1997) *Das Wiener Pflege- und Betreuungskonzept der ambulanten Pflege- und Sozialdienste*. Wien: MA 47.

MedTogether. *Schnittstellenmanagement zwischen ambulanter und stationärer Versorgung*. (http// www.medtogether.at).

Mutschler, R. (1998) 'Kooperation ist eine Aufgabe Sozialer Arbeit: Zusammenarbeit und Vernetzung als professionelle Verpflichtung – Regionale Arbeitsgruppen als Standard beruflicher Sozialarbeit', *Blätter der Wohlfahrtspflege* 3+4: 49-52.

Nemeth,C./Pochobradsky, E. (2002) *Pilotprojekt: Qualitätssicherung in der Pflege*. Bundesministerium für soziale Sicherhheit und Generationen.

Oelschlägel, D. (2000) 'Vernetzung und Ressourcenbündelung im Gemeinwesen', *Theorie und Praxis der Sozialen Arbeit* 1: 16-20.

Österreichisches Bundesinstitut für Gesundheitswesen (ÖBIG) (1993) *Integrierte Gesundheits- und Sozialsprengel. Handbuch zur Umsetzung von IGSS*. Wien: ÖBIG.

Österreichisches Hilfswerk (2001) *Hilfe und Pflege daheim. Die mobilen Gesundheits- und Sozialdienste des Hilfswerks*. Wien: Österreichisches Hilfswerk.

Patientenorientierte integrierte Krankenbetreuung (Wien 14.-17) (http://www.univie.ac.at/pik).

Pelikan, J. M/Stacher, A./Grundböck, A./Krajic, K. (1998) *Virtuelles Krankenhaus zu Hause – Entwicklung und Qualität von Ganzheitlicher Hauskrankenpflege*. Wien: Facultas.

Petzl, D. (2003) 'Pflegevorsorge – ein statistischer Überblick', *Soziale Sicherheit*, Nr. 5: 240-251.

Pfeil, W. (1994) *Neuregelung der Pflegevorsorge in Österreich*. Wien: Kammer für Arbeiter und Angestellte (Rechts- und sozialwissenschaftliche Schriftenreihe, Band 11).

Pratscher, K. (1992) 'Sozialhilfe: Staat – Markt – Familie', S. 61-95 in: Tálos, E. (Hg.), *Der geforderte Wohlfahrtsstaat. Traditionen – Herausforderungen – Perspektiven*. Wien: Löcker Verlag.

Pratscher, K./Stolitzka, B. (1999) 'Sozialhilfe 1997', *Statistische Nachrichten* 4: 264-270.

Rosenmayr, L./Majce, G. (1998) *Was können Generationen einander bieten? Zweifel und Hoffnungen für das kommende Jahrhundert*. Wien: Bundesministerium für Umwelt, Jugend und Familie.

Rotes Kreuz Wien (2001) *Daheim gesund werden. Weiterführende Betreuung durch Ganzheitliche Hauskrankenpflege* (http://www.redcross.or.at/mains/dienste/forschung/Endbericht/ KurzDaheimGesundWerden_09072001.pdf).

Rubisch, M. (1998) 'Die Umsetzung der Pflegevereinbarung zwischen Bund und Ländern', *Soziale Sicherheit* 12: 941-945.

Rubisch, M./Philipp, S./Wotzel, W./Enge, I. (2001) *Pflegevorsorge in Österreich*. Wien: Bundesministerium für Soziale Sicherheit und Generationen.

Schaffenberger, E./Jurasovich, B./Pochobradsky, E. (1999) *Dienste und Einrichtungen für pflegebedürftige Menschen in Österreich. Übersicht über die Bedarfs- und Entwicklungspläne der Länder*. Wien: Bundesministerium für Arbeit, Gesundheit und Soziales.

Schmidt, B. (2002) 'Organisationskultur im Wandel – von der krankenhauszentrierten zur gemeindenahen integrierten Versorgung', *PflegeManagement* 1: 12-28 (http://www.pr-internet.com).

Statistik Austria (2004) *Statistisches Jahrbuch 2004*. Wien: Statistik Austria.

Wild, Monika (2002) 'Ambulant vor stationär – Quo Vadis?', *Österreichische Pflegezeitschrift*, 5/ 02: 22-26.

130

Annex: Selected Model Ways of Working

A1 Social Care and Health District Hartberg

Example for an extramurally organised model way of working based on the concept of *Integrated Health and Social Care Districts* **(see 3.3.1)**

Name	Integrierte Sozial- und Gesundheitssprengel in Hartberg (ISGS-Hartberg)
Provider	In 1989 the Integrated *Social Care and Health Districts in Hartberg* was established. The social care and health organisations "Red Cross", "Caritas" and "Volkshilfe" work together in this field and since 2000 there is also a co-operation with the district hospital. The principal task is to coordinate the network between the different social and health care providers in a district.
Objectives	• To offer patients in need of care the possibility to stay at home, • to improve and guarantee the offer of health and social care organisations in a district, • to help patients and their families to find the appropriate organisation for their needs, • to start and develop care programmes for relatives.
Target group	In 2002 941 elderly received care services in the districts.
Number of staff involved	55 persons (managers, nurses, family and home helpers) plus volunteers work in the district. In 2002 they worked a total of 48,319 hours whereas 28,696 hours were for care and 2,536 hours for case management.
Methods	The *Social Care and Health District* in Hartberg is a regional organisation for coordination and cooperation of health and social care organisations in a district. The concrete work of a *Social Care and Health District* is guided by the regional situation. They analyse the provision situation of a district, guarantee the provision of health and social care organisations in a district and they are the partners of the patients and their families to look for special organisation(s) for their needs. They offer home nursing, family care, meals on wheels, visiting services and health prevention.
Strengths and weaknesses	*Strengths* • The *Social Care and Health Districts* in Hartberg extend the health and social care systems in a region for the elderly in need of care at home.

131

- They improve the quality of care because the continuity of care is secured and the services are more in line with each other.
- They have preventive and rehabilitative health programmes to prevent and to delay the necessity for care.
- The *Social Care and Health District* in Hartberg cooperates with the district hospital.
Weaknesses
- The Social Care and Health Districts are basically associations, where different providers get together and provide services. This leads to the question whether clients in one district have enough choice of providers.

Results of evaluation/keywords	The *Social Care and Health District* in Hartberg is a specific model way of working in one province of Austria. It is a good practice example to start a model way of working on the provincial level and to start a political programme for a better care provision or better cooperation between different social service organisations and a district hospital.

A2 Organisation of Patients' Care between the Donau Hospital and the Health and Social Centre Donaufeld

Example for a vertically integrated intramurally organised model way of working

Name	Organising patient care between the "Danube" Hospital and the Health and Social Centre "Donaufeld" (GSZ 21/22) (LBI, 2000a)
Provider	*Donau hospital*, Health and Social Centre *Donaufeld*. Based on the cooperation agreement between The Hospital System of Vienna (Wiener Krankenanstaltenverbund (KAV) and the Local Government Department of Vienna for care at home (MA 47, Betreuung zu Hause)
Objectives	• To develop concrete structures between the *Donau* hospital and the mobile organisation Health and Social Centre *Donaufeld* to guarantee the continuity of provision for elderly in need of care, • to limit the number and length of hospital stays, • to intensify the offer of information, advice and care.
Target group	Older patients needing complex mobile provision
Number of staff involved	A working group of hospital doctors, family doctors, managers of social care organisations, social workers and local government officials.

Methods	The working group regularly met every month from 1997 to 1999 to develop relevant structures for discharge management and to transfer the results into their practical work.
Strengths and weaknesses	*Strengths* • The working group evaluated the output of their meetings as being effective. The regular working group meetings between hospital, family doctors, and mobile care organisation improved the concrete cooperation between the different actors in the care system. The exchange of experience helped the involved staff to understand the process of organisation of the other involved actors in care provision of the elderly in need of care and the working plans they developed helped to coordinate discharge management for elderly in need of care. • This model way of working is a first step to start a co-operation between regional health and care systems. *Weaknesses* • The weaknesses of this model way of working are the complicated structures of the Austrian Health System (see 2.1-2.5) and the missing legal framework for these model ways of working.
Results of evaluation/keywords	• A regional working group with different actors from the health and social care systems is regarded as a first step to start cooperation. • The intensive exchange of experience improves the acceptance of the different ways of working in hospitals and social care services. • The cooperation agreement is an important basis to improve the cooperation between health and social care organisations.

133

A3 Discharge Management in the "Hartmann" Hospital: A Cooperation Project between the Viennese Red Cross and the "Hartmann" Hospital

Example for a vertically integrated extramurally organised model way of working

Name	Discharge Management in the Hartmann Hospital
Provider	Wiener Rotes Kreuz (Viennese Red Cross), Hartmann Hospital
Objectives	• It is a follow-up project of the model project Recovering at Home (Daheim gesund werden) of the Viennese Red Cross and the Hartmann Hospital, • to foster cooperation between hospital and home care service providers to guarantee the continuity of provision for the elderly in need of care, • to offer individual services in the hospital (before discharge) for elderly in need of care at home, • to limit the hospital stay.
Target group	Patients needing complex provision at home
Number of staff involved	In 2002, there were 389 inquiries, on average the number amounts to 32 consultations per month One discharge manager plus a substitute
Methods	The discharge management takes place in different wards of the hospital and the heads of wards refer the patients to the discharge managers. They accept the responsibility for organising and coordinating the provision of home care for the patients while they are still in hospital.
Strengths and weaknesses	*Strengths for patients and their families:* • The patients and their families receive a "made-to-measure" maintenance schedule for care at home from the discharge manager. • The discharge manager works in cooperation with patients, families, hospital and social care services. The personal confidence between discharge manager, patients and their families helps to reduce the fear and the insecurity caused by the new personal situation of elderly in need of care and their families at home.

134

Strengths for the hospital:
- The cooperation between hospital and discharge managers demonstrates the limits and possibilities of mobile social care services and promotes the bilateral understanding of hospital and social care services.
- The discharge managers relieve the hospital employees in their work and the duration of the patients' stay in the hospital becomes shorter.

Strengths for the home care organisations:
- The social care service receives detailed information from the discharge manager on the need for care. Thus, the social service providers have enough time to prepare special services for the elderly in need of care at home.

Strengths for the health system:
- The cooperation agreement between hospital and social care service (local level) is an important basis for the continuity in the provision of integrated health and social care for older persons.

Weaknesses:
- The high standards of the discharge management: discharge managers need to have knowledge about the medical sector, the mobile care services and have to organise the network between different systems and persons (hospital employees, social care employees, elderly in need of care and their families).
- The high standards of the cooperation agreement between hospital, discharge manager and social care system are a prerequisite for an effective network.

Results of evalua-tion/keywords	• High contentment of the patients and their families. • Enough time for the social care organisation to prepare the care at home. • The stay in the hospital is shorter and thus the hospital costs are reduced. • The intensive exchange of experience improves the acceptance of the different ways of working of hospitals and social care services.

135

A4 Patient-Oriented Integrated Care in Vienna, Districts 14-17

Name	Patient-oriented integrated health care (in Vienna 14.-17.) [pik] (www.univie.ac.at/pik) / July 2002 – December 2004
Provider	Viennese Health Insurance Agency (Wiener Gebietskranken-kassen) and the local government of Vienna
Objectives	*Patient orientation:* • to assess the needs of the patients • to develop an information system of mobile care for the patients • to include the patients in developing their care programmes • to help the patients to be active partners in their care programmes *Integrated care:* • to provide a bridge in health and social care in difficult phases (e.g. a hospital stay is necessary for a person, the discharge of a patient from a hospital, home care is needed) • to improve networking and communication between the professionals and the patients
Number of staff involved and target group	*The following groups work together in a district:* • patients, their families and their other social contacts • hospitals • medical practitioners • social care organisations • therapists • pharmacies
Methods	• a project team with regular meetings supports the work • an evaluation team accompanies the project • the LBI's feasibility study will be validated through this project • an interactive website for information exchange
Strengths and weaknesses	*Strengths:* • The important point of the project is to include the patients and their families and to install a focus group. *Weaknesses:* • The project only tries to improve the management level between the different partners and does not link the health and social organisations and truly integrates them.

A5 "MedTogether" – Management between Outpatient Care and Hospital Care

Name	MedTogether – Schnittstellenmanagement zwischen ambulanter und stationärer Versorgung "MedTogether" – Management between outpatient care and hospital care October 2002 – 2004 (www.medtogether.at)
Provider	Federal Structural Funds
Objectives	• to improve the management between social care and health provision • to improve the care of the patients • to optimise the admissions and the discharge of patients in a hospital • to increase the satisfaction of the patients and the health care providers • to optimise the length of stays in hospitals • to slow down cost increases in the hospital
Target group	Hospitals, social organisations and patients and their families in a region build a network
Number of staff involved	The project is focused on the whole of Austria
Methods	• a regional project team is the basis • task forces have the overlapping function to build a network between the regional project teams • a discussion forum for all involved persons • the project coordinator and the controlling team lead the project • the project is structured according to people with specific diseases, e.g. diabetes, cardiac infarction, aberrant mamma, apoplectic stroke
Strengths and weaknesses	*Strengths:* • It is the first model way of working that will be planned and implemented throughout Austria. *Weaknesses:* • It is only a project to improve the cooperation between the different health and social care systems concerning the involvement of patients and their families. The focus of the project is not to integrate health and social care systems in one.

137

CHAPTER 4

Providing Integrated Health and Social Care for Older Persons in Denmark

Ellinor Colmorten, Thomas Clausen, Steen Bengtsson

1   Introduction

In the course of the 20th century the public sector in Denmark has been developed continuously to secure the welfare of citizens. In the beginning of the 20th century the public sevices mainly concerned economic security in case of loss of income while in the second half of the century the provision of services has increased as public services were provided to improve citizens' living conditions. This development has also concerned the elderly.

In Denmark, health and social care are available on a universal basis depending on need and not age or ability to pay. If an older person is in need of care, it is accepted and underwritten by legislation that the public assumes responsibility for the care services required (Blackman et al., 2001). Health service, hospitals and social care are provided at no cost to the elderly and financed through general taxation (Wagner, 1994).

Due to the fact that, in Denmark, the rate of women participating in the labour market is one of the highest in Europe, and that people retire earlier the nature and scope of informal family care have changed. Families have no legal obligations to care for elderly family members. Assistance given by family members or relatives is considered additional input to the assistance provided by the public services, rather than a substitution. Although there continues to be a culture of additional support provided by family members, in particular by children of older people, family care rarely substitutes for public care (Blackman et al., 2001).

The development of Danish policy on older persons has, in the course of the 20th century, been characterised by incremental changes and adaptations to different socio-economic challenges and public demands. These developmental trends in the Danish policy on elderly led to an increasing awareness that the various policies concerning older persons lacked internal coherence and in many cases policies in one area contradicted policies in another. Against this background the Commission on Elderly was constituted in the late 1970s. The objective of the commission was to formulate coherent visions and objectives for the Danish policy on elderly. One of the main recommendations of the Commission on Elderly was to aim at an increasing level of integration of the services provided to senior citizens. According to the commission *"a higher level of coherence must be considered a central means to achieve tangible improvements in the living conditions for the individual older person, while ensuring that this is achieved without an extreme rise in expenditure"* (Ministry of Social Affairs, vol. 3, 1982: 30; our translation). In subsequent years the following developments have characterised the Danish policy on elderly.

During the 1980s and until the end of the 1990s an increasing part of the elderly population has made use of the possibility of receiving services provided by the public (Ministry of Social Affairs, 2000). Most of the period the Danish economy has been characterised by stagnation. Consequently it has been difficult to meet growing needs of care for older people by a similar growth in the use of economic resources. Instead the growing need for elderly care has been met through restructuring and innovation, for example in the form of a shift from institutional care to home care along the lines of the recommendations of the Commission on Elderly. At the same time the municipal organisation of services and the use of staff have changed (Ministry of Social Affairs, 1995). These developments have resulted in an increasing level of integration of the health and social care services provided by the local – municipal – level of government.

This process of integration, however, has until now to a large extent eluded the health services of hospital services that are provided by the regional level of government. As will be discussed in the following, the boundaries between local and regional government, thus, appear to constitute a significant barrier in terms of integrating the health services provided by the regionally administered hospitals with the health and care services provided by the municipalities.

In the second half of the 1990s, however, changes in public policy resulted in a reduction of public services, first of all in the area of care for the elderly. Economic considerations combined with an increasing request for home help had as a consequence that the municipalities gave priority to personal care at the expense of the emphasis on practical assistance. Altogether, this meant less time for practical assistance. At the same time there has been a change in measuring the services. Before, the help was given and measured according to the total need, while it is now measured according to a detailed description of needs. For the citizens it appears that the help provided is less generous (Hansen, 2000).

However, in the following decades the Danish welfare state will increasingly be confronted with the challenges of coping with an ageing population. The challenges associated with an increasing proportion of potential recipients of elderly care, thus, put the tax-financed Danish model of universal provision of elderly care under pressure.

The presentation will focus on the following issues in the organisation of elderly care in Denmark. After a brief presentation of basic concepts in Danish elderly care the attention will be directed towards a description of the structure of health and social care services. This description will focus on who are providing and who are provided with health and social care. Furthermore, this description will discuss the conflicts between the actors involved in the provision of health and social care services. The subsequent section will discuss model projects that aim at solving various problems in the existing system through innovation of new ways of working. Finally, the presentation will focus on the lessons that can be learned from the model projects and from the aggregate experiences of providing health and social care services in Denmark.

141

2 Basic Principles and Concepts in Danish Elderly Care

The Commission on Elderly[1] announced the principles in policy for older persons in the beginning of the 1980s. The general objective of Danish ageing policy is to improve the individual's possibility of living at home or to ease his/her everyday existence and improve his/her quality of life. Danish ageing policy is based on the general principles of (i) ensuring continuity in an individual's life, (ii) making use of older people's own resources, (iii) preserving older people's self-determination, and (iv) sustaining older persons' ability to influence their own circumstances.

The philosophy behind these principles is that (i) older persons do not make up a homogeneous group with uniform needs, (ii) the provision of services to older persons shall not be provided as a package solution in nursing homes, but be given in accordance with the individual need for aid, and (iii) residents of nursing homes – as other older persons – should have influence on their own economy and daily lives (Ministry of Social Affairs, 1982).

The concept of Danish ageing policy presupposes that a broad and varied range of services and activities is available to the elderly. The services concerning integrated health and social care are home help, home nursing, rehabilitation and nursing homes[2] (Ministry of Social Affairs, 1998).

The central government lays down the general legislative framework for the provision of services for older persons but the municipalities decide on and are responsible for the range and organisation of the services provided. It is furthermore the responsibility of the municipality to provide coherent services to the individual as well as to monitor that resources are used in an effective way. Even though the services will vary from one municipality to another the cooperation between home nurses, home helpers and other social and health services is a central requirement.

2.1 Integrated Care at the Municipal Level

The aim of Danish elderly policy is to enable older persons to live a life as close to the normal life as they want it. The key phrase is *"in your own home as long as possible"*. It presupposes that a varied range of services is available to the elderly. Only in cases of actual illness treatment will be given in hospital. When an older person no longer needs treatment, the local authority assumes responsibility for care and services. Apart from nursing homes, Denmark has almost no institutions outside the hospital system taking care of the frailest elderly. Their needs are met through integrated health and social care within municipalities. Integration between home help and home nursing means that in practice the two professions, social and health care, are formally working together in integrated teams. The service also includes physiotherapists and occupational therapists.

With the social reform of 1976 social security and some health and social services were united in municipalities. The idea was that citizens only had

142

to contact a single authority instead of several, as was previously the case. But in the municipalities social services were spread over several departments: One for home nursing, one for home help, one for health, one for nursing homes and one for social work for the elderly. Each department had its own budgets, management and employees. This diversion entailed that an elderly citizen might have several case managers and cooperation between the departments was not always flexible.

During the period of economic stagnation in the 1980s the social services were under pressure for more effectiveness. There was almost no discussion about competitiveness or of involving the market as in the UK or later in Sweden. Instead, the focus was on gearing the municipal health and social care units for a more effective use of resources. The result was, among other things, a re-organisation of health and social services for elderly.

The aim was an integrated health and social care. The integrated health and social services imply that the services are provided to all elderly – independent of where they live – by integrated teams of home helpers, home nurses ect. Each elderly person in need of support has a case manager in the municipality, who is the individual counsellor of the older person applying for support. The case manager coordinates the efforts and cancels when the elderly is hospitalised, on vacation or visiting relatives. The decision to support is made on request from GPs, hospitals, the elderly or relatives.

As services are provided without regard to type of housing, no distinction is made between nursing homes, adapted dwellings and independent housing for the elderly. The 24-hours assistance services are accessible for all elderly in need. By providing personal assistance at all hours of the day this service contributes to reducing the demand for nursing home places, handling early discharges from hospital, and preventing some incidents of socially induced hospitalisation.

According to the Act on Housing for Older People it must be possible to call in speedy assistance at any time of the day or night to all sheltered housing. In addition, ready assistance may be made available for other types of dwelling. If an ordinary telephone does not provide an adequate means of calling, an emergency call system may be installed (Ministry of Social Affairs, 1995).

Many local authorities cooperate on measures of prevention and rehabilitation for the elderly, with the aim of enabling older people to remain in their homes as long as possible. In addition, practical and personal assistance is supplied by local authorities, which employ physiotherapists or occupational therapists.

143

As regards discharge of older people from hospital, there are no regulations or standards to ensure coordination, although in some counties the hospitals and municipalities have reached their own agreements on coordination. The problems with the integration of health and social services are often connected with discharge from hospital. The decrease in the average number of bed days at hospitals results in an increasing demand for domiciliary care. The process of integration of health and social care, thus, appears to be most advanced at the municipal level. As will be discussed later, the bulk of the problems in terms of integration occurs at the interface between the regionally administered hospital system and the municipally administered health and social care services.

2.2 The Concept of Self-care

The provision of integrated health and social care for older persons is based on the concept of self-care. The concept of self-care includes the acceptance of the human being as a free, independently thinking and acting individual with the ability to make decisions about his/her life. According to Orem's concept of self-care, the role of health care personnel is consultative and their professional skills should be used to ensure that each member of the community receives the assistance s/he requires to continue being responsible for his/her life (Wagner, 1994).

To a wide extent, Danish policy for older persons is founded on making use of older people's own resources, to preserve older people's self-determination and influence on their living conditions and to ensure continuity in older people's lives. The services are governed by the principle of help to self-help and are therefore to be performed together with the older person insofar as this is possible, so that the skills of the recipient are maintained or retrained. The home help may support the older person in maintaining social contacts and areas of interest (Bierring et al., 1987).

The concept of self-care has among other things resulted in a change for elderly in nursing homes. Nursing home staff are not supposed to take over responsibility for the life of individual residents. Each resident is to decide what services s/he wants to make use of. Staff are responsible for treatment, care and supervision.

Since 1993 all residents at nursing homes have to manage their own pensions and pay rent, electricity, health and for services such as meals, hairdressing, shaving etc. When older persons have to pay directly for the services, their incentives to do things themselves increase as well as their self-determination (Ministry of Social Affairs, 1995).

3   Provision of Health and Social Care in Denmark

3.1   *Who Are Receiving Health and Social Care Services?*

Health and social care services constitute the largest single area of municipal services. In 2001 roughly 180,000 persons aged 67 or over received home help from the municipalities. Thus, in Denmark 24% of older persons over 67 years of age receive public home help – the highest rate in Scandinavia (Social Appeal Board, 2001; Daatland, 1997; Rostgaard/Fridberg, 1998). In total more than 212,000 persons received home help in 2001. 112,000 of them received less than four hours of help a week. Furthermore, 28,000 persons lived in nursing homes in 2001, another 57,000 were attached to a day-care centre and 63,000 adapted dwellings had been established. Finally, the municipal expenditures on elderly care amounted to 3 billion euros in 2000. In 2000 the overall direct transfers in cash or kind to elderly citizens in Denmark amounted to 10,6% of the GDP.

145

According to figures on who does the work in the households of elderly people, however, it does not seem that responsibilities are handed over to the municipalities just because one has reached a certain age. A study from the end of the 1980s shows that two thirds of all elderly aged 70 years or more and living at home do not receive home help (Platz, 1990). Another study from the middle of the 1990s shows that among persons between 80-100 years more than 40% do not receive home help (Hansen/Platz, 1995).

Still, more than one third of all hospitalised persons are over 65 years and are using more than 50% of the total amount of bed days in all hospitals. Over the latter years hospitals have been run more effectively, which has resulted in a decrease in the average amount of days patients stay at the hospital. This means that also older persons are discharged earlier, thus requesting more services from the municipality once back home which again puts emphasis on the provision of integrated care (The National Association of Local Authorities in Denmark, 2000; Felbo/Søland, 1996).

3.2 Who Provides Health and Social Care Services?

Health and social care are characterised by an extensive delegation of responsibilities to politically elected regional and local authorities. Regional (16 counties) and local (275 municipalities) authorities administer health and social policy respectively. The Ministries (Health and Social) are responsible for overall control and for establishing the broad legislative and financial framework of health and social policy.

An important feature of Danish legislation on health and social welfare is that it only provides the general framework. The local authorities determine the actual contents and organisation of the health and social care services provided. As a consequence of the decentralisation of responsibilities to counties and municipalities, there are variations in the services provided to older persons depending on where they live.

- *The Ministry of Interior and Health* is responsible for primary health services and hospitals.
- *The Ministry of Social Affairs* is responsible for pensions for and care of the elderly.

As noted above the responsibilities of implementing health and social policy have been delegated to the counties and municipalities.

3.2.1 Counties

The 16 counties administer hospitals, including geriatric rehabilitation services, primary health care (except home nursing) and health promotion initiatives. Long-term care is not in general a county health authority responsibility, but older people with mental illnesses, such as dementia, may be referred for care at specialised units. Counties are therefore responsible for the running of hospitals and for the coverage of general practitioners (GPs) (Blackman et al., 2001). Hospitals and GPs are financed through general taxation, which means that the users do not pay directly for services provided by hospitals and GPs. The charges for medicine are subsidised to a high degree.

3.2.2 Municipalities

The 275 municipalities administer pensions, nursing homes and adapted dwellings for older persons, home nurses, psychotherapists, occupational therapists[3] and social care as home help. The referrals of all aids to older persons that are not in hospitals, are coordinated in the municipality by the health visitor, who is also the case manager.

The municipalities have a statutory duty to offer home help for both practical and personal assistance, home nursing and provide housing for disabled persons – including adapted dwellings, nursing homes and attached day care facilities. Care is delivered free of charge to the recipient irrespective of the type of housing of the recipient. Other social services provided are: transport for people requiring treatment, day centres, which may offer recreational activities as well as rehabilitation, loan of equipment and aids and, finally, meals on wheels, for which there is a charge.

The municipalities are the main provider of services, but some of the nursing homes and attached day care facilities are run by voluntary organisations. These organisations have contractual agreements with the municipality. The municipalities, however, remain responsible for standards in the home, admission criteria, and the setting of rents and services charges. In all practical ways, there is no distinction between nursing homes and day care facilities run by the municipality and those run by voluntary organisations (Blackman et al., 2001).

147

3.3   *What Kinds of Health and Social Care Services Are Provided?*

This section will provide a brief outline of the components of the health and social care services that are provided in Denmark. With two exceptions the services that are described below are fully provided by the municipalities. The general practitioners are organised at the county level and the rehabilitation services can be provided either by the county or the municipality, depending on whether the older person has received hospital treatment or not. As the contents of the health services provided by the hospitals appear fairly self-evident, these will not be described below.

Over the past decades there has been a drive in Danish elderly policy to integrate the services provided at the municipal level. The individual kinds of services described below are thus provided in concert depending on the need of the individual user. The actualities of the services provided may differ from municipality to municipality, as the municipalities are individually entitled to organise the services provided on the basis of the perceived need profile of the community.

3.3.1 24-Hour Health and Social Care

The municipal health and social services are accessible 24 hours every day. Persons in acute need of help can, thus, call in assistance in case of need. In special cases and for shorter periods a carer might stay in the home of a very ill person day and night. This 24-hour home care system made it possible to care for very dependent people in an ordinary dwelling (Hansen, 2001). Many elderly remain in their own homes even in case of heavy care needs and the demand for 24-hour service has risen sharply (Social Appeal Board, 2001).

The most recent developmental trend is the introduction of "integrated schemes" comprising both staff in nursing homes/adapted dwellings and social and health staff working in the community. There are integrated staff-units of this kind in 86% of the 275 municipalities, while in the remaining municipalities staff may work in integrated teams but formally still belong to their individual professional group. The integrated teams consist of eight to ten persons, who are responsible for the care of older people in a local area, i.e. the two sets of professionals provide home care together (Blackman et al., 2001). The integrated teams primarily consist of home-helpers and home nurses. The services provided by these two professional groups will be presented below.

3.3.2 Home Help

The aim of the municipally organised home help is to provide (i) personal care and assistance, (ii) assistance or support for necessary practical work in the home, and (iii) assistance in maintaining physical or mental skills. Home help services are provided by trained staff.

An applicant for home help is entitled to an individual assessment of his/her need for personal care and practical assistance. A nurse, a home-helper or a home help manager normally visits the applicant in his/her home to assess the need for care. Provision of care does not take into account the help that could be provided by adult children or other family members living outside the household. The range of services available to meet needs, the entitlement or eligibility criteria applied, and the number and type of hours of help allocated are all dictated by the budget and political preferences of the local municipality (Blackman et al., 2001).

Since 1998, the majority of municipalities tended to be less generous when assessing for home help for domestic tasks. Instead, home help is more likely to be targeted on the most dependent elderly in need of personal care. Some municipalities may be evading the law by withholding home help for domestic care (Blackman et al., 2001).

3.3.3 Home Nursing

Home nursing is provided free of charge either following referral from a GP or in cooperation with the home help services. The home nurse often plays a key role in terms of supporting the home help and assessing the individual senior citizen's need for assistance. Home nursing is often carried out on short-term basis following discharge from a hospital to ensure that the treatment the older person has received at hospital is sustained. The home nursing services are organised and administered by the municipalities.

3.3.4 Preventive Home Visits

All municipalities have been obliged to conduct at least two preventive home visits a year by social and health workers for older people aged 75 years or more. The aim of the preventive home visits is to reduce risk factors for elderly. This might be reducing falls, social isolation, suicide, traffic accidents and to improve physical activities. The visit is made on acceptance by the older person (Rostgaard/Fridberg, 1998) The municipality may also decide to make exceptional visits in relation to the death of a spouse, serious illness or discharge from hospital. The person (often a nurse) making the visit must have thorough knowledge of general social as well as health issues.

A recent investigation into the municipal activities with regard to the preventive home visits shows that in 85% of the municipalities the elderly are offered preventive home visits twice a year. For various reasons 15% of the municipalities do not meet their obligations in this regard (Social Appeal Board, 2002).

3.3.5 Nursing Homes and Adapted Dwellings

Denmark no longer builds conventional nursing homes. Separate dwellings individually adapted to the needs and capacities of the elderly are replacing institutions, which are considered to limit the independence of the elderly. Such dwellings may be integrated into existing housing or constructed separately (Ministry of Social Affairs, 1995).

During the last 20 years the availability of nursing home places has been reduced from approximately 40 places to approximately 20 places per 100 persons aged 80 or more. In their place independent adapted dwellings have been built, but they are not all staffed and are therefore not all as fully supportive care units as the conventional nursing homes.

The municipalities have the responsibility for assessing people's needs for adapted housing. The municipality is obliged to ensure that those who cannot remain at home, even if they receive home assistance or personal care, can be admitted to a nursing home or another care facility such as different forms of adapted dwellings, staffed around the clock (Blackman et al., 2001).

3.3.6 General Practitioners

For many older persons the general practitioner often constitutes the primary link between the elderly and the health and social care services provided by the municipalities as the GP refers persons who experience loss of functions or trouble in handling everyday domiciliary tasks to the municipal services. The GPs may also participate in preventive home visits and promote preventive measures in their consultation after agreement.

GPs are self-employed but their activities are highly regulated through agreements between their professional organisations and the counties' Health Insurance Negotiating Committee. Using the GP in municipal work depends on the specific contracts between the municipality and GPs. Because of the stipulations of these contracts – and the many GPs involved – formalised cooperative relations between the GPs and the municipalities appear troublesome in many cases.

3.3.7 Rehabilitation

Rehabilitation is part of a continuous treatment at hospitals, while maintenance training typically is a municipal service. In a Danish context *rehabilitation* is defined as conscious and goal-oriented training, which aims at restoring the patient's earlier functional level, before the accident or illness took place, whereas *maintenance training* is defined as conscious training to prevent loss of function and to maintain or improve the functions of the individual.

As will be discussed in further detail below, however, the division of labour with regard to rehabilitation is the cause of significant conflict between the municipalities and the counties. As a result of a long-lasting debate about lack of sufficient rehabilitation and an unclear division of labour in the field of rehabilitation the ministries of Health and Social Affairs have passed legislation in order to clarify the responsibilities of the counties and the municipalities. Thus, the *municipalities* are responsible, when elderly become ill without hospitalisation, but need rehabilitation. This effort is connected to the existing maintenance training. The *counties*, however, are responsible that discharged patients have a carefully arranged plan of rehabilitation. The act may ensure that all patients, who need it, have a continuing coherent rehabilitation plan, no matter who has the responsibility.

3.3.8 Other Services

Other types of municipal services for older persons are: centres of social activities and maintenance training, day care in nursing homes, meals-on-wheels, gardening services, technical aids, alarm systems, adaptation of housing, short stay and/or night care in nursing centres.

151

3.4   *Problems and Solutions in the Provision of Health and Social Care*

Even though health and social care appears to be fairly well integrated at the municipal level the problems persist in coordinating the activities of the municipalities and the counties.

The main problems concern (i) patients who cannot take care of themselves after hospitalisation and therefore may have to wait at the hospital for a place in an adapted dwelling or a nursing home, (ii) cooperation between the hospital and the municipality to ensure home nurses and home help in relation to discharge from hospital, and (iii) rehabilitation at hospitals and after discharge from hospital.

The collaboration and the division of labour between hospital and health and social care units vary from municipality to municipality and from one hospital department to another. This is due to the fact that decision-making in this field is decentralised and, thus, not based on governmental guidelines or centralised legislation.

A study from 1992 in four municipalities, concerning elderly with massive health problems and/or social problems shows that policy on ageing mostly works. But there appears to be room for improvement, however. The health and social services are often provided too late, which means that the preventive potentials of the health and social care services are not fully utilised. Most of the elderly do not know the possibilities of services and the social workers and decision-makers often do not know the elderly well enough to provide sufficient proactive services. In almost all studied cases there are unsolved problems, which may be due to the fact that the capacity is too scarce, for example too few adapted dwellings, or that the health and social workers are too busy or not well enough qualified. In the following, the main problems concerning integration between hospitals and municipalities will be discussed.

3.4.1 Bottlenecks in the System

One problem concerns patients who are not able to take care of themselves upon discharge from hospital and are therefore waiting for a place in a nursing home or an adapted dwelling. These patients cannot be discharged due to the lack of nursing homes or other municipal efforts. The problem has existed for years (The Association of County Councils in Denmark/The National Association of Local Authorities in Denmark, 1991; Ministry of Health, 2001).

The counties administer and finance the hospitals, while the municipalities administer and finance the measures concerning elderly discharged from hospitals. The municipalities thus have an economic incentive to prolong the stay of elderly citizens at the hospitals (The Association of County Councils in Denmark/The National Association of Local Authorities in Denmark, 1991). One of the solutions has been to make the municipalities pay for patients at hospitals who have finished their treatment. From 1993 onwards the counties are enabled to make municipalities pay per day for patients waiting for admission to a nursing home. Thus, since 1993 there has been a decrease in the amount of elderly somatic patients at hospitals waiting for a place in nursing homes (Ministry of Health, 2001).

Until now the experiences with payment shows that patients in counties with payment have shorter waiting intervals than in counties without payment (Ministry of Health, 2001). Other solutions for municipalities have been to establish temporary places in nursing homes or other places for elderly who will recover after a shorter period and return to their homes.

3.4.2 Discharge from Hospitals and Coordinating Efforts

The decrease in the average number of bed days for elderly patients in hospitals requires an extended cooperation and dialogue between the hospital, the general practitioners and the health and social care units in the municipalities to ensure that the patients are in "safe" hands upon discharge. Discharge from a hospital can be described as an upheaval for the elderly. Returning to one's own home can be experienced both as a relief and a load. In any case there will be a need for follow-up in the home with the purpose to clarify and solve problems concerning, e.g. home help, aids and medicine. Experiments show that following-up after discharge will reduce the amount of elderly, who later need living in nursing homes (Hansen et al., 1994).

There are, however, different understandings at the hospitals and in the municipalities of central concepts when patients are discharged. They mainly disagree about when a patient has finished treatment. The hospital alone has the competence to make decisions about the discharge of patients. According to municipalities, however, elderly patients are often discharged without having finished their treatment. The municipalities experience a development where they have to take over more and more tasks from hospitals – without general planning or more resources (Felbo/Søland, 1996).

Information and communication is another area causing problems. The municipalities express problems with no or late warnings when a patient is discharged. Beside that, exchange between the hospital and domiciliary care regarding results achieved at hospital or changes in use of medication is lacking for elderly receiving home help. Furthermore, there are disagreements about the patients' needs in their own homes when they are discharged from hospital. The experience of municipal home helpers is that upon discharge the patient sometimes can manage less than reported by hospital officials. This may be explained through different understandings of "autonomy", as hospital staff often does not consider architectural barriers or other problems occurring in patients' homes that are not equipped for long-term care. Also the GP often misses information about the results achieved by the hospital treatment, because s/he receives the discharge report long after the patient had been discharged (Feldbo/Søgaard, 1996).

153

3.4.3 "Getting the Municipalities into the Hospitals"

One way of solving discharge problems is to develop cooperation models between hospitals and municipalities where staff from the municipality participate in planning the discharge from hospital. This can be done by (i) the home nurse who sometimes visits the elderly at the hospital and thus also gets information from the hospital staff or (ii) by inviting the home nurse to meetings concerning the discharge of an older patient.

One solution on the problem might be to employ a visiting nurse, visiting all citizens above 65 years that are either admitted to hospital, losing a spouse or moving into the municipality. The purpose with visiting the elderly at hospital is to build bridges between hospital and home and to deal with questions and problems – before they arise. There have, however, been problems with the cooperation model caused by the rules of professional secrecy (Feldbo/Søgaard, 1996).

Another solution has been discharge-meetings with staff from hospital and municipality to strengthen coherence in the effort. It is inconvenient when the hospital discusses social efforts with the patient without involving the municipality. The reason is that hospital staff not always know about the range of care services provided and the assignment criteria in the municipalities, which might result in expectations from the elderly that cannot be fulfilled (Hansen et al., 1991).

3.4.4 "Getting the Hospital to Work with the Municipalities"

Another way of strengthening cooperation in connection with discharge from hospital is to provide the hospital staff with outgoing functions. Two typical solution models are home visits and geriatric teams.

Home visits after discharge from hospital take place in cooperation between hospital, municipality, the elderly and relatives, if possible. The purpose of the visit is to arrange a rehabilitation plan close to the daily practice in the home and to estimate the need for aid, changes in the home and specific care efforts. Because of the shortening of the average number of bed days at hospitals and the increasing number of patients coming through hospitals, the pressure on occupational and physiotherapists, which often is the group with outgoing tasks, has increased. Often there will be waiting times for home visits which either extend the time at hospital or the discharge will be without a home visit (The National Association of Local Authorities in Denmark, 2000).

To ensure a coherent treatment and follow-up after discharge from hospital, some hospitals have established *geriatric teams*. A geriatric team can be
formed made up of staff from hospital, for example a doctor, a nurse, secretary and occupational and physiotherapist, social workers or others. The aim
of the team is to treat the elderly in his/her own surroundings and prevent
(re-)admission to hospital. The team is supposed to ensure coordination of
the effort for the elderly between the two sectors. The target group for the
geriatric teams are elderly with complex health problems and/or loss of function.

The efforts of the geriatric teams concerning discharge have resulted
in a rapid growth in the access to municipal services, mostly home help, home
nurse, day-centre, meals on wheels, changes in the home and aids. It is not
possible to measure how many of these services would have been offered
without the geriatric effort. In one municipality that cooperates with geriatric teams it is estimated that the teams have contributed to uncover needs
which otherwise would have remained hidden (The National Association
of Local Authorities in Denmark, 2000).

3.4.5 Cooperation between Hospital, General Practitioner
and the Municipality

The GP also has a role connected to the discharge from hospital. The GP
mostly becomes informed about the medical condition of the patient when
the patient is discharged. The GP subsequently has to carry on treatment,
monitor rehabilitation and carry out the necessary control (Hansen et al,
1994).

As discussed above formal barriers often hinder cooperation between
the GP and the municipality. The GPs, thus, rarely participate in formalised
cooperation with either the hospital or the municipality in case one of their
patients is discharged from hospital and requires further treatment in the
subsequent period.

One development project which involved GPs and the home nurse in
a systematic follow-up on elderly patients discharged from hospitals shows
that it is possible to prevent institutionalisation of elderly persons through
follow-up visits. In the project, a district nurse visited the elderly persons in
their homes the day after discharge from hospital and two weeks later the
general practitioner visited the discharged patients (Hansen et al., 1994).

Most hospitals have gradually established warning systems to inform
the municipality. It might be warnings about patients, who are to be dis-

charged to their own homes or patients who are discharged to a nursing home. For example, at the hospital in Herning there is a cooperation contract which stipulates that the domiciliary care has to be notified at least three days before a discharge, if the discharge concerns a patient who needs municipal health or social care. The purpose is to avoid hasty discharge and the following problems in the municipality when a patient with needs for services is discharged without prior notification.

3.4.6 Rehabilitation

The county and municipal services concerning rehabilitation have been discussed for several years. The discussion concerns both the coherence in the service and the division of labour between counties and municipalities (Ministry of Health, 2001). One of the impediments for sufficient rehabilitation is the division of responsibility between counties and municipalities which has not been clearly clarified.

156

Until recently the boundary between health and social rehabilitation has not been laid down in the legislation neither in the Social Act nor in the Health Act (Ministry of Health, 1994).

It is difficult to make a clear delimitation between rehabilitation in the health system (counties) and maintenance training and prevention of loss of function in the social system (municipalities). A gradual shift from the specialised rehabilitation at hospitals to the rehabilitation that is normally carried out in the municipalities appears to be taking place. Between the two sectors there is a so-called grey area where patients can get jammed insofar as none of the rehabilitative bodies accepts responsibility for a given patient. The problems of delimitation between the two sectors in connection with the obligation to continue or to start training are typically related to discharge from hospitals.

The municipalities have stated that discharged patients are frailer and less self-reliant than earlier due to the shortening of hospital stays. Therefore municipalities have to provide increasingly specialised efforts of rehabilitation, which is straining their economy. The municipalities claim that the boundaries between counties and municipalities have shifted. The counties claim that the methods of treatments have become gentler and it is therefore not necessary to use as many resources for rehabilitation on each patient as before (Felbo/Søland, 1996). From the perspective of the municipalities the counties appear to shift the economic burden of rehabilitation to the municipalities, and a conflict of interest with regard to the financing of rehabilitation upon discharge, thus, becomes evident at the interface between the hospitals and the health and social care units.

A study in two hospitals and four municipalities concludes that there has been a displacement of tasks from hospitals to municipalities as the hospitals in the study do not adequately meet the patients' needs for rehabilitation. Patients living in municipalities with inadequate rehabilitation schemes thus risk falling into a void if neither the hospital nor the municipality provide the rehabilitation needed upon discharge from hospital (Engberg/Tang, 2000).

Projects in several municipalities show that coherent rehabilitation efforts reduce the economic expenditures of health and social care. The reduction in expenditures is held to be caused by fewer re-admissions, and a decreasing need for home nurses, home help and aids. A project in the municipality of Vejle shows that a goal-directed and limited rehabilitation effort in the citizen's own home offers both better quality of life for the elderly and reduces the use of home care – especially when the rehabilitation effort has started as early as possible (The National Association of Local Authorities in Denmark, 2000).

It is necessary that counties and municipalities cooperate on the issue of rehabilitation. An improved cooperation and coordination between county and municipality can, among other things, be furthered by increasing communication, cooperation contracts and contracts specifying who is doing what. In these ways they obtain more coherence in their efforts towards citizens and a better use of resources (Ministry of Social Affairs, 1998). The counties and municipalities are not able to reap the full rewards of well-planned rehabilitation due to the conflict of interest in terms of the financing and division of labour with regard to rehabilitation.

4 Overcoming the Barriers: Model Projects and Experiments

The different kinds of services that are provided in Danish elderly policy have been developed over a long period. A large part of the developmental impetus stems from model projects and experiments in individual municipalities. These projects are often carried out in collaboration with the Ministry of Social Affairs. In this section the focus will be on five model projects that have contributed to the evolution and improvement of health and social care services in Denmark over the past 20 years.

The experiences gained from these and other model projects and experiments are pooled in, e.g. the Ministry of Social Affairs, the Ministry of Health, the Institute for Service Development and the National Association of Local Authorities in Denmark, in order to provide all counties and municipalities with inspiration for the evolution of health and social care services provided at the regional or local level.

The first project presented has had a major impact on the provision of integrated health and social care in Denmark, as it was one of the first experiments with the provision of health and social care services around the clock in Denmark. The discussion above has made it clear that the primary problem in terms of integrating health and social care in Denmark appear at the interface between regional and local authorities. The four other projects concern initiatives to overcome the barriers and difficulties inherent to the coordination of the efforts of hospitals and municipalities.

4.1   Developing 24-Hour Integrated Health and Social Care

The municipality of Skaevinge started a project in 1984 with the purpose to create a more dynamic and flexible provision of services for elderly persons. All categories of staff working with elderly persons were involved, together with actual and potential elderly users.

The starting point was a traditional municipal organisation with (i) a nursing home, (ii) a department for home nursing, (iii) a department for home help, (iv) a department for health, and (v) an office for social work for the elderly. These different departments all had their own budgets, management and employees (Wagner, 1994).

The objectives of the Skaevinge project were:

- To separate housing from health and social care and introduce 24-hours integrated health and social care. All citizens are eligible and should have equal access to health and social care, irrespective of living at home or in an institution.
- To evolve a common professional understanding between the health and social care workers through working with the concept of *self-care* as a basis for health and social care.
- To provide early and individual care in order to obtain better health statuses and prevent admissions to hospitals in the target group.

- To organise service provision in autonomous teams with the responsibility and competence to plan actual health and social care services provided without a delaying hierarchical structure.
- To integrate the traditional health and social care sectors and bring them together in one common department in order to obtain a better utilisation of the pooled resources (Wagner/Mogensen, 2001).

4.1.1 The Results of the Project

The project has produced a host of results of which the most significant will be mentioned below. The former nursing home was converted into individual apartments in order to provide residential units that resembled the type of housing that the residents were accustomed to before requiring sheltered housing. At the same time a health centre was established, putting together home nursing, public health nursing and day centre under one roof. Here, the various professional and technical groups closely worked together for the first time. The centre directs its attention towards all potential older users in the municipality regardless of their housing status.

   Due to the availability of the 24-hour service throughout the municipality and improved information on self-care and possibilities for help in their homes, many older persons have chosen to keep on living in their own homes instead of opting for residence in nursing homes or adapted dwellings. The day centre in the former nursing home has also been extended and work has been further developed and systematised, particularly in identifying potential clients in the community in need of support (Wagner, 2000).

   Furthermore, the project shows that it is important to be aware of professional and cultural differences in the health and social sector when collaboration is to be established. Staff in the health sector suffers from the "maid servant syndrome", as they are being paid to be on duty eight hours per day and have acquired some deep-seated habits of "helping" and "taking care of" instead of encouraging patients to do as much as possible themselves. And patients expect these services since the nurses are being paid to perform them. On the other hand, staff in the social sector appears to be more accustomed to the principle of self-care where the citizen plays an important role in the provision of services. The social sector builds on the use of older persons' own resources to preserve their self-determination and influence on their living conditions in order to ensure continuity in their lives (Wagner, 1994).

An evaluation of the Skaevinge project was conducted in 1997. The evaluation showed that:

- The older persons estimate that their health statuses had improved. They were asked in 1985 and again in 1997.
- Even though the number of persons with 75 years or more has increased by 30%, the operational expenditures have decreased.
- There is the same amount of staff in 1996 as there was in 1986.
- The preventive efforts have entailed a surplus of capacity, which among other things has been used to establish acute beds and rehabilitation places in the community to prevent unnecessary admissions to hospitals.
- The use of bed days at hospitals has been reduced by 30-40% for all citizens in the community.
- For 10 years, the municipality has not had waiting days at hospitals for older people having finished treatment.
- There is no waiting time for apartments in the health centre or for home help.
- The use of and expenditure for national health insurance is less than in the rest of the county.

The results of the project thus provide a compelling argument for the provision of integrated health and social care, as it not only appears to have improved the well-being of the users but also – in line with the reasoning of the Commission on Elderly – produced these results in an economically efficient way. According to Wagner (2000), these results were obtained because the municipality has put weight on prevention, flexibility and individual health and social care.

As already mentioned, the most significant result from the project is that all 275 municipalities provide integrated health and social efforts and 24-hours health and social care services along the lines of the Skaevinge project.

4.2   Acute Rooms as a Substitute for Hospitalisation

Acute rooms administered by the municipality are an alternative to hospitalisation for the elderly who do not need specialised treatment at the hospital and where the GP can take on responsibility for the treatment. Acute rooms are established in municipality centres for elderly or at nursing homes.

Referrals to acute rooms will take place in consultation between the GP or the doctor from the emergency service and the health and social care unit, relatives or the elderly themselves. The acute rooms have 24-hours nursing attention. The GP or the doctors from the emergency service provide medical service (Felbo/Søland, 1996).

In 1992 the municipality of Roedding made an agreement about cooperation with the county concerning the establishment of acute rooms financed by the county and the municipality. The interest of the county was to avoid expensive and unnecessary admissions to hospitals among older persons. The municipality wanted to improve their elderly service and to avoid unnecessary spells of hospitalisation.

4.2.1 The Results of the Project

Along with a reorganisation of the service for the elderly the municipality of Roedding reserved ten of the earlier rooms at three nursing homes. Removal to an acute-room happens in situations with acute illness, e.g. pneumonia, fever or fall accidents. According to the municipality both professional staff and the elderly users find that the acute rooms are a success. During the stay at the acute rooms the elderly receive service from their own home helpers, home nurse and GP. The elderly are pleased that they can receive service from staff they already know instead of being treated by a new team at the hospital. Another important factor is that the elderly remain in the local community with enhanced possibility for visits from relatives and friends (Feldbo/Søland, 1996).

The elderly from the municipality of Roedding are not hospitalised as much as elderly in the neighbour municipality and the differences have increased over the years. Elderly citizens who used the acute rooms in the period from autumn 1995 to spring 1996 (six persons) were satisfied with the assessment and the service they received during their stay. They were especially satisfied to be helped through an acute crisis and that it could take place in their homes or close to their homes (Hansen et al., 1997). The stay first of all has helped the elderly through a critical phase while medical treatment and rehabilitation were individualised.

The question is whether the elderly have received an optimum treatment through the acute stay or whether some elderly would have been better off if they had been hospitalised. During the stay at the acute room, the patient is observed by the GP and – if needed – it is also possible to draw

161

upon more specialised medical knowledge – for instance through ambulant treatment at a hospital or visits from medical specialists to the acute room. The possibilities of engaging specialised medical officers serve to ensure that the elderly patient receives a proper medical treatment during the stay at the acute room. However, from the evidence cited it is not possible to conclude if treatment in acute rooms from a strictly medical point of view constitutes a superior or inferior alternative to the treatment available at hospitals (Hansen et al., 1997).

4.3 Evolving "Good Cooperation" between Hospital and Municipality

Admission to hospital and discharge are critical phases in a treatment, because the responsibility is handed over from one sector to another. Different projects have aimed at improving the communication between the hospitals and the health and social care units, so that information on the patient in one sector is passed on to another sector with the consent from the citizen in order to ensure a coherent treatment. Cooperation and communication have been in focus in the latest years and different projects have been started in that respect.

Several municipalities have thus entered a contract with the counties concerning cooperation in case of admission and discharge from hospital. As an example, in the following the contents of a contract of the hospital of Skive with several municipalities will be described.

The background for the contract was that it was often difficult to coordinate and establish the necessary municipal measures prior to discharge of patients in need of support, which resulted in waiting time for patients prior to discharge. Waiting time prior to discharge unnecessarily extends hospital stays for patients who have finished treatment. Furthermore, readmissions occurred that could have been avoided.

Against the background of an analysis of the interaction between the sectors, a working group with nurses of hospital departments and district nurses from five municipalities prepared information material about "Good cooperation practice" and a checklist that could be used as a tool to control that all guidelines were followed. The purpose of the contract was to ensure quality and continuity in treatment, care and rehabilitation of the patient in the event of admission to and discharge from hospital.

One of the cornerstones in the cooperation between hospital and municipality is "The citizen booklet". It is an open communication system in writing for citizens, municipality staff and hospital staff. The booklet belongs

162

to the citizen and follows the citizen if s/he accepts it. The booklet is established when a citizen receives home help or home nurse. The booklet is supposed to ensure that the citizen receives information and participates in decisions concerning treatment, training and care. The staff can use the booklet as a tool (information about the condition of the citizen and information from one colleague to another) and documentation for the provided services (Hansen et al., 1997).

Issues in the contract are:

- The ideal communication between the sectors is a dialogue between staff at the hospital and in the municipality. The amount of care is estimated and provided by the municipality according to the resources and needs of the citizen.
- The therapist at the hospital contacts the health and social care department in the municipality if the patient is in need of a home visit, in case of changes in the home, aids, follow-up or continuous rehabilitation administered by the municipality.
- If the functional level of the citizen has changed dramatically compared to the status prior to admission to hospital, staff from the municipality visits the home to clarify needs for changes in the home and aids. The main rule is that citizens cannot be discharged before necessary aids and changes in the home are prepared, guaranteed or installed and the necessary services have been arranged.

163

4.3.1 The Results of the Project

A precondition for "Good cooperation practice" to work is that the contract is essential for admission to hospital, that the contract is followed in practice and that the booklet is used. According to an evaluation of the project, the case records show that the documentation of the items in the cooperation contract has not been fulfilled sufficiently. In the evaluation only one patient has brought the booklet to the hospital, which means that it has not had any influence on the selected admissions to hospital. The municipalities are normally not informed about hospitalisation of citizens and it is not relevant if the citizens do not receive services from the municipality; but even if they do receive services, they are not systematically informed (Hansen et al., 1997).

The result of the contract of "Good cooperation practice" has been that the staff at the hospital and the staff in the municipality normally are in contact in order to clarify the need for services after discharge. Home transport, aids and changes in the home are normally arranged before discharge. A common understanding has been developed; when a patient is discharged, it is a common task for hospital and municipality to find a solution, if there are problems. This understanding forms a basis for developing a better practice in the future and it is concluded that citizens are not discharged, without information being given to the municipality prior to discharge, if there is need for services (Hansen et al., 1997).

4.4   Coordinating the Provision of Rehabilitative Measures

Insufficient rehabilitation measures provided by counties and municipalities have been discussed since many years. The largest impediment for sufficient rehabilitation has been a vague legislative definition of the responsibilities between the counties and municipalities. Hospitals are responsible for finishing the treatment of patients but it is not clear whether rehabilitation is part of the treatment – and therefore a task for hospitals. Neither have the responsibilities of the municipalities been clearly defined and therefore the rehabilitative measures differ quite a lot between them. As discussed above the division of labour with regard to rehabilitation is the cause of tension between counties and municipalities – not least in terms of which of the branches are obliged to carry the financial burdens associated with rehabilitation.

New legislation about rehabilitation from 2001 gives the citizen the right to a rehabilitation plan upon discharge from hospital. The right to municipal rehabilitation comes into play when the illness is not treated at a hospital. The new legislation strengthens the demand for formal cooperation concerning rehabilitation and for making arrangements with exact instructions for referrals.

A developmental project running for several years with the purpose of preparing a general model focusing on the citizen's needs of rehabilitation, has been started parallel with the new legislation. The objective is to develop a model which municipalities can use, including the demands for a rehabilitation plan as legislation demands from hospitals. According to legislation all hospitalised patients with an identified need for rehabilitation are entitled to a plan outlining the goals for and contents of the rehabilitation efforts. The hospitals (counties) are responsible for preparation and implementation of the action plan (Ministry of Social Affairs, 2002).

The model for municipalities includes the same demands for action plans as the legislation demands from hospitals. As the model includes the possibility for expressing both actual and potential profiles of functional ability of citizens, it can be used in cooperation between the two sectors. The tools developed in the model can contribute to the description of the relations of cooperation between county and municipality and as a concrete tool in the daily distribution of work between the parties. The use of the tools also has an additional effect, in relation to defining the division of labour between the counties and municipalities.

A total of eight municipalities have participated in developing and testing the model. Four municipalities have been in charge of the developing work. Subsequently four other municipalities have contributed to quality control and testing of the developed tools. The model aims at:

- Ensuring a simple and coherent rehabilitation process for the individual even though several services may be involved (e.g. training, domiciliary care, aids).
- Ensuring sufficient and equal services for all citizens where the citizens' own requests and priorities of rehabilitation efforts are included in the basis for referral.
- Ensuring unambiguous definitions and delimitation of the contents of services to be used in the practice of rehabilitation as well as in relation to other departments in the organisation (e.g. domiciliary care, hospitals, GP, physiotherapists).
- Creating a basis for a goal-oriented effort and an aggregated evaluation. The citizens' actual functional ability is supposed to be documented as well as the potential function capacity might be estimated.

The project is under progress and concrete experiences with the use of the model within the municipality are not expected until the beginning of 2003. Therefore the project has not yet been evaluated.

4.5 *Overcoming Communication Problems: MedCom*

A great part of the problems of integrating the services provided by the hospitals and the health and social care units concerns communication problems related to admission to and discharge from hospital. The problems concern both the communication between hospital and GP and between hospital and the municipal health and social care units (Wagner/Olsen, 2000).

MedCom is a project, involving cooperation between municipalities, hospitals, general practitioners and private companies linked to the health sector. The purpose of MedCom was to develop nationwide standards for the most common communication flows between medical practices, hospitals and pharmacies: referrals and discharge letters, laboratory requests, results and prescriptions. All counties, hospitals, pharmacies, two thirds of medical practices (GP), one thirds of specialists and 16 local authorities use the Danish Health Care Network – MedCom (MedCom / The Danish Healthcare Data Network, 2001). The next step in the project, which took place in the period 2000-2002, concentrated on communication flows between hospitals and the social and health care sector within municipalities.

The first phase of the MedCom project makes it possible for the hospital to warn the municipality when a citizen is hospitalised or discharged. The messages contain information about where and when a patient is hospitalised or discharged and the status of the patient. This information is useful for the municipality when planning the services that are to be provided to the individual upon discharge.

166

The second phase of MedCom is testing communication between care reports and warnings messages between hospital and municipality. The health and social care unit in the municipality gives information about practical assistance and need for personal care, aids and use of medicine. The care report can be sent from the municipality immediately after admission to hospital and provides information to the hospital about care and treatment of the patient as well as medication.

Before the patient is discharged the hospital sends a warning to the municipality, which uses the information to prepare an assumed responsibility for the patient. After discharge the hospital sends an updated care report to the health and social care unit to ensure that important information for further treatment is not being lost (e.g. information about medicine) when the patient is removed from hospital to the municipality. One municipality has asked for hospital admissions and discharge warnings for all older persons of more than 75 years of age. All elderly who do not receive home help or home nursing, have been contacted after discharge in order to monitor the need for health and social care on a more systematic basis.

4.5.1 The Results of the Project

The second phase has not yet been evaluated, but the preliminary report from the participating municipalities shows that citizens receive better services and that hospitals and health and social care units avoid wasting time. The earlier experiences were that communication between the two sectors could fail. The home helper visited the citizen and found out that s/he had been admitted to hospital. Or a citizen who needed help was alone for several days because the health and social care unit was unaware that the citizen had been discharged from hospital. The project ensures that information is given immediately. The aim of the project is to make as many counties and municipalities as possible use MedCom.

5   Conclusions and Perspectives

In Denmark the provision of health and social care is integrated in all municipalities. These processes of integration started in the beginning of the 1980s on the basis of the recommendations expressed by the Commission on Elderly. At first, model projects were established in a few municipalities and the experiences from these were used to develop models for integrated care. However, integrated health and social care schemes have not been implemented in all municipalities until the end of 1990s. Due to an extensive delegation of powers to the local authorities integrated health and social care has been managed in different ways in the municipalities.

    The development of integrated care is connected to the liquidation of traditional nursing homes. The result of this process of de-institutionalisation has been that the services that were earlier exclusively provided in the nursing homes are now provided to all elderly regardless of their housing status. Due to the fact that integrated care builds on the concept of self-care, de-institutionalisation has resulted in a strengthening of the emphasis on the older persons' own resources in order to preserve their self-determination.

    At the same time the developments at hospitals have been to intensify and improve productivity with an increasing weight on intensive, short and ambulant treatment. Elderly patients are thus discharged earlier from hospitals with increasing needs for sustained treatment and care in the local setting. The decrease in the average number of stay-days at hospital has thus resulted in an increasing demand for integrated health and social care in the municipalities.

    Even though integrated care exists in all municipalities, problems still remain in terms of integrating the efforts of hospitals (counties) and health

167

and social care units (municipalities) when older persons are discharged from hospitals. Some of the main problems concern (i) elderly who cannot take care of themselves after treatment at hospital and therefore wait for a place in an adapted dwelling or a nursing home, (ii) cooperation between hospital and municipality to ensure home nursing and home help when patients are discharged from hospital, and (iii) rehabilitation.

A variety of factors – professional, cultural, organisational and financial – constitute barriers to the process of genuine integration between the health and social care services provided by the counties and the municipalities. Many projects have been developed with the intent to solve the problems at this interface between hospitals and health and social care units. These problems partly stem from the fact that legislation comes from two different ministries and furthermore is administered and financed by different regional and local authorities, namely the counties and the municipalities. The scarcity of economic resources and the priorities within the counties and municipalities might have the result that disagreements about responsibilities arise in some areas at the interface between hospitals and health and social care units. One result might be that municipalities do not provide adapted dwellings to elderly at hospital whose discharge is dependent on adapted housing, because – economically – it can make sense for the municipality to prolong the period of hospitalisation of elderly citizens. Another result might be that hospitals discharge elderly patients before treatment is actually finished and, thus, pass the buck to the municipalities in terms of rehabilitation.

Another impediment in integrating health and social care services in municipalities as well as at the interface between hospitals and municipalities might stem from cultural, professional and organisational differences between the sectors. The differences in culture between health and social care staff can result in different views on the citizen's need for services when discharged from hospital. The staff at hospital might overestimate the need for services and the patient's expectations will be influenced accordingly, while the municipality subsequently will tend to provide less service than expected. The result may be users who are discontent with municipal services. When cooperation between hospitals and municipalities is established, it is important to be aware of the differences and to find common conceptions concerning the need for services. The modes of care also appear to differ between health care and social care staff.

168

Furthermore, one has to be aware that cooperation does not just arise without support or supervision. When cooperation is being established it is important that all persons involved know what the cooperation implies and with whom to cooperate. It is important that all staff involved participate in courses or education with the aim of obtaining a common understanding of what kind of service the hospital can provide and what the municipality can provide; to know when and what to cooperate on and be motivated to cooperate. It is also important that the different professions are involved in the decisions about how the cooperation is organised and what it implies. Finally, it is important to note that cooperation is implemented by the managers and that the management, thus, reorganises the organisation according to the implemented patterns of cooperation.

Also the organisation of health and social care at the regional and local level influences cooperation, i.e. both the organisation of hospitals and the organisation of municipalities. Some hospitals have established geriatric departments where the treatment of elderly is holistic whereas others have stuck to a more departmental structure. In the geriatric departments the elderly patients are treated for several diseases in the same department instead of being moved from one department to another. When patients are moved from one department to another, information is often lost and one has to start from the beginning to collect information about the patient.

169

To sum up, there appear to have been very favourable conditions for developing an integrated system of health and social care services for elderly people in Denmark. The institutional structure has eased this process of integration because institutional elderly care in nursing homes and home help and home nursing in the elderly persons' own home were managed by the same agency – the municipality – before the processes of integrating the services got under way. The integration of all types of permanent care has thus been possible within the municipal institutional framework. Unsurprisingly, the most significant stumbling block towards the provision of truly integrated health and social care services by counties and municipalities in concert, thus, appears to be bridging the organisational gaps between the local and regional levels of government.

One of the lessons to learn from the Danish experience is that collaboration between hospitals and municipalities can be organised in many ways, depending on motivation and existing cooperation. It is not possible to emphasise the best practice or the best model for cooperation or to expect that a general model can be implemented in all counties and municipalities. The parties involved can learn from each other's experiences, but not always directly copy a model developed by others because the organisation of and access to services are different.

A more radical solution might be to unite health and social care in one ministry or to let either counties or municipalities organise and administer both health and social care services. The problem of organising the levels of decentralised government has been discussed for years – including the organisation of the health service. The government has appointed a committee, which within two years will put forward a proposal for a new organisation of the decentralised levels of government and the health service. One proposal has been to abolish the counties and to centralise health services. However, if such a solution is implemented the problems of integrating health and social care services provided by hospitals and municipalities will still remain.

5.1   The Political Debate on Elderly Care in Denmark

In spite of what might be expected, the issue of elderly care has been strongly contested on the political scene in Denmark in the past decade. In conjunction with the resource situation of hospitals the issue of elderly care has been crucial to the electoral vote cast in the last three general elections (cf. Borre et al., 1999: 122).

The history of the development of elderly care in Denmark, however, appears to be a textbook example on how to generate public discontent. From the 1950s onwards, the old people's homes got more staff with care functions so that they gradually developed into nursing homes and a home help service was established for elderly persons in need of domestic services. From the 1960s onwards and especially in the 1970s, this development gathered momentum. In 1960 about 15,000 received home aid, ten years later this number had more than doubled, but during the 1970s the number of home aid receivers more than quadrupled to about 150,000. However, since then the number of home help receivers has not grown as fast as the number of elderly.

The massive expansion of home help in the last part of the 1970s can also be regarded as an employment project as most municipalities were in need of creating jobs – especially for women. The system, thus, developed faster than the need. In some cities every pensioner who wanted, could get a home help in these years. As the problems of financing this system grew and persisted during the 1980s and 1990s, the criteria for getting home help were tightened in order to reduce public spending on elderly care. This caused a great deal of press debate, where many elderly stood up for and told they had received home help since "god knows when" where they were quite able, but now where they really needed assistance, it was either reduced or taken away.

Since the beginning of the 1990s when parts of elderly care in Sweden were being contracted out, a discussion has been ongoing as to whether this should be done in Denmark as well. The opinions have been strongly polarised with the bourgeois parties as proponents and the centre-left parties as opponents. In practice, however, the municipalities have opted for a more pragmatic stance. Only few bourgeois municipalities have actually opted to contract out municipal health and social care services, and some Social-Democratic municipalities have used this instrument to create more value for money in elderly care. Until now, contracting out has not proven a success, as most of the private enterprises that hitherto have entered the market have found themselves incapable of competing with the publicly provided services in terms of price and quality.

Recently the bourgeois government has passed legislation obliging the municipalities either to contract out or to provide their users a choice between public and private providers of health and social care services. The majority of the municipalities are expected to choose the latter model. In order to make contracting out easier legislation also demands that the municipal administration of elderly care has to be divided into two parts, with one part of the administration acting as the customer, and another part of the administration acting as the supplier of services. With this transformation of the public administration some of the preparations that will be necessary if the municipalities want to contract out are already made in any case. The municipalities only have to replace "the providing" office with the private company that wins the tender.

In the general perception of many Danes, elderly citizens are – often mistakenly – perceived as a "weak" social group. A number of press reports that have pointed to cases of neglect in nursing homes and in the home help service, have sounded the political alarm bells of central government, which has led to a demand for the municipalities to upgrade the level of service provided to elderly citizens in need. Furthermore, the Danish elderly care has been criticised for organisational slack and an increasingly "Fordist" work ethic. According to the critics home help appointments are often cancelled without prior notice, and the intensification of the workload of the staff has accordingly reduced the services of the home helpers to that of cleaning rather than caring (cf. Rold Andersen, 1999).

Such debates and calls for improvements in the services provided – in order to provide a more dignified service – have persisted, in spite of a vast majority of receivers of health and social care expressing high levels of satisfaction with the services provided. Against the background of the apparent public discontent on the issue, the municipalities have thus been imposed by central government to increase the level of service – and, thus, spending – even though their budgets are highly constrained through the general spending agreements between local and central government. In order to accommodate the requirements of the central government the local authorities now have to cut the budgetary cake anew.

The current drive in Danish elderly policy, thus, appears to point to increased spending in the field, and although the political debate pays tribute to the problems associated with an ageing population this seemingly does not have much effect on the political priorities in terms of promises of increased spending.

The current political debate and priorities on elderly care in Denmark thus appear to be more focused on providing better quality in services provided rather than bracing the welfare state for future pressures that are to be expected due to an increasing number of potential recipients of health and social care services over the coming decades.

Notes

1   The Commission on Elderly – appointed by the Danish government – worked from 1979 to 1982. The aim was to formulate a coherent Danish ageing policy.
2   In 1988 new legislation was implemented on dwellings for dependent elderly and this legislation was directly inspired by the recommendations of the Commission on Elderly. According to this legislation municipalities could no longer build nursing homes according to former legislation. Adapted dwellings with 24-hour assistance service replace the nursing homes. 24-hour assistance services are provided to all elderly independent of where they live.
3   The objective of occupational therapy is to restore or maintain the patients' physical and mental abilities.

172

References

Bierring, A./Bjørn, A./Christensen, B.W. (1987) *Fremme af sundhed og egenomsorg hos ældre* (To promote health and self-care among elderly). Copenhagen: Dansk Institut for Sundheds- og Sygeplejeforskning.

Blackman, T./Brodhurst, S./Convery, J. (2001) *Social Care and Social Exclusion – A Comparative Study of Older People's Care in Europe*. Hampshire: Palgrave.

Borre, Ole et al. (1999) *Vælgere med omtanke – en analyse af folketingsvalget i 1998* (Considerate voters – an analysis of the general elections in 1998). Århus: Systime.

Due, P./Holstein, B.E./Almind, G./Holst, E. (1992) *Hvad sker der, når gamle får brug for hjælp?* (What happens, when elderly need help?). Copenhagen: University of Copenhagen, Institute for Social Medicine.

Daatland, S.O. (ed.) (1997) *De siste årene. Eldreomsorgen i Skandinavia 1960-95* (The latest years. Elderly care in Scandinavia). Oslo: NOVA-rapport 22/97.

Engberg, L./Tang, K. (2000) *Genoptræning af ældre i kommunerne – baseret på 6 interviews* (Rehabilitation of elderly in municipalities – based on 6 interviews). Copenhagen: DSI (Institut for sygehusvæsen/The Danish Institute for Health Services Research).

Felbo, O./Søland, A.M. (1996) *Ældre og sundhedsvæsenet – Hvordan bliver vi bedre?* (Elderly and the health system – How can we be better?). Copenhagen: Akademisk forlag.

Fyns Amt/MedCom (2000) *Omsorgssektoren på sundhedsdatanettet* (The care sector on health data net). Odense: Fyns Amt/MedCom (internetudgave).

Hansen, E.B. (2000) *Social Protection for Dependency in Old Age in Denmark. Modernising and Improving EU Social Protection: Conference on Long-Term Care of Elderly People in the EU and Norway*. London: Department of Health Publications.

Hansen, E.B. (2001) *Home Care for Dependent and Ill People in Denmark* (unpublished paper). Copenhagen, Amternes og Kommunernes Forskningsinstiut

Hansen, E.B./Platz, M. (1995) *80-100-åriges levekår* (80-100 years old's living conditions). Copenhagen: Amternes og Kommunernes Forskningsinstitut & Socialforskningsinstituttet.

Hansen, E.B./Eskelinen, L./Sejr, T./Wagner, L. (1997) *Ældrevenlige behandlingsforløb – analyse af fem indsatstyper* (Elderfriendly treatments – an analysis of five types of efforts). Copenhagen: Amterne og Kommunernes Forskningsinstitut, Dansk Institut for Sygehusvæsen/FOKUS.

Hansen, F.R./Schroll, M./Spedtberg, K. (1991) 'Behov for samarbejde (Need of cooperation)', *Sygeplejersken* 32.

Hansen, F.R./Spedtberg, K./Schroll, M. (1994) 'Follow-up Visits to Elderly Patients after Discharge from Hospital', *Ugeskrift for læger* 156: 3005-11.

MedCom-The Danish Healthcare Data Network (2001) *The Healtcare Communication of the Future*. Funen: Danish Centre for Health telematics.

Ministry of Health (1994) *Mellem to stole* (Between two chairs). Copenhagen: Ministry of Health.

Ministry of Health (1999) *Regeringens Folkesundhedsprogram 1999-2008* (The Government's Public Health Programme 1999-2008). Copenhagen: Ministry of Health.

Ministry of Health (2001) *Rapport om den ældre medicinske patient* (Report on the elderly medical patient). Copenhagen: Ministry of Health.

Ministry of Social Affairs (1982) *Ældrekommisssionsrapporter, delrapporter 1,2 og 3* (Reports from Commission on Elderly, part 1,2 and 3). Copenhagen: Ministry of Social Affairs.

Ministry of Social Affairs (1995) *Social Policy in Denmark*. Copenhagen: Ministry of Social Affairs.

173

Ministry of Social Affairs (1998) *Vejledning. Sociale tilbud til ældre m.fl. Lov om social service* (Guidelines on Social effort for elderly et al, Act on Social Service). Copenhagen: Ministry of Social Affairs.

Ministry of Social Affairs (2000) *Nøgletal på det sociale område. December 2000. Ældrepleje.* (Key Statistics in the Social Policy Area. December 2000. Elderly Care). Copenhagen: Ministry of Social Affairs. http://www.sm.dk/netpublikationer/noegletal_de2000/kap8.html

Ministry of Social Affairs (2002) *Rundt om kommunernes træningsindsats* (Around the rehabilitation in municipalities). Copenhagen: Ministry of Social Affairs.

Platz, M. (1990) *Gamle i eget hjem. Bind 2: Hvordan klarer de sig* (Elderly in own home. Volume 2: How do they managed?). Copenhagen: Socialforskningsinstituttet.

Plovsing, J. (1991) *Udviklingen i kommunernes serviceydelser til ældre in Social Forskning* (The development in municipal services in social research). Copenhagen: Socialforskningsinstituttet.

Rold Andersen, Bent (1999) *Ældrepolitik på afveje : en gammel socialdemokrats refleksioner over udviklingen på ældreområdet i Danmark* (Elderly politics ...Reflections by an old social democrat on the development in elderly policy in Denmark). Kbh. : Fremad.

Rostgaard, T./Fridberg, T. (1998) *Caring for Children and Older People – A Comparision of European Policies and Practices.* Copenhagen: The Danish National Institute of Social Research (Social Security in Europe 6).

Social Appeal Board (2001) *Sociale Danmarkskort 2001, Kommunernes beslutninger om ældreplejen* (Social map of Denmark 2001, Municipal decisions on elderly care). Copenhagen: Social Appeal Board.

Social Appeal Board (2002) *Kommunernes administration af reglerne om forebyggende hjemmebesøg* (The municipal administration on the rules on preventive home visits). Copenhagen: Social Appeal Board.

The Association of County Councils in Denmark & The National Association of Local Authorities in Denmark (1991) *Ventepatienter på sygehusene* (Patients waiting at the hospital). Copenhagen: Amtsrådsforeningen.

The National Association of Local Authorities in Denmark (2000) *Ældrevenlige behandlingsforløb – Om samarbejde mellem kommunerne, sygehusene og de praktiserende læger* (Elderfriendly treatments – About cooperation between municipalities, hospital and general practitioner). Copenhagen: Kommunernes Landsforening.

Wagner, L. (1994) *Innovation in Primary Health Care for Elderly People in Denmark.* Gothenburg: The Nordic School of Public Health.

Wagner, L. (2000) 'Ti år efter – aktionsforskning anvendt i udvikling af ældres pleje og omsorg (Ten years after – action research used in development of health and care for elderly)', in: Gress, N./Graugaard, K. (eds.), *Klinisk Sygepleje 1, 2 og 3 – Praksis & Udvikling (Clinical nursing 1, 2 and 3 – Practice & Development).* Viborg: Akademisk Forlag.

Wagner, L./Mogensen, T. (2001) 'Hjemmeplejens bidrag til forebyggelse og sundhedsfremme (The domiciliary cares contribution to prevention and health promotion)', in: Avlund, K., et al. (eds.), *Forebyggelse i alderdommen* (Prevention in old age). Copenhagen: Dafolo Forlag og Dansk Gerontologisk Selskab.

Wagner, L./ Olsen, L. (2000) *Inerti i den kliniske hverdag* (Inertia in daily clinical practice). Copenhagen: Universitetshospitalernes Center for Sygepleje- og omsorgsforskning (The University Hospitals Centre for Nursing and Care Research).

Annex: Model Ways of Working

A1 The Skaevinge Project

Name	The project of Skaevinge (24-hours care with integrated health and social care)
Provider	Ministry of Social Affairs and the municipality of Skaevinge
Objectives	• To integrate the traditional health and social care departments in one department to obtain a better utilisation of the united resources. • To obtain a common understanding through working with the concept of self-care. • To introduce 24-hours integrated health and social care. • To change the organisation of the services by introducing autonomous groups with more responsibility and competence for each employee and a better planned health and social care without delaying hierarchic structure.
Target group and number of clients	• Older users • Elderly citizens
Number of staff involved	All categories of staff working with the elderly (home help, public health nursing, home nursing and nursing homes)
Methods	• Action research theory. • The staff's and citizens' active involvement. • Self-care approach, building on the acceptance of the human being as a free, independently thinking and acting individual. • 24-hours service regardless of type of dwelling.
Strengths and weaknesses	*Strengths:* • Access to 24-hours health and social care service irrespective of living at home or at an institution has the result that many older persons have chosen to remain at home. • The former nursing home was converted into individual apartments and a health centre was established – putting together home nursing, public health nursing and day centre. The centre directs its attention towards all pensioners in the municipality. *Weaknesses:* • The consequences of intervention on the health status of the older people were not examined in these studies, and some clinical-empirical studies would be needed to show if health status has improved among the elderly • It would have been obvious to discuss the cause and the effect of the intervention, but due to its multi-factorial

175

	nature it would be almost impossible to draw conclusions regarding single items as too many confounding factors would have to be considered.
Results of evaluation/keywords	The evaluation of the project 10 years after (1997) shows among other things that: • The operating expenditures have decreased even though the number of persons of 75 years or more has increased by 30%. • The use of bed days at hospital has been reduced by 30-40% for all citizens in the municipality. • During 10 years there have been no waiting days for older persons who have finished treatment at hospital.

A2 Acute rooms in the Municipality of Roedding

Name	Acute rooms in the municipality of Roedding
Provider	The municipality of Roedding and County of Soenderjylland
Objectives	• To reduce inappropriate admission to hospital. • To intensify observation and care of elderly. • To facilitate returning to one's own home.
Target group and number of clients	• Elderly citizens who, in an acute situation, need more care and treatment than can be provided at home. • Elderly citizens who might be discharged within 2 weeks. • 20-25 elderly use the service during a year.
Number of staff involved	GPs, doctors from emergency service, home nurses
Methods	Corporation between the GPs, emergency service and home nurses. A nurse observes the elderly in the acute-room
Strengths and weaknesses	*Strengths:* • The elderly were satisfied with the service. They were pleased to be helped in an acute situation and to stay close to their homes. • During the stay the home nurse could observe the older person's need for help in the future and plan future services. *Weaknesses:* • One could question whether the elderly had the optimal treatment or would be better off at a hospital.
Results of evaluation/keywords	The project has not been evaluated. But the results have been so positive that the project has been extended and prolonged. The elderly from Roedding are less often hospitalised than the elderly from the neighbouring municipality and the difference has increased over the last years. But it cannot be proved that the acute rooms caused the difference.

176

A3 Good Cooperation Practice

Name	Good cooperation practice
Provider	The management of nurses at the hospital of Skive and five municipalities: Fjends, Sallingsund, Skive, Spoettrup and Sundsoere.
Objectives	• To ensure quality and continuity in welfare, caring and rehabilitation courses when patients are hospitalised and discharged. • To reduce waiting time at hospitals for patients who have finished their treatment. • To reduce the number of re-admissions.
Target group and number of clients	Elderly citizens (70+ years) at the hospital of Skive (between 1,000 and 1,200 a year).
Number of staff involved	GPs, doctors from hospital, nurses, home help, home nurses
Methods	A working group with nurses from hospital departments and nurses from five municipalities prepared a contract. A checklist according to discharge. A booklet belonging to the patients used to provide information to all involved staff.
Strengths and weaknesses	*Strengths:* • There has been an increase in the dialogue between hospitals and municipalities. *Weaknesses:* • The booklet is not used in all cases or used as intended. • The checklist is not always followed.
Results of evaluation/keywords	The result of the contract of "Good cooperation practice" has been that staff at hospitals and staff in municipalities normally are in contact by telephone or arrange meetings about the needs for help after discharge. If there is need for services, the patients are not discharged without information given to the municipality prior to discharge. There is a common understanding about the need for a better practice in the future. At the time for evaluation the reduce in re-admissions was not observed because of a lack of data.

177

A4 Rehabilitation

Name	Around municipal rehabilitation
Provider	Ministry of Social Affairs and eight municipalities: Hjoerring, Esbjerg, Broendby, Soelleroed, Skagen, Fjerritslev, Dronninglund and Hobro
Objectives	• To develop a general model to ensure rehabilitation with focus on the citizen's needs for rehabilitation. • To ensure a simple and coherent process for the citizen also when several actors are involved. • To ensure unambiguous definitions and delimitation of each service's contents, to be used in the practice of rehabilitation as well as in relation to other departments in or outside the organisation (e.g. domiciliary care, hospitals, GP, physiotherapists). • To ensure sufficient and equal service for all citizens, where the citizens own requests and if any priority of rehabilitation efforts are included in the basis for referral.
Target group and number of clients	All older persons in need of rehabilitation.
Number of staff involved	Practical and administrative staff in eight municipalities and the relevant counties.
Methods	• Four municipalities have been in charge of the developing work. • Four other municipalities have contributed to quality control and testing the developed tools.
Strengths and weaknesses	*Strengths:* • The citizen gives priority to different functional abilities and this priority is part of the documentation together with the professional assessment of rehabilitation possibilities. • There is quality control and testing of the developed tools. *Weaknesses:* • A well-tested model is not enough to ensure older people's rehabilitation. Use of the model presupposes that the municipalities allocate economic resources to rehabilitation as well as educate their staff in using the model.
Results of evaluation/keywords	The developmental project is not finished and the concrete experiences with the use of the model within the municipality are not expected until the beginning of 2003.

178

A5 MedCom

Name	MedCom – The Danish Healthcare Data Network
Provider	Ministry of Health, Ministry of Social Affairs, The National Board of Health, Association of County Councils in Denmark, The National Association of Local Authorities in Denmark, Copenhagen Hospital Corporation, Copenhagen and Frederiksberg Local Authorities, Danish Pharmaceutical Association, Danish Dental Association, Association of Danish Doctors, Kommunedata, Tele Danmark, Dan Net
Objectives	• Developing Communication standards for the most common communication flows between local authorities and hospitals. • Expanding communication between medical practices, hospitals and pharmacies. • Expanding basic communication between hospitals and local authorities.
Target group and number of clients	All hospitals, pharmacies and laboratories, all medical practices, local authorities.
Number of staff involved	Potentially all staff in all counties, hospitals, pharmacies, two thirds of the GPs, one third of medical specialists and 16 municipalities.
Methods	• Establishing pilot projects. • Developing and testing care reports and warning messages between hospital and municipality. • Dissemination of experiences.
Strengths and weaknesses	*Strengths:* • The project facilitates the communication between hospital, medical practices and local authorities. • The information is given immediately. • The citizens receives better service. • The hospital and the domiciliary care can avoid wasted time. *Weaknesses:* • Not all medical practices and local authorities use the system.
Results of evaluation/keywords	The developmental project is not finished and the concrete experiences with the use of the model within the municipalities are not expected until the beginning of 2003. A preliminary report from the participating municipalities shows that the citizens receive better service and the hospitals as well as the domiciliary care avoid wasted time.

CHAPTER 5

Providing Integrated Health and Social Care for Older Persons in Finland

Paula Salonen, Riitta Haverinen

1   The Development of Health and Social Care Services

Equality, social integration, economic independence and safety plus fair treatment are the values underlying old-age care policy in Finland, and its aim is to promote the well-being and functioning ability of ageing people, and to ensure that they get good care and service when they need it (Ministry of Social Affairs and Health, 1999a). The national policy sets prerequisites for local policies carried out in municipalities, and the task of municipalities is to respond to local needs in accordance with the national legislation and with municipal priorities and resources (Vaarama et al., 2002: 76). Finland is thus representing the Nordic social welfare state model (Sipilä, 1997; Mäkinen et al., 1998: 28) the central features of which are the principle of universality (a statutory right to social welfare in accordance with need), a strong public sector, tax funding, equal treatment and social benefits of a relatively high level (Ministry of Social Affairs and Health, 1999b).

The development of health care and social services[1] took place separately until the 1990s (Järvelin, 2002). The development of the health care system began in the 1940s, but progress took place mainly during the 1960s and the 1970s. At the end of the 1980s there existed both primary health care provided by municipal health centres, including e.g. primary medical care, preventive services, home nursing and rehabilitation, and a network of high-standard specialised hospitals (Ministry of Social Affairs and Health, 1999c;

Järvelin, 2002). During the last decades a system of personal physicians has been introduced in some health centres, the aim of which is to simplify access to general practitioners and ensure the continuity of care. In some municipalities there is a multiprofessional team responsible for the health care in a defined geographical area (Järvelin, 2002).

Since 1950, and especially during the 1980s the social services developed rapidly. In 1984, the care of older people was finally included in the government subsidy arrangement, as until then it had been practised outside the laws. At the end of the 1980s Finland had a social service system – planned and directed by the state and enacted by the municipalities (Kröger, 1996) – that encompassed social work, home help services, housing services, institutional care and support for informal care (Ministry of Social Affairs and Health 1999b). These welfare services covered all classes of society and all regions in Finland (Kröger, 1996).

Finland disposes of a joint Ministry of Social Affairs and Health and several state agencies subordinate to the Ministry emerged, e.g. the National Agency for Medicine and the National Research and Development Centre for Welfare and Health (Rintala et al., 1997: 2; Järvelin, 2002: 13, 14, 19).

A large-scale development between the social and health sectors was begun in the year 1991, when the Ministry set up a working group to make a proposal for an action programme to help improve the service structure. The programme recommended, for instance, the improvement of cooperation between social and health care services by uniting the municipal health and social service committees and respective agendas (Seiskari, 1997: 149). However, until 2000 only 38% of Finland's municipalities (N = 448) had followed this recommendation and even in that case health care and social welfare services continue to be separately arranged on the practical level (Järvelin, 2002: 4, 19).[2]

In the 1990s, for reasons of economy as well as quality, there was a shift in emphasis towards non-institutional health care and social services, and away from institution-oriented care. According to the policy on ageing, the goals of the non-institutional services were set to provide appropriately gradated services, integrated care chains and coordinated service packages for older persons (Ministry of Social Affairs and Health, 1999a). Regardless of these goals, outpatient services for the elderly have been diminished and the loss of institutional care has been compensated by housing services (Vaarama/Lehto, 1996: 55). However, the situation is not unambiguous. On the one hand the integration of social and health care services has been discussed, while on the other hand differentiation has taken place, e.g. cleaning services have at least partly been outsourced in some municipalities. One possible future trend is that the providers of social welfare services in the private sector will specialise and concentrate on the provision of core services of their own (Partanen, 2002).

2 Legal and Structural Framework: The General Discourse on (Integrated) Care Provision

2.1 The Legal Framework on Health Care and Social Welfare Services

In Finland, people's basic rights are laid down in the Constitution Act of Finland of the year 2000. According to this Act the government must provide each person with sufficient social and health services (Finlex, 1999), and promote public health (Ministry of Social Affairs and Health, 2001a), in accordance with the provisions enacted elsewhere (Ministry of Social Affairs and Health, 1999a). The government's duty is more precisely defined in the Finnish legislation on social welfare and health care (Ranta, 2001). The Constitution Act also includes the principle of equality and stipulations forbidding discrimination, meaning, e.g. that everyone has the same right to receive the needed services regardless of his/her age. There is no separate legislation on the care for older people (Ministry of Social Affairs and Health, 2001a); instead, their rights to services are prescribed in the general national legislation and in observance of international agreements (Ministry of Social Affairs and Health, 1999a). However, home care for older people is dealt with in several different acts and decrees (Ministry of Social Affairs and Health, 2001a), e.g. in the Primary Health Care Act it is declared that the physician in charge of a health centre decides on the arrangement and content of the patient's medical treatment and nursing care, e.g. home nursing (Ranta, 2001: 151). In the Social Welfare Act home help services and the grounds for receiving these services are defined (Ranta, 2001: 90).

The Primary Health Care Act and the Act on Specialised Medical Care contain general provisions on the duty of municipalities to provide health care, medical care and activities related to the care (Ministry of Social Affairs and Health, 2001a). Care can be provided at health centres as non-institutional care, or in health centre wards, or in the form of home nursing.

Specialised medical care means health care services involving prevention, examination, treatment and rehabilitation of medical conditions within the specialised fields of medicine. There is no detailed legislation on the required scale and quality of care, but the municipality is responsible for ensuring that people receive the specialised care they need (Ranta, 2001: 149, 160). Specialised medical care can be purchase by the municipality from the hospital district to which it belongs, from another hospital district or from private providers (Järvelin, 2002: 23). The Act on the Status and Rights of Patients regulates the status of users of health care services (Ministry of Social Affairs and Health, 2001a).

As regards social welfare, the general legislation consists of the Social Welfare Act, and the newer Act on the "Status and Rights of Social Welfare Clients" which entered into force in 2001. These acts set the principles that apply to all social welfare services and to the provision of general social services, while defining the main procedures to be used in client services and data protection. Social work, home help services and support for informal care are included in the statutory social services (Ministry of Social Affairs and Health, 2001a). Social work means that professional social welfare staff gives guidance, advice and help in solving social problems, and it includes support measures that help individuals to cope and to maintain and improve their security. Home help services are provided for those who need help with everyday chores and tasks because of, e.g. reduced functional capacity, illness or disability. Support for informal care is a form of financial and supportive service available for private individuals looking after someone at home, the terms of the support being detailed in a care and service plan (Ranta, 2001: 90, 92, 93).

The provision of most social welfare and health care services is statutory, meaning that there are laws requiring the municipalities to provide certain services. Although the legislation does not set detailed requirements for the extent, content or method of provision, definition is made on how access to services must be ensured in practice. Depending on local conditions and the specific needs of the local population there may be variations in the operations of different municipalities. While the responsibility for providing social welfare and health care services for residents lies with the municipalities, they may choose to provide other services, too, as part of their own operations, through membership in a joint municipal board, or by purchasing services from other municipalities or private providers (Ministry of Social Affairs and Health, 2001a), meaning private companies or non-governmental organisations (Ministry of Social Affairs and Health, 1999b). The respective quality recommendations to support the municipalities' quality management efforts are not legally binding (Ministry of Social Affairs and Health, 2001a; 2001b).

The provision and supervision of social welfare services in the private sector are strictly regulated by the Act and Decree on the Supervision of Private Social Services (Partanen, 2002; Ranta, 2001: 128, 129) and the Decree on formal qualifications for social welfare personnel (Ranta 2001: 293, 294). Especially requirements for the educational standards of the providing organisation and employees, work premises (Partanen, 2002), and home help services (Ranta, 2001: 129) are defined. The provision and supervision of private health care services are covered by the Private Health Care Act and Decree (Ranta, 2001:173-175), and the competence of health care staff is defined in the legislation on vocational practice (Ranta, 2001: 295, 296). This legislation also applies to services that municipalities purchase from private service providers and to employees in the public sector (Ministry of Social Affairs and Health, 2001a).

2.2 *The General Discourse on Care for Older Persons: Policies and Steering Mechanisms towards Seamless Service Chains*

Social welfare and health care services are mainly steered through legislation. In addition, national guidelines to help local authorities to develop their service systems were recently published. The Target and Action Plan for Social Welfare and Health Care for 2000–2003 (Ministry of Social Affairs and Health, 1999d) approved by the Government (Ministry of Social Affairs and Health, 2002: 48) contains the targets set for care and actions, and recommendations and instructions to reach the targets (Ministry of Social Affairs and Health, 2001a). The Plan focuses on the services in non-institutional care, stating that the elderly should be given a possibility to receive services at home instead of institutions, whenever non-institutional care is justified. It further suggests that the Ministry of Social Affairs and Health ought to change the fee systems to provide better financial support to non-institutional services. The programme requests that independent performance and maintenance of the functional capacity should be supported, and all services and care should incorporate a preventive, promoting and rehabilitating aspect (Working Group Investigating the Significance of Non-Institutional and Institutional Care, 2001: 44). According to the governmental act on services for the elderly, attention should be paid especially to home nursing, home help services, supported living at home and possibilities for rehabilitation. As development targets, the Action mentions subjects such as the creation of effective and functional care chains, suited gradation of care, use of new technology, as well as increasing home services and offering preventive home visits to all over-80s. Also the seamless and customer-oriented chain of care and services are included in the recommended actions (Viitala, 2000).

The "National Framework for High-quality Care and Services for Older People" (Ministry of Social Affairs and Health, 2001c) is part of the new target and action plan. The Framework was designed to help local authorities to plan and evaluate their own activities. It sets national guidelines for developing good services for older people, and requires that local authorities should base their future care and services on local needs and conditions. For this purpose the municipalities should draw up plans for their policy strategy related to concrete development of services for the care of the elderly. Implementation of the set targets should be systematically monitored and evaluated with quality indicators. In the year 2000, 39% of the municipalities had prepared this document and 27% were in the process of doing so (Vaarama et al., 2002: 77).

According to the Framework, the main emphasis is laid on home care, service housing and residential care. Living at home will be supported with rapid-access professional social and health care services, the focus points being, e.g. in the arrangement of high-standard and well-timed care, to support a good quality of life and the right to self-determination and independent life, regardless of the individual's functional capacity. Services should be ethical and based on user needs, using rehabilitation as an integral element; they should rely on applying evidence-based procedures and recommended care practices, be specified in written service plans or care agreements, and implemented in smooth cooperation between the various service providers and the client's family. People employed to care for older people should be suited to the job and they should ideally possess a qualification that meets the requirements (Ministry of Social Affairs and Health, 2001c).

A new special Act, applied at first in seven municipalities, on Experiments with Seamless Service Chains in Social Welfare and Health Care Services and with Social Security Card, entered into force in 2000 (Ranta, 2001: 274, 275). The purpose of the Act is to gain experience in arranging seamless service chains, and in ways of optimising the use of information technology so that it responds to the needs of the clients of social welfare and health care services, and in establishing how to allocate information technology resources in these activities in a sensible way (Ministry of Social Affairs and Health, 2000). Seamless service chains are defined as an operating model, where the services received by a client and forming part of a service context within the social welfare and health care services and other social protection are integrated into a flexible entity which will satisfy the client's needs regardless of which operating unit provides or implements the services (Ranta, 2001: 274, 275).

The idea of seamless service chains emerged as one of the most essential definitions in Finnish national policy at the end of the 1990s. In the service chains, cooperation between social and health care organisations is emphasised, to which both public and private providers equally contribute their know-how. The central areas for definition in the national policy have been the aspirations to reorganise the production of services, development of customer orientation, multi-professional teamwork and networking. Further core issues are the improvement of cooperation between clients and professionals, clients' possibilities to influence decision-making, and seamless chain of services (Ruotsalainen et al., 2000: 5-6; Ruotsalainen, 2000: 14). Consequently, the experimental use of seamless service chains will expand when other regions, e.g. Finland's largest cities, adopt this form of service chains (Working Group Investigating the Significance of Non-Institutional and Institutional Care, 2001: 33).

2.3   Financing of Health Care and Social Welfare Services

Municipalities finance their services with tax revenues (70%), state subsidies (20%) and client fees (10%) (Vaarama et al., 2002: 98). Government subsidies are paid according to the cost of the service, including the size, age structure and morbidity of the population, unemployment, and remoteness of the municipality's location (Ministry of Social Affairs and Health, 2001a).

As public health care services are financed mainly either with tax revenues or with state subsidies, the fees charged from clients who use public health care services form only a minor part (about 10%) of the total costs of the service, with most annual fees for medical treatment in health centres being € 20-25, and with no charge for preventive health care. There is some variation in the sum and collection of the fee in different municipalities. The average charge for a home visit by a general practitioner to a person in temporary home nursing (about 1-5 visits per month) is about € 8, and by other health personnel about € 5. A monthly charge can be applied for continuous home nursing depending on the quality and quantity of services, gross income of the person involved and of his/her family, and size of the family. A visit to a hospital outpatients' department costs approximately € 17, and a daily charge for inpatients is approximately € 21 both in health centre hospitals and in specialised care hospitals. This charge covers examination, treatment, medication and full board. However, recently the percentage of all health care expenditure funded out of the public purse has diminished, while the role of households in financing has correspondingly risen, being almost a quarter of the total funding in 1996. At the same time central government funding has been cut, while the proportion funded by local authorities has slightly risen (Ministry of Social Affairs and Health, 1999c). One reason for this development may be the increasing share of persons who use private medical treatment and care services (Tervala, 2002).

188

In public health service there is a payment limit, to the effect that if the client fees exceed a certain amount during 12 months (in 2001 the limit was about 588 €), s/he needs to pay for no further costs. All other health service fees are included in this payment limit, except the fees for long-term institutional care (periods over three months), dental care and home nursing services. Even after the payment limit is fulfilled, the municipality is, however, allowed to charge about 12 € per bed-day for short-term institutional care (Working Group Investigating the Significance of Non-Institutional and Institutional Care, 2001: 31).

The system of national health insurance administered by the Social Insurance Institution supplements the public health care system by refunding some of the costs incurred when the customer uses private care services or medicines prescribed in outpatient care. Employers and insured employees fund this insurance system through compulsory contributions (Ministry of Social Affairs and Health, 1999c).

Municipal taxation accounts for 64% of the total financing of social welfare services, and the share of state subsidies is about 24% while clients' fees cover about 12% of the costs (Ministry of Social Affairs and Health, 1999b). For temporary home help services (1–5 visits per month at the client's home) the municipality itself sets the fee. For regular home help services maximum amounts are defined, e.g. in 1999 for a person living alone the fees could rise to a maximum of 35% of the client's gross income exceeding € 420 (Ministry of Social Affairs and Health, 1999a). For support services, such as cleaning and transport, the municipality can charge without considering the income level of the client, for as long as the fee does not exceed the total costs of the service. In long-term care (over 90 days) the clients pay 80% of their net incomes regardless of the provider (Working Group Investigating the Significance of Non-Institutional and Institutional Care, 2001: 31).

2.4 *Process of Care Provision*

SUPPLY AND DEMAND

In Finland nine out of ten older persons (75 years of age or older) suffer from some chronic disease or disability, the most prevalent being cardiovascular diseases and musculoskeletal diseases, together with diabetes and dementia. Especially the number of people with dementia increases among older age groups. Most of older people, however, manage on their own or with the support of their family. Some sort of assistance from the formal or informal sector is received by 36% of those over 60 years of age (Ministry of Social Affairs and Health, 1999a). Persons most commonly providing assistance are spouses; according to the elderly barometer in 1998 the percentage of care providers who were spouses was 49% (Vaarama et al., 2000: 84), followed by care providing children, and then by municipal home help services or home nursing services (Ministry of Social Affairs and Health, 1999a). In 1998, spouses acted as caregivers twice as often as was the case four years earlier (Vaarama et al., 2000: 84).

According to national and international estimations, 30-50% of persons over 75 need at least some help, and 25-30% need regular help. The need of help increased with age so that half of those over 85 needed assistance (Vaarama et al., 2002: 79). About 12% of those over 75 receive home help services and/or home nursing services on a regular basis (National Research and Development Centre for Welfare and Health, 2000). Almost half of the clients received only home help services, a quarter received only home nursing services and the rest received both home help and home nursing services (Vaarama et al., 2000: 83). Long-term care in health centre wards has increased by 15% during the past decade (Vaarama et al., 2002: 83). In 1997, people over 65 accounted for 85% of all care days in health centre hospitals and wards (Ministry of Social Affairs and Health, 1999c).

189

During the 1990s services for the aged were cut even though the proportion of ageing people in the population increased. The cuts affected mostly home help services, where the ten-year trend shows that the coverage has been reduced almost to a half of the 1990 level, and consequently there is a tendency to turn to less expensive solutions in long-term care (Vaarama et al., 2002: 79, 83). In 1997, home care (integrated home help service and home nursing) was received by 55,000 older persons, 10,000 below the number for 1995. Although many local reports have shown an increased number of home visits by home help services, the duration of these visits has decreased (Vaarama et al., 2000: 78, 81, 84, 97). In many municipalities staff have been moved from non-institutional care to service housing, thus diminising the availability of non-institutional services for those elderly who live at home (Vaarama et al., 2002: 83, 94).

There are regional and municipal variations in the present public system, which present problems regarding the level (quality or quantity) and availability of care for older persons (Ministry of Social Affairs and Health, 2001c: 33), as well as the arrangement of services (Ministry of Social Affairs and Health, 2002: 170). The demand and supply of elderly care services meet each other poorly (Vaarama et al., 2000: 97). The availability of care depends on factors such as size, wealth, and age structure of the municipality, state of health of residents, and number of personnel (Ministry of Social Affairs and Health, 2002: 115, 162-169). The most modest supply of non-institutional care, in relation to the size of the elderly population, is in towns, and the most substantial supply is in the countryside and in Helsinki, the capital city of Finland (Vaarama et al., 2000: 77). The main problem is the difficulty in finding permanently employed certified physicians, especially in small municipalities, because of a general lack of medical doctors. This tendency seems to be spreading also among other professionals due to the baby-boom generations now approaching retirement age, and the fact that there are not enough younger trained professionals to enter these positions. The trend is already seen among social workers. Another difficulty is that the distances between homes of clients vary considerably in different municipalities. While the distances between clients in larger cities remain within a few kilometres, they may in other areas, like Northern Finland, be as much as 200–400 kilometres (Ministry of Social Affairs and Health, 2002: 55-58, 163-168). Also, private social and health services have concentrated primarily in the larger municipalities (Ministry of Social Affairs and Health, 1999c; Partanen, 2002: 16).

190

Table 1:   Coverage of Services for the Elderly, 1990-2001 in Finland

Year	Regular home care services	Service housing	Old-age homes	Health centres	Psychiatric wards	Other health care
	Clients as a percentage of the population aged 65 and over					
1990			4.0	2.0	0.4	0.3
1995	7.3	2.0	3.2	2.0	0.1	0.1
2000		2.9	2.7	1.8	0.1	0.1
2001	6.6	2.9	2.6	1.7	0.0	0.1
	Clients as a percentage of the population 75 and over					
1990			7.8	4.0	0.6	0.6
1995	13.8	3.4	6.5	4.1	0.2	0.2
2000		5.1	5.2	3.4	0.0	0.1
2001	12.1	5.1	5.0	3.3	0.0	0.1

Sources: Care Registers for Social Welfare and Health Care, STAKES; Statistics on Municipal Finances and Activities, Statistics Finland, SOTKA; Note: Home care services per 30 November, all other data per 31 December of the given year.

Table 2:   Service Structure in Care for the Elderly, 1990-2001 in Finland

End of year	Regular home care services	Service housing for the elderly	Old people's homes	Health centres, long-term inpatients	Psychiatric wards, long-term inpatients	Other health care, long-term inpatients
	Clients, aged 65 and over					
1990			26,634	13,383	2,907	2,013
1995	53,277	14,661	23,088	14,573	987	757
2000		22,189	20,674	13,706	416	461
2001	52,353	22,710	20,547	13,615	373	522
	Clients, aged 75 and over					
1990			22,180	11,258	1,689	1,582
1995	41,284	10,197	19,535	12,175	474	545
2000		17,226	17,618	11,580	167	374
2001	42,231	17,843	17,509	11,524	153	417

Sources: Care Registers for Social Welfare and Health Care, STAKES; Statistics on Municipal Finances and Activities, Statistics Finland, SOTKA

MAIN SERVICE TYPES

The main service types for older people are support, home help, home nursing, and health centre services that in many municipalities are also provided
in the evenings and on weekends. Home nursing services include giving
care, taking samples and performing tests. For this purpose health centres
employ separate personnel trained as public health nurses, specialised
nurses, registered nurses or practical nurses. Another aspect of home nursing services is to support family members, especially during terminal care
(Ministry of Social Affairs and Health, 1999a).

Support services promote coping in daily activities and social interaction, and may include meals on wheels, day activities, transport and escort
services, various emergency telephones, laundry and cleaning services, etc.
Commonly the municipalities, produced by trained home helpers or home
aids, or by practical nurses in the social and health care system, but also
associations and parishes, provide home help services. The home help
worker assists the client with everyday chores and personal care, monitors
the state of health of the client, and also provides guidance and advice in
questions pertaining to services. Today there are signs that the work has
increasingly concentrated on personal assistance and care (Ministry of Social Affairs and Health, 1999a).

Due to financial incentives the number of service housing facilities as
a form of non-institutional care has increased rapidly during the 1990s
(Working Group Investigating the Significance of Non-Institutional and
Institutional Care, 2001: 52, 53). These services are organised by public,
voluntary non-profit and by commercial providers. Usually they consist of
a block of service flats, a group of service homes, or as an individual small
service home. Living in a service home is targeted to older people who need
support and assistance on a daily basis, as it includes both dwelling and
provision of services. The resident pays a rent (a rental agreement is common practice) or a maintenance fee for his/her home, selects the services
needed and pays for them separately in accordance with the use. The basic
services of a municipal service home are the responsibility of the home help
and home nursing services, or they are the responsibility of the service
home's own staff (Ministry of Social Affairs and Health, 1999a).

With the action programme that was launched in the beginning of the
1990s, major changes have taken place in the service structure, most nota-
bly concerning elderly people being placed in service homes, together with

the fact that the supply of services has significantly improved in these homes (Järvelin, 2002). On the other hand, the supply of services has not improved among outpatients living in their own homes. At the same time, it has become clear that the level of services does not fit personal needs, nor do the care or services support independent initiative, especially in service homes. The objective of changes in the service structure can therefore not yet be said to have come true to a sufficient extent, especially in the services and care for persons living in their own homes. As one solution, it has been suggested that preventive home visits should cover all persons 80 years or older, and that after the first home visit the situation should be followed up. With the help of preventive interventions, such as with sufficient home care services and with proper technical aids or improved facilities at the client's home, the need of institutional care can be postponed (Working Group Investigating the Significance of Non-Institutional and Institutional Care, 2001: 52-65).

Of the health services provided in the year 2000, 81% were arranged by the public sector, 3% by non-governmental organisations and 16% by private companies. Approximately every sixth service was produced by the private sector. The number of private companies has increased during the last five years; the net increase was 30% during the period 1995–2000. The main role of the private sector has, until now, been to supplement the public supply and to even out the peak hours of the public service supply. In the future the demand for health services will, however, continue to increase, and the service purchases from the private sector by municipalities is estimated to increase likewise (Tervala, 2002: 3, 4).

Home nursing services have developed into one link in the chain of care, the other links being primary health care, specialised health care, health centre wards or hospitals, and the home of the client. For instance, health centre inpatient ward and home nursing are jointly increasingly responsible for the terminal care of cancer patients (Ministry of Social Affairs and Health, 1999a).

The provision of social services has traditionally been the responsibility of the public sector, but new legal grounds and the growing number of older persons who need more services have increased the demand for services provided by the private sector, especially in the 1990s. In 2000, 78% of social services was arranged by municipalities, 17% by non-governmental organisations and 5% by private companies (Partanen, 2002). Home help services are still mostly provided by the public sector (Ministry of Social Affairs and Health, 1999a), but even in this area the number of private pro-

193

viders has increased recently. Home help services, which are some of the most typical services needed by the elderly, were the most commonly provided services purchased by municipalities from private companies. Also, the law concerning the support for domestic work (a tax exemption for citizens) has enabled citizens to buy more services directly from private companies (Partanen, 2002). It seems that the tendency towards private provision of social services will continue, because the demand for these services is growing more rapidly than their supply by the public sector (Ministry of Social Affairs and Health, 2002: 162–172).

FAMILY MEMBERS AS CAREGIVERS

Also in Finland family members are an important source of support and assistance for older people, as well as important cooperation partners. There has even been speculation that the service contribution, which by social legislation is today the responsibility of society, has to be moved back to the family members (Mäkinen et al., 1998: 52). At any rate, the responsibility of family members as caregivers will increase (Ministry of Social Affairs and Health, 2002: 115). The municipality can support the person providing care by paying a fee for the care and/or by arranging diverse social welfare and health services that support the care-giving. The municipality and the caregiver draw up an agreement, including a plan on care and services, to support informal care. The caregiver has the right to at least one day off per month, and the municipality is responsible for providing the care during the statutory free time. In recent years, cooperation between family members, volunteer workers, the public sector and service-producing organisations has intensified (Ministry of Social Affairs and Health, 1999a).

2.5 Towards an Integrated Health and Social Care System?

HOME CARE AS A FORM OF INTEGRATED HEALTH AND SOCIAL CARE SERVICES

In Finland, social and health care services are commonly implemented by two different organisations, but cooperation between home help and home nursing services has become more common, especially in those municipalities that have multiprofessional teams for defined areas. In some municipalities, home help service and home nursing have been combined to form a home care unit, and an entity of care given by this unit is called home care. Home care means that a client lives most of the time at home while receiving various services. The main purpose of home care is to enable the client to cope by supporting his/her functional capacity, especially after illness or disability. Home care includes help with everyday tasks and support of social relationships together with medical care and nursing. The clients of home care are mainly 75 years of age and older, a great part of them being 85 or older. Eight out of ten clients have a cardiovascular disease, half of the clients have a musculoskeletal disease and every fifth client suffers from moderately severe or severe dementia (Mäkinen et al., 1998: 10, 12, 23, 29).

ARRANGEMENT OF HOME CARE FOR OLDER PERSONS DISCHARGED FROM HOSPITAL

Care can be given in specialised care hospitals, regional hospitals, health centre hospitals or wards, or hospitals specialised in geriatric or psycho-geriatric disorders. Further, it can be part-time, short-term or long-term care. The purpose of short-term and periodic institutional care is to help older people cope at home and to give respite to family members who normally provide the care, while at the same time preventing the need for permanent institutional care. Institutional care can alternate with living at home (Ministry of Social Affairs and Health, 1999a).

   Overall, the arrangements for home care or home help services and home nursing services vary in different municipalities, decisions on the social welfare services needed by clients are commonly made by individual municipal civil servants (Ministry of Social Affairs and Health, 1999a), e.g. by the head of the home help service in the social welfare unit (Mäkinen et al., 1998: 35). Usually the arrangements begin with the hospital sending the patient's medical history to the health centre physician, whereby also the responsibility for further medical care is transferred. Also the client's personal nurse from the hospital sends her referral to the home care unit or to the home nursing unit. This includes information about the patient's illness and medicines, how s/he copes with everyday tasks, and instructions for treatment. After receiving the information, the need for and decision on home care is prepared in a working group which usually consists of a general practitioner, social worker, home help worker and health visitor, but the size and tasks of the group may vary (Ministry of Social Affairs and Health, 1999a). The physician makes the decision concerning home nursing together with the client and his/her relatives (Mäkinen et al., 1998: 25).

195

After the decision, an individual care and service plan will be drawn up by a civil servant together with the client and his/her relatives. The plan also serves as an action plan and contract on arranging the care and services. It includes a combination of home help and home nursing services that best suits the client's present situation. The individual care and service plan includes an assessment of the client's situation, and specification of targets, implementation of the plan, evaluation of the implementation, and evaluation of how the targets have been fulfilled. At the same time the possibilities and prerequisites for family members and volunteers to take part in providing care will be determined, and the information about the division of labour between the different care providers will become part of the plan. The overall accountability for the care of the client rests with the worker under whose scope of responsibility the client's primary need for services falls (Mäkinen et al., 1998: 105-116; Ministry of Social Affairs and Health, 1999a).

196

CO-OPERATION BETWEEN PUBLIC AND PRIVATE SECTORS IN ARRANGING ELDERLY CARE

Given the legally defined public responsibility to provide social welfare and health services the production of services is based on a close cooperation between the central state and local municipalities. Local municipal councils, however, hold considerable autonomy in deciding on their service policy (Sipilä, 1997: 5). Municipalities can provide health and social care services independently or jointly, or buy them from private non-profit or commercial service-providers (Ministry of Social Affairs and Health, 1999b; Ministry of Social Affairs and Health, 1999c). Voluntary non-profit health and welfare organisations provide mainly sheltered housing for elderly people. Finland's Slot Machine Association is the main sponsor of these volunteer organisations' capital investments (Järvelin, 2002: 21, 26).

Private health care services are located primarily in the larger municipalities in which private medical services (Ministry of Social Affairs and Health, 1999c), medical doctor's practices and physiotherapy units are the most typical providers. Private health care comprises mainly outpatient care, although a few private hospitals exist which give both outpatient and inpatient care. Inpatient care provided by the private sector accounts for about 3-4% of all inpatient care. Recently there has been a slight increase in the use of private care (Järvelin, 2002: 21), as well as in the externalisation of social services (Partanen, 2002: 3).

Cooperation between public and private sectors in health care has a longer tradition compared with cooperation in social care. Specialist consultations and special medical examinations are the most typical services that smaller municipalities usually purchase from private providers.

STILL LACKING CO-OPERATION BETWEEN ORGANISATIONS AND
    OCCUPATIONAL GROUPS

It has been become evident that home care requires cooperation between many professionals and networks. At the moment, however, the situation still varies greatly in different municipalities. In some municipalities cooperation has been successful both between social and health care sectors as well as between them and other service-producing providers, while in other municipalities cooperation has been poor. Generally speaking, cooperation works well when home help and home nursing units cover either the same area or the same population. Difficulties appear especially when members of a joint municipal board have one common health centre and home nursing service, but every municipality has a social office and home help service of its own (Mäkinen et al., 1998: 30). Other reasons for the difficulties in cooperation, besides the organisational structure, may be factors of competition and defence of professional territories between different occupational groups, arising perhaps of a fear that new or other occupational groups might "rob" work from the incumbent group (Parviainen/Pelkonen, 1997: 33). In particular, resistance appears when the change threatens relations between different professionals (Lehto, 2000: 45). Other reasons may be attitudinal, meaning that it is not easy to recognise that one does not work alone. It is important to understand the tasks, way of working, and skills and needs as well as the way of thinking of those with whom care is provided (Mäkinen et al., 1998: 32).

There are some strong rational arguments to explain why social care systems and especially health care systems have been divided into separate units and parts. To accommodate the constantly increasing stocks of knowledge in these broad fields calls for specialisation, especially in health care. Often a chain of services is developed only between physicians, general practitioners and medical specialists. This is a very narrow perspective – other professionals should be included in the chain as well (Lehto, 2000: 33, 41, 42).

Generally in Finland, a professional strategy has been adopted that relies on full-time staff and requires all employees, including home helpers, to be educated for their particular jobs. The work of health care profession-als, including permission to nurse and perform medical tasks, is strictly regulated by the Act Concerning Health Care Professionals, as a consequence of which employees in home nursing, registered nurses, enrolled and aux-iliary nurses, undergo specific education. Today, however, there is also a new profession of less-educated home helpers for elderly people (Sipilä et al., 1997: 36, 50; Ministry of Social Affairs and Health, 1999b).

The basic and professional curricula for social and health care work-ers were reorganised in the beginning of the 1990s (Mäkinen et al., 1998: 34), which may solve some problems between different professional groups, especially at the practical basic level. The new curriculum for practical nurses for social and health care replaced the earlier training for enrolled nurses and trained home helpers, among others. The education lasts between 2 and 3 years depending on the basic education of the student. This new curricu-lum is aimed at giving broad competence to perform basic-level assistant duties in social and health care, since practical nurses have an essential po-sition in home care working teams. There are also shorter courses for home aides, who perform basic duties such as cleaning and laundry services at the client's home. The field practice for home help services is supervised by service managers, who can be trained home helpers with several years of practical experience, or social workers with degrees in social work either at the polytechnic (Bachelor of Social Services, length of education: 3.5 years) or academic (M.Sc. in Social Work, 4–5 years) level (Mäkinen et al., 1998: 34, 35; Pirkanmaa Polytechnic, 2002a).

The redesigned curricula also had an impact on the education of reg-istered nurses and public health nurses. Nowadays the education at the polytechnic level takes 3.5 years (Bachelor of Nursing) or 4 years (Bachelor of Public Health Nursing) (Pirkanmaa Polytechnic, 2002a), but most of the registered nurses and public health nurses working in home nursing have the earlier college-level degree. The physicians in home care are either gen-eral practitioners or specialists in general practice. The basic education for physicians takes about 6 years, and specialisation usually takes 5 more years (Mäkinen et al., 1997: 36, 39, 42). In the future, the development targets in social and health education include, e.g. increasing education in both social and health areas as well as in cooperation between different professionals (Risikko, 2000: 195). The status and salaries of different professionals gener-ally vary linearly with the length and level of education, with salaries being a little bit higher among health care personnel than among social welfare personnel (Tilastokeskus, 2001).

THE QUEST FOR CO-OPERATION AND SYNERGIES

Well-arranged home care can yield different kinds of benefits and interests for political, professional and user groups. Improved health status and functional capacity promote coping of the elderly at home and in non-institutional care. The use of more effective medicines and rehabilitation, and the development of technical aids and equipments as well as of support services have improved the capacity of non-institutional care. Diversification and gradation of the social and health services have narrowed the difference between institutional and non-institutional care. Nowadays it is possible to give more demanding treatment and care even in non-institutional settings. Consequently, the average length of institutional care periods has been reduced (Ministry of Social Affairs and Health, 2002: 115).

As the work in home care is versatile and demanding, and requires independent yet cooperative work, the possibility for workers to improve their professional skills is important. Workers especially experience their work as rewarding and meaningful when it brings benefit, help and joy to the client. Well-arranged home care enables the elderly to live at home longer, while at the same time the autonomy of the person is better preserved (Mäkinen et al., 1998: 16, 200–202).

199

The aim to transfer older persons from institutional care to non-institutional care has brought along the challenge to seek for new ways of organising services as the number of people with care needs is increasing and the level and availability of services has been reduced (Ministry of Social Affairs and Health 2001c: 33, 36). At the municipal level this results in the attempt to find synergies in closer collaboration between social care and health care (Parviainen/Pelkonen, 1997: 25).

The differences in old-age care service provision among municipalities have raised national concern. Especially the study results concerning the development in the 1990s, like Vaarama and others (2002) have addressed the equity issue, the main question being how to keep up the service production in line with the community-based care policy. The national steering by information strategy of the Ministry of Social Affairs and Health has addressed the quality issues by providing the National Framework for High-quality Care and Services for Older People (The Ministry of Social Affairs and Health, 2001b) and recommendations for quality improvement (National Research and Development Centre for Welfare and Health, 2001). The National Framework (The Ministry of Social Affairs and Health, 2001b) is part of a general national standards project under the government-approved

Target and Action Plan for 2000-2003 (The Ministry of Social Affairs and Health, 1999d). It is a new way of steering by recommendations and knowledge and calls for development and evaluation of good practices.

3 Model Ways of Working: Developing Coordination and Integration of Health and Social Services

Scientific research concerning home care, or integrated home help and home nursing services for the elderly has been published to a lesser degree until now. After the Target and Action Plan for Social Welfare and Health Care (Ministry of Social Affairs and Health, 1999d) and the National Framework for High-quality Care and Services for Older People (Ministry of Social Affairs and Health, 2001b) were introduced, the Ministry of Social Affairs and Health together with other organisations has started development projects on elderly services. Preventive home visits, quality of care for demented people, as well as recommendations for care and service planning are the key issues of these projects (Ministry of Social Affairs and Health, 2002: 116).

Projects and research have also been started or carried out on the municipal level concerning subjects such as case management in the integration of social welfare and health services (Ala-Nikkola/Valokivi, 1997), organisation of home care (Sinkkonen, 1995) and its consequences (Sinkkonen et al., 2001), and quality of home care (Karhula, 2000). The Mix Project, carried out in four municipalities, surveyed the existing service structures and made recommendations in order to develop services for the elderly (Rajaniemi/Sonkin, 2002). The Home Care 2005 project (Pirkanmaa Polytechnic, 2002b), as well as projects on preventive home visits (Häkkinen, 2002) are ongoing research projects or planned projects. The evaluation of elderly services is one of the study themes in a large ongoing research programme on ageing by the Academy of Finland, coordinated by the University of Tampere (2002).

All these activities are certainly geared to improve or solve some major shortcomings in the continuity of care, in coordination mechanisms and eventually the integration of health and social care systems. In the following, we shall analyse some of these shortcomings and provide information on evidence-based solutions that have been developed in Finland during the past decade.

3.1   Discharging from Hospital to Home Care

As already mentioned, a successful discharge process from hospital to home care was identified as an essential factor to ensure the coping at home and the continuity of care. This first case describes how successful discharging could be implemented.

In 2000, the biggest city in Finland, Helsinki, started an elderly care project concerning the discharge of elderly patients from hospital to home, with the purpose to develop cooperation between hospital and home care (Heiskanen et al., 2001). A working group, including nurses from hospitals and home care, made an operations model that could be applied in different working units in social and health care. The aim of the description of the discharge process was to develop older patients' discharge by improving customer-orientation, safety and flexibility. The description also helps the staff to realise that discharge actually begins when patients leave their homes for hospital.

The concepts used in the discharge process in this project are home care, "hospital at home", discharge nurse, multiprofessional team, great region and intensified home care. Home care means care and services, which are arranged by home help service and home nursing for clients with impaired functional capacity living either at home or in service homes. "Hospital at home" gives treatment at hospital level and replaces treatment given in hospital acute wards. A discharge nurse is either a registered nurse or a public health nurse who works in a hospital. She coordinates and arranges safe discharge and follow-up treatment after specialised care for a patient who needs plenty of assistance and support. The multiprofessional team comprises different professionals from hospital and non-institutional care work, for instance, a physician, a personal nurse, a discharge nurse, a physiotherapist, an occupational therapist, a social worker and a head of the social care service. The city of Helsinki is divided into seven geographical areas, called great regions. Every great region has its own social centre and health centre, and these centres work together in home care, including discharge. Intensified home care means special care and support given on a round-the-clock basis for persons who need plenty of assistance and treatment because of impaired functional capacity or serious disease. This differs from traditional home help service and home nursing in that it is concentrated on the frontier between institutional and non-institutional care. Moreover, it is based on strong medical treatment given by a physician, with the purpose to give periodic treatment, and to replace hospital care and care at an old-age home, as well as to support and speed up discharge. Intensified home care is meant for persons who need various kinds of assistance and support, whose coping at home is on balance, who have repeatedly been in acute wards, who are waiting for a place in an intensified service housing or in long-term institutional care, who need special treatment because of a serious disease, or who receive terminal care.

During the discharge the main focus is on supporting patients to reach optimal independency with the help of their relatives. A working pair including the nurses in charge of home care and in hospital is the key solution. The operations model includes the phases of a discharge process and the content of every phase, meaning operations, functions and instructions for those in charge of a particular task, and how the documentation and flow of information are checked. The phases and functions of a discharge process are the decision of going to a hospital, anamnesis at the hospital, contact between home care and hospital; setting targets for discharge, treatment and rehabilitation at the hospital, assessment of coping at home, ensuring follow-up treatment, discharge from hospital, and evaluation and follow-up of client's well-being and coping at home. The phases may partly follow an individual order, according to a patient's needs. Particularly important is that all needed phases will be done according to planning and everyone participating in the process knows his/her duties.

During the year 2002 the data system of client and patient work in the health office in Helsinki will be reformed. After that all manually written sick and health records will be transferred in computerised forms which creates opportunities for a quick and reliable exchange of information and smooth cooperation between the professionals in various units of health care.

The discharge process occurs at the same time with the rehabilitation process for elderly patients called geriatric rehabilitation. The process includes: anamnesis, setting targets, treatment and rehabilitation, compensation, meaning e.g. technical aids, arrangement of follow-up treatment and follow-up.

3.2   Multiprofessional Care and Service

Developing multiprofessional care and services is an essential step towards an integrated health and social care system. A developing programme for elderly care recommended by the Government is one of the measures to reach the goal. In the next case it will be described how care and services were developed in one of Finland's largest cities.

The social and health affairs of Espoo were united in 1993, and at the same time five regional social and health centres were created with the aim to produce all non-institutional social and health services in the regions of patients themselves (Siltari, 1998). In 1993, the board of social and health affairs in Espoo challenged all regional social and health centres with the task of preparing regional development programmes for elderly care. This report describes the development programmes in one of Espoo's regions, Leppävaara. The programmes were drawn up by a multiprofessional working group of elderly care of Leppävaara's social and health centre. The first programme lasted for the period 1994–2000 (The elderly working team of Leppävaara's social and health centre, 1994), and the second will last 2001–2005 (Lindström, 2000).

The first programme included basic information and targets for the development of elderly care during the period 1994–2000. In the second programme, there were parts that reflected the changes and events during the past years. Some of the targets set for the previous development period have also been evaluated. The main purpose of the second development programme, however, was to clarify the most essential problems, challenges and development needs in current elderly care. Here, only those parts from the second programme concerning the evaluation of the first programme are described.

3.2.1 The First Development Programme for Elderly Care (1994–2000)

The purpose of the first development programme (The elderly working team of Leppävaara's social and health centre, 1994) was to estimate Leppävaara's situation in 1994, and to propose changes that the future seemed to call for at that time. Although the programme was directed at the year 2000, it also aimed to consider the following decade so that it would be easier to respond to challenges that the year 2010 might bring along.

Functional cooperation had been developed multiprofessionally and the work had been planned more closely with clients and their relatives. Home care workers made home visits when needed, and drew up care and service plans together with clients and their relatives. Population-based care had reached also the medical care services by improving the availability and quality of services. The personal physician and the nurses were able to es-

203

tablish long care relationships with patients. The oldest people, most of whom had several diseases, benefited most from the continuity of care and multiprofessional care. If, in case of impaired health condition and follow-up treatment, a need for home care existed, the personal doctor participated in the treatment together with home care staff. The continuity of treatment had brought persistency to care plans and expediency to service use, including also laboratory and X-ray examinations as well as physiotherapy and psychological services.

Home care had been available on every weekday, evening services, however, were only provided to those with a very difficult treatment situation, and night services to just some persons in terminal care. In home care, the so-called Joensuu's gradation of care was in use. With the help of this method, it was possible to clarify both the level of coping with basic and instrumental activities, and of difficulties, e.g. in movement and home work, and relate them to seven grades from A to G. According to this classification a person who was classified as an A-client needed services no more than every other week, whereas a G-client needed services at least three times every day. Most of the clients in Leppävaara were placed in grades D and E, needing services 2-5 times per week or services on a daily basis but less than three times a day.

In 1994, even though Leppävaara's municipal services were already many-sided, there was concern over how the future service needs of a growing number of older people could be met to a sufficient and proper extent.

Because the resources of home care had been small compared to the age structure of the population, the principles of home care had to be re-estimated. Consequently, services had to be focused more accurately on using care and service plans and gradation of care as a help.

WHAT SHOULD BE DEVELOPED

SWOT analysis was used as a basic instrument when drawing up the development programme for elderly care for the period of 1994–2000. In the analysis, possibilities, strengths, weaknesses and threats in elderly care in Leppävaara have been discussed and recorded. In the development of operations, special attention had been paid on the removal of weaknesses and utilisation of strengths.

As Leppävaara's elderly people mostly lived at home with relatively high-quality equipment, the principle was to arrange services in such a way that older people could continue to live independently at home for as long as possible by using normal services targeted to all population. The purpose was to further develop non-institutional and institutional services, in order that they would form a service entity, which could respond to the life situation and service needs of an aged person. Elderly care should, however, be arranged as non-institutional care with the emphasis on customer orientation. Furthermore, expensive investments should be avoided in favour of non-institutional care services and the lightening of institutional care. It was necessary to develop sufficient cooperation between various organisations of elderly care and private providers, and actively implement such cooperation, because the public sector will not be able to respond to all needs of an increasing number of elderly people in the future.

Further, a larger proportion of all non-institutional services should be targeted to the elderly population, as well as gradation of specialised medical care, institutional care and non-institutional care should be developed to improve flexibility in meeting individual care requirements.

205

3.2.2 The Second Development Programme for Elderly Care (2001–2005)

The second development programme for elderly care was drawn up for the period of 2001–2005, taking into account also the next three years (Lindström, 2000).

EVALUATION OF THE FIRST DEVELOPMENT PROGRAMME

The first development programme and its implementation were evaluated in 1997 at the level of municipal authority and in Leppävaara's social and health centre. The report covered all elderly services provided by the city of Espoo or by acquired services or other elderly services used. Also the central services that support other elderly services were included in the evaluation. In order to fulfill the service strategy and its goals, binding profit targets were set for home care. The goal was that 90% of all persons aged 75 or older should live at home and 10% of this age group would be in institutional care. In the year 1999, only 5.7% of this age group were in institutional care. Leppävaara's social and health centre had actively and purposefully developed regional elderly care following the goals set by the city, but emphasising, however, the issues which had come up from their own development needs.

As principles of working procedures, issues such as the following had been pointed out:

- To produce customer-oriented and individual services in multi-professional and population-based care.
- To try to determine recourses of clients, to support independent initiative and independent coping at home.
- Cooperation with relatives and friends of clients.
- Safety and integration of care.
- Economy of operations.

As the health status of home care clients continued to deteriorate, the need of demanding medical treatment services given by home nursing continued to increase, resulting in a decrease of pure ordinary home help services by the end of the 1990s.

Most of the basic services were further produced by the municipality, even though part of the support services, such as transport and shopping services, meals on wheels, home cleaning, safety phones and laundry services, were arranged as purchasing services. Also the use of private doctor's clinics together with private examinations and care had increased.

The second development programme was drawn up during the year 2000. The second SWOT analysis produced the following issues as serious threats: labour shortage, insufficiency and unavailability of current labour force, insufficiency of present institutional beds and intermediate care services, and a strong increase in the number of elderly people, which is associated with the fact that the number of demented persons is still growing.

3.3 Merging Home Help and Home Nursing Services: Developing the Quality of Home Care

Since the beginning of the 1990s there have been studies on home care from various points of view at the university of Kuopio. The Kuopio project is a large project, the purpose of which is to evaluate how the merging of the social and health sectors takes places, and to determine its effects on the quality and content of home care (Sinkkonen, 1995). The social welfare and health care organisations had merged in 1993–1994, and were then reorganised in 1998 (Sinkkonen et al., 2001). A sub-study called "Content and quality of home care in Kuopio in 1994" was part of the Kuopio project. This study examined the quality and content of home care, as well as the problems and solutions in home care as evaluated by the elderly, their relatives and the staff involved (Hyvärinen et al., 1995). A second study about the home care received explored the perceptions of elderly living at home, and the importance of living at home and of home care (Hirvonen, 1995). A third study examined the information flow between the staff involved in home care and nursing homes, and some other forms of cooperation. The ways of organising home care and the opportunities for the staff to contribute to their own work were also investigated (Laitinen et al., 1995). Content and organisation of home care have been studied also later (Sinkkonen et al., 2001).

3.3.1 The Quality of Elderly Home Care in 1994 and in 1997

In this connection, one of the sub-studies of the Kuopio project called "The quality of elderly home care in 1994 and in 1997" (Rissanen et al., 1999) was chosen as a sample, which evaluated how the merging of home help service and home nursing affected the quality of home care as evaluated by clients, their relatives and staff involved.

207

PURPOSE OF THE STUDY

The main purpose of this study was to assess the effects on the quality of home care after the merging of home help service and home nursing from two points of view: To assess the quality of home care in relation to the quality objectives which were set for the integration by the organisation and to assess the quality of home care in relation to the expectations of elderly clients, their relatives and staff.

In the study, goal and expectation-based assessments were applied.

SUBJECTS AND METHODS

The subjects (two samples) were home care clients aged 65 or older, mostly widows above 75 years living on their own, and their relatives, mostly children of the clients, as well as the staff directly involved or in interaction with these clients on a regular basis. Part of the subjects participated in both studies. The clients were interviewed with structured questions and information from relatives and staff was collected with structured questionnaire forms.

Quality of home care included:
1. Adequacy of help and care
2. Relevance of help and care
3. Adequacy of time given to clients
4. Guidance, advice and information
5. Continuity of care

Information concerning adequacy of help and care as well as continuity of care was based on separate questions. The other three were composed of various questions, which were formed into factors, on which factor analysis was applied.

MAIN RESULTS

The elderly clients considered the adequacy of help and care to be slightly better in 1997 than in 1994. The employees estimated that help and care were slightly less sufficient in the follow-up year in almost all help forms, and especially in medical care. The relatives considered the adequacy of help and care to be slightly poorer in both years than the elderly did. Especially cleaning help had impaired during these years, and it was also a form of service that the elderly clients reported as having not received when asked if they had received all services they had asked for. An effort had been made to reassign the municipal cleaning service to other service providers. All respondents complained of insufficiency of moments of conversation and the lack of help in moving about at home.

Division of working hours had changed only slightly. The employees who traditionally had belonged to the home nursing unit still used most of their working hours in special treatment and discussions with clients. Those employees who traditionally had been in home help service still mostly performed tasks belonging to home help services, even if they used a little bit more time for discussions, medical care and special treatment, and slightly less time for assistance with eating in 1997.

All respondents, and especially the clients, considered the essential areas of help and care as good. Adequacy of time appeared as the critical factor that was also assessed as the most deficient and mostly worsened issue over the years. Especially impairment had occurred insofar as employees did not make home visits at times that clients had wished for. The urgency of employees had still increased over the years.

The continuity of care was also considered to be worse in 1997. Most of the elderly clients wished that the same worker would visit them at their home.

The effects of the merging of home help service and home nursing on the quality of home care were rather minor. In some aspects of quality, the level had increased a little. The quality objectives of the organisation were mostly reached. The clients and relatives estimated that there were no changes in the competence of employees to recognise clients' needs; the employees, on the other hand, assessed that this observation was slightly impaired. The small amount of changes in the quality of home care is quite reasonable, because the working hours and the duties have remained almost unchanged.

3.4   Discharge Management: The Laatuvanttu Project

209

Laatuvanttu was an elderly development project carried out in 1994 and 1995 in five Finnish municipalities: Forssa, Hämeenlinna, Janakkala, Lammi and Tuulos. The common purpose of this project was to produce a description of the estimation of quality in elderly care, and to develop tools for the estimation of quality in practice. Social and health personnel together pondered on good quality of municipal elderly care. Every municipality chose its development targets, which were closely linked with challenges related to changes in service structure, such as non-institutional development needs, a decrease of institutional care and supporting living at home (Autio, 1996). In this connection a project carried out in Lammi and Tuulos will be examined more closely.

BASIC INFORMATION ON LAMMI

Lammi is quite a small municipality (number of inhabitants 5,685) and there are different organisations for social welfare and health care services. Home service, including service and care work done by home helpers, is among Lammi's social services. Meal service, day centre, safety phone and informal support services are included in the support services. Those clients who only need cleaning or shopping help are guided to other providers (Lammin kunta, 2002). Health care services, including health centre and home nursing, are arranged together with Tuulos through membership in a joint municipal board in Lammi and Tuulos (Lammin-Tuuloksen kansanterveystyön kuntayhtymä, 2002).

THE PURPOSES OF THE PROJECT

- To find out how the timing of discharge from a health centre ward could be optimally planned.
- To think over the ways that could best support elderly people's coping at home (Suoninen, 1996).

The project group included workers and managers from social welfare, the elderly home organisation, and the health centre of the federation of municipalities in public health work in Lammi-Tuulos, as well as a researcher and a consultant.

THE STEPS:

(1) The first step was to consider contributory factors that influence safe living at home of elderly people and successful discharge from hospital. To find out about the opinions of elderly people and their relatives, a questionnaire was prepared. According to the results of the interviews with elderly people (living at homes or in service homes or in an old-age home or health centre ward) and their relatives, contributory factors were defined.

The contributory factors concerned safe living at home, successful discharge, methodological cooperation, safety and realism.

The idea was to realistically estimate client's resources, ability to move and function, and on the grounds of estimation to choose the most suitable alternative for place and discharge time of follow-up treatment

(2) During the second step, obstacles to smooth discharge and flow of information were talked over in the mixed group consisting of employees from home help service, home nursing, the health centre and the old-age home and day centres. It appeared that, among the home help service employees, there was a high threshold to visit the client in a health centre ward, and in order to lower this threshold they were invited to visit the health centre. This step eased the visits and nowadays the employees go to see their clients in the ward whenever they have the time.

(3) After discharge from a health centre ward, a client partly turns from a health care client into a social care client. During the third step, to help smooth the flow of information, employees make a checklist of discharge.

The checklist is on the back page of the care and service plan, to ensure that all essential discharge phases have been completed.

IMPROVEMENTS DURING AND AFTER THE PROJECT

The charge nurse has traditionally taken care of discharge, but nowadays the personal nurse undertakes this process. After the project, home nursing at staff administrational level was merged with the health centre ward. During this phase, cooperation between the different partners has been eased, also between the ward and home nursing. Both discharge from ward and transition from home to ward are easier nowadays.

Cooperation between home nursing and home help service has also improved. Common meetings are arranged in small groups and, for instance, care and service plans are made together. Employees in home service and home nursing work very independently and their responsibility has increased, which makes working more meaningful. Cooperation between the social worker and health centre ward's personnel has become tighter. The social worker visits the ward once a week, on which occasion preconditions for discharge, such as adaptations at a client's home will be discussed. The home help service receives the information of discharging well in time, in fact at the point when the discharge planning begins. A few days before the discharge the health centre personnel contacts the home help service to ask if they can help with the discharge. In Lammi there are also trained volunteers, coordinated by the parish, who support clients during the discharge process.

Home nursing and home service increasingly work together regarding evenings so that the home help service makes the evening shifts at the beginning of the week, and the home nursing takes care of the remaining evenings. A new thing is that ward personnel also makes home visits before discharge together with the client and the parties involved in care.

Other actions supporting elderly people's living at home are the increasing number of safety phones, meal services, and interval care that have also been arranged for clients who are taken care of by relatives.

After the project, the change of patients has increased enormously. As there is no queue from the central hospital to the health centre ward, it is possible to receive a patient nearly immediately after receiving transfer information. Likewise, it is also possible to promise elderly persons at the time of discharge that they can come back to the ward if they cannot cope at home.

211

3.5   Case Management to Support Patients with Dementia and Their Caregivers at Home

Case management is one of the tools to improve coordination and integration of care and services needed by the clients. Support and help is especially important in the case of demented persons and their caregivers. The last description examines how case management can be arranged.

OBJECTIVE AND DESIGN

The objective of the study was to determine whether community care of demented patients could be prolonged by a 2-year support programme based on nurse case management (Eloniemi-Sulkava et al., 2001) that was part of Eloniemi-Sulkava's doctoral thesis (2002). The study was a randomised controlled intervention study with a 2-year follow-up (Eloniemi-Sulkava et al., 2001).

212

SUBJECTS AND METHODS

The study population comprised 100 demented patients, age 65 and older, living at home in five Finnish municipalities: Kuopio, Iisalmi, Siilinjärvi, Maaninka and Vehmersalmi. Caregivers were family members who primarily supported the patients. The main diagnosis causing dementia was Alzheimer's disease both in intervention patients and control patients. The Mini-Mental State Examination was used to assess the severity of dementia.

INTERVENTION

Intervention consisted of a 2-year support programme based on nurse case management and carried out by a dementia family care coordinator, later called coordinator, who was a registered nurse with a background in public health. The coordinator took responsibility for the care of demented patients, coordinated their care and services, solved problem situations, and supported the families. The holistic responsibility for the demented patients as well as the availability and reliability of the nurse were characteristic of the operation. The main focus was to quickly react to situations that threatened the continuity of home care. A good relationship between the coordinator and the patient's physician was essential, because the expert knowledge of the physician was often needed in problem situations.

The intervention was based on the patients' needs and wishes, the control groups received the usual services provided for geriatric patients in community care by the municipal social and health care system or the private sector. Patients in the intervention group and their caregivers were provided with a support programme, in which, during two years, they received systematic and comprehensive support given by the coordinator. The coordinator provided: advocacy for patients and their caregivers; comprehensive support for patients and their caregivers; continuous and systematic counselling; annual training courses for patients and their caregivers; follow-up calls; in-home visits; assistance with arrangements for social and health care services; 24-hour-per-day availability by mobile telephone.

The frequency of contacts varied from once a month to five times a day depending on the situation. The number of contacts concerning problematic situations and phases threatening the continuity of community care varied greatly. In these situations, the coordinator tried to find solutions to issues such as health problems of patients or caregivers, behavioural and psychological symptoms of patients, or caregivers' stress and burden, and in interventions; measures were used, such as: diagnosis of the cause of a problem and arranging intervention accordingly, consultation with a physician in the study, arranging other medical care, physiotherapy or rehabilitative measures, systematic support for the caregiver, arranging rest periods for the caregiver, counselling the caregiver to find out ways to manage problematic behaviour, helping the caregiver to find proper medical care and giving health advice to the caregiver.

Three annual training courses lasting 5-10 days were provided for patients and their caregivers. The purpose of these courses was to support the functional abilities and adaptation of patients and caregivers. They included a medical check-up and psychological assessment of the patient, various kinds of physical, mental and social activities, as well as separate group meetings for patients and caregivers, and lectures for caregivers. During the courses, a service plan was made for each family, and the coordinator then arranged the planned services.

The occurrence of two endpoints (after one year and after two years), placement in long-term institutional care and death at home, were registered. The main outcome measure was the time of institutionalisation, meaning the period in community care, from the enrolment of patients in the study to their placement in long-term institutional care.

213

Main Results

During the first months, the rate of institutionalisation was significantly lower in the intervention group than in the control group. The benefit of the intervention, however, decreased with time. The intervention was especially beneficial to patients with severe dementia and those who had problems, such as behaviour disorders or problems in functional capacity, threatening the continuity of community care.

Conclusions of the Study

It is possible to defer the placement of demented patients in long-term institutional care with the support of the programme based on nurse case management. The research group suggested that intervention by a dementia family care coordinator should be targeted especially at patients with problems threatening the continuity of community care, or at patients with severe dementia. Based on their experience, the study group suggested that one dementia family care coordinator is able to support 50 demented patients and their caregivers.

4 Conclusions: Lessons to Learn

In Finland the integration of health and social care for older persons has emerged as an actual topic during the 1990s, but only since the end of the 1990s with the National Target and Action Plan (Ministry of Social Affairs and Health, 1999d) and the National Framework (Ministry of Social Affairs and Health, 2001b) being launched, more attention has been paid to the respective issues in many municipalities. After the National Framework (Ministry of Social Affairs and Health, 2001b) had been introduced, some municipalities started to draw up policy strategies, while others are preparing one. Because the issue is new, many development projects and studies on integrated care or dementia service or hospital discharge are still waiting to be done.

The fact that cooperation between different professionals and units is quite a new issue in Finland is best reflected in the project called "Discharging from hospital to home care" (Heiskanen et al., 2001) which has the purpose to develop cooperation between hospital and home care with the help of a new operational model developed by persons who are actually occupied in elderly care. The report clearly displays how confused the situation was in Helsinki before the project. One of the most important matters in this report was that concepts were determined so that according to the description of the model everyone who participates in elderly work knows the basic concepts and issues. The other, maybe the most essential part of this project consists of a new operations model which can be used in different settings, and with the help of which practical work becomes easier, more flexible, safer, and presumably cheaper. Following the model and its instructions will benefit all providers involved in the discharge process and home care, as well as discharged patients.

The situation, as it existed in Helsinki, may be generalised to many other municipalities, too. The operation model or a similar instrument would also benefit other municipalities, even if they already have some working model for the discharge system and follow-up care. Anyway, the situation is not so deficient in all municipalities; in some smaller municipalities, e.g. in Pirkkala (number of inhabitants: 13,280), cooperation between home help service, home nursing, health centre wards and hospitals works well. In Pirkkala, health care and social welfare services are arranged separately in an "old-fashioned way", in spite of elderly care being teamwork with different professionals, and at present they make multiprofessional (including a physiotherapist, a social worker, a head of home help service, a physical education instructor from the bureau of exercise, a home nurse, and a nurse from an old-age home) home visits to all clients (n=150) who are already customers of regular home care. Dental care also takes part in this ongoing project. In Pirkkala, the physician has an essential role in elderly care. Changes at administrative level have not been considered as necessary.

The development programmes of Leppävaara represent another aspect of elderly care (The elderly working team of Leppävaara's social and health centre, 1994; Lindström, 2000). These programmes included various factors, such as operations, functions, tasks, providers and administrative sectors, which are involved in elderly care, and which have been formulated according to governmental recommendations. Leppävaara programmes probably belong to the best development programmes drawn up in Finnish municipalities. The first development programme well met its expectations, and it was well-planned and useful containing the most important development areas and issues in elderly care. The monitoring and evaluation results after

215

its first development period were implemented, followed by new development targets being discussed and recorded in the second development programme. The main emphasis has been to focus on activities concerning the elderly with the worst health status that, accordingly, need plenty of services and care.

In the university of Kuopio many projects related to home care have been conducted. One of their main issues is quality in home care (Rissanen et al., 1999). Quality is also one of the main issues in the national framework (Ministry of Social Affairs and Health, 2001b). The Kuopio studies are good examples of studies concerning the effects of the merging of two organisations, like in Kuopio, since as a consequence of the integration of the social welfare and health care organisations, home help service and home nursing were united in one home care unit. The Laatuvaara project conducted in Lammi and Tuulos (Suoninen, 1996) is another example concerned with quality. In this project there were concrete practical targets and as a result the change of patients has enormously increased and the number of long-term beds has rapidly decreased, showing that goals have been reached. The fact that, at least in 1996, there was no queue from the central hospital to the health centre ward confirms that improvements had occurred. These were notable findings even if they were not defined as development targets.

Dementia research is a good example of studies on intervention in which the effects on support interventions directed both at demented patients and their caregivers have been examined (Eloniemi-Sulkava et al., 2001). The results of the study are promising. According to these results it is possible to prolong demented patients' living at home through a support programme based on nurse case management.

CONCLUDING REMARKS

Even on a larger scale there are several home-service development pilots going on at different stages at the local level. The field of service provision is varied and in constant change, with no standard practices. A number of different concepts are being used. It can be foreseen that the intensity of services provided to persons aged 75 and older is increasing, and demands are voiced for a more efficient integration of social and health services on a client-centred basis. The national target is to support older people's living at home as long as possible. The challenge is to be able to develop a variety of service housing arrangements and, in particular, to increase the range of services provided for persons with impaired memory. In any case there is an increasing emphasis on the requirements expected of professional skills in the field of care-giving.

As conclusion it can be stated that in Finland, because of a rapidly growing number of aged people, the main concern is how all the needed care and services can be arranged. In the Finnish elderly care system the proportion of institutionalised persons is quite large with respect to the number of old people. A large part of them is placed in hospital for long-term care. It is obvious that in the future, municipal resources are simply not adequate for providing all elderly care, including both institutional and non-institutional care. Many municipalities have already been initiated to develop co-operation with other care providers. Services are also partly becoming outsourced, whereby part of the services is acquired from private companies that are bound to extend their offer. A part of services, like cleaning, transport and escort services, which traditionally have been provided by municipalities, have been cut down during the 1990s. Consequently, the role of family members and other relatives as providers of informal care has been increased and will further increase in the future.

There are, however, other important issues, such as cooperation between municipal sectors and sub-sectors, which have to be solved. It is also relevant to develop integration between social and health care as well as inside the health sector as has been done for instance in Helsinki. The projects described above are good examples of efforts to improve elderly care, and could be useful also for other municipalities wishing to develop their elderly care.

217

Notes

1   In the Finnish literature there is no officially endorsed concept of social care; however, the concepts of social services and social welfare (Nygren et al., 1997: 13) are covering this area.

2   One reason for this low figure is that over half of the municipalities are members of the Federation of Municipalities of Public Health Work, which in itself hampers the integration of social and health affairs (Sinkkonen et al., 2001).

References

Ala-Nikkola, M./Valokivi, H. (1997) *Yksilökohtainen palveluohjaus käytäntönä. Loppuraportti sosiaa-lija terveydenhuollon palvelujärkestelmää ja yksilökohtaista palveluohjausta (case management) koskeneesta tutkimuksesta Hämeenkyrössä ja Tampereella* (Case management as practice. The final report of a study conducted in Hämeenkyrö and Tampere into service provision and individualised case management in social welfare and health care). Helsinki: Reports of National Research and Development Centre for Welfare and Health, 215.

Autio, T. (1996) 'Laatua vanhustyöhön Hämeessä' (Quality for elderly work in Häme), *Vanhustyö* 4: 19–22.

Eloniemi-Sulkava, U./Notkola, I-L./Hentinen, M./Kivelä, S-L./Sivenius, J./Sulkava, R. (2001) 'Effects of supporting community-living demented patients and their caregivers: a randomized trial, *Journal of the American Geriatrics Society* 49: 1282-1287.

Eloniemi-Sulkava, U. (2002) Supporting community care of demented patients (dissertation). University of Oulu. Abstract of the doctoral thesis. Retrieved 2 August 2002 from the World Wide Web: http://www.uku.fi/tutkimukset/vaitokset/2002/ISBN951-781-879-3ueloniemisulkava.htm.

Finlex (1999) Oikeus sosiaaliturvaan (The right for social security). Retrieved 19 June 2002 from the World Wide Web: http://finlex1.edita.fi/dyna.../@ebt-link?showtoc=false;target=IDMATCH(id,19990/31.sd.

Heiskanen, L./Lamppu, M./Luomaala, T./Mustonen, S./Pasanen, M./Pilvinen, J./Schleifer, P./Tuomikoski, E./Valvanne, J. (2001) *Kotiutuminen sairaalasta kotihoitoon* (Discharging from hospital to home care). Helsinki: City of Helsinki, Social Office, Health Office.

Hirvonen, R (1995) 'Kotihoidon merkitys vanhuksille: Laadullinen tutkimus vanhusten kokemuksista' (The importance of home care for elderly people: A qualitative study on experiences of aged people), pp. 79-90 in Sinkkonen, S. (ed.), *Kotihoidon sisältö ja laatu Kuopiossa 1994* (Content and quality of home care in Kuopio in 1994). Kuopio: Kuopio University Publications E, Social Sciences 30.

Hyvärinen, S./Laitinen, P./Hirvonen, R./Sinkkonen, S. (1995) 'Kotihoidon sisältö ja laatu vanhusasiakkaiden, heidän omaistensa ja työntekijöiden arvioimana Kuopiossa 1994' (Quality and content of home care, as well as problems and solutions in home care as evaluated by the elderly, their relatives and staff involved in Kuopio in 1994), pp. 45-76 in Sinkkonen, S. (ed.), *Kotihoidon sisältö ja laatu Kuopiossa 1994* (Content and quality of home care in Kuopio in 1994). Kuopio: Kuopio University Publications E, Social Sciences 30.

Häkkinen, H. (2002) *Ehkäisevät kotikäynnit vanhuksille. Kuntakyselyn tulokset sekä kotimaisia ja ulkomaisia käytäntöjä* (Preventive home visits for the elderly. Results of a national survey, national and international experiences). Helsinki: The Association of Finnish Local and Regional Authorities.

Järvelin, J. (2002) *Health Care Systems in Transition. Finland*. European Observatory on Health Care Systems 4 (1).

Karhula, S. (2000) *Kotihoidon laadun arviointi ja asiakaspalautejärjestelmän kehittäminen* (Assessment of quality in home care and development of system for customer feed-back). Jyväskylä: City of Jyväskylä, Reports of Social and Health Centre.

Kröger, T. (1996) 'Kunnat valtion valvonnassa?' (Municipalities under state supervision?), pp. 23-85 in Sipilä, J./Ketola, O./Kröger, T./Rauhala, P.L. (eds.), *Sosiaalipalvelujen Suomi* (Finland of social services). Juva: WSOY.

Laitinen, P./Taskinen, H./Hyvärinen, S./Jalava, E.L./Sinkkonen, S. (1995) 'Koti- ja laitoshoidon työntekijöiden välinen tiedonkulku ja kotihoidon organisointi Kuopiossa 1994' (The information flow between the staff involved in homecare and nursing homes, and the ways of organising home care in Kuopio in 1994), pp. 93-114 in Sinkkonen, S. (ed.), *Kotihoidon sisältö ja laatu Kuopiossa 1994* (Content and quality of home care in Kuopio in 1994). Kuopio: Kuopio University Publications E, Social Sciences 30.

Lammin kunta (2002) Retrieved 9 August 2002 from the World Wide Web: http://www.lammi.fi.

Lammin-Tuuloksen kansanterveystyön kuntayhtymä (2002) Retrieved 9 August 2002 from the World Wide Web: http://www.htk.fi/asteri/lam/terv/03/33sivu1.htm

Lehto, J (2000) 'Saumaton palveluketju mosaiikkimaisessa järjestelmässä' (Seamless service chain in a mosaic-like system?), pp. 33-48 in Nouko-Juvonen, S./Ruotsalainen, P./Kiikkala, I. (eds.), *Hyvinvointivaltion palveluketjut* (The chain of services of welfare state). Helsinki: Kustannusosakeyhtiö Tammi.

Lindström, C. (2000) *Leppävaaran vanhustenhuollon kehittämisohjelma II 2001–2005 (2008)* (Leppävaara's second development programme 2001–2005 [2008]). Espoo: City of Espoo; Leppävaara's social and health centre.

Ministry of Social Affairs and Health (1999a) *Policy on Ageing.* Helsinki: Brochures of the Ministry of Social Affairs and Health 1999:4eng.

Ministry of Social Affairs and Health (1999b) *Social Welfare in Finland.* Helsinki: Brochures of the Ministry of Social Affairs and Health 1999:6eng.

Ministry of Social Affairs and Health (1999c) *Health Care in Finland.* Helsinki: Brochures of the Ministry of Social Affairs and Health 1999:13eng.

Ministry of Social Affairs and Health (1999d) The Target and Action Plan for Social Welfare and Health Care. Retrieved 17 July 2002 from the World Wide Web: http://www.vn.fi/stm/suomi/julkaisu/julk01fr.htm

Ministry of Social Affairs and Health (2000) Act on Experiments with Seamless Service Chains in Social Welfare and Health Care Services and with a Social Security Card. No. 811 (issued 22.9.2000). Retrieved 17 July 2002 from the World Wide Web: http//www.vn.fi/stm/english/tao/publicat/makro/act811.htm.

Ministry of Social Affairs and Health (2001a) *Statutory Social Welfare and Health Care Services.* Helsinki: Brochures of the Ministry of Social Affairs and Health 2001:7eng.

Ministry of Social Affairs and Health (2001b) *National Framework for High-quality Care and Services for Older People.* Helsinki: Handbook of the Ministry of Social Affairs and Health; Association of Finnish Local and Eegional Authorities 2001:6.

Ministry of Social Affairs and Health (2001c) *Sosiaali- ja terveyspolitiikan strategiat 2010 – kohti sosiaalisesti kestävää ja taloudellisesti elinvoimaista yhteiskuntaa* (Strategies for social protection 2010 – towards a socially and economically sustainable society). Helsinki: Publications of Ministry of Social Affairs and Health 2001:3.

Ministry of Social Affairs and Health (2002) *Sosiaali- ja terveyskertomus 2002* (Report on Social Affairs and Health 2002). Helsinki: Publications of Ministry of Social Affairs and Health 2002:11.

Mäkinen, E./Niinistö, L./Salminen, P./Karjalainen, P. (eds.) (1998) *Kotihoito* (Home care). Porvoo: WSOY.

National Research and Development Centre for Welfare and Health (2000) A count of clients having regularly home care services on 30 November 1999. STAKES/Stakes Information. Welfare and Healthcare Statistics. Retrieved 4 June 2002 from the World Wide Web: http://www.stakes.fi/stakestieto/PDF/palaute2.pdf

National Research and Development Centre for Welfare and Health (2001) *Whole Municipality Working Together for Older people, Perspectives on the Development of Elderly Peoples´s Independent Living, Care and Services*. Saarijärvi: Gummerus.

Nygren, L./Andersson, M./Eydal, G./Hammarqvist, S-E./Rauhala, P-L./Warming Nielsen, H. (1997) 'New policies, new words – the service concept in Scandinavian social policy', pp. 9-26 in Sipilä, J. (ed.), *Social care services: The key to the Scandinavian welfare model*. Aldershot/Brookfield USA/Hong Kong/Singapore/Sydney: Avebury.

Partanen, I. (2002) *Toimialaraportti 2002. Sosiaalipalvelut* (Report on social services of line of activities 2002). Kauppa- ja teollisuusministeriö; TE-keskus.

Parviainen, T./Pelkonen, M. (1997) 'Muuttuva hoitotyö ja Terveyttä kaikille –ohjelma' (Changing nursing care and Health for all – programme), pp. 25-36 in Parviainen, T./Pelkonen, M. (eds.), *Yhteisöllisyys – avain parempaan terveyteen* (Communality – the key for better health). Helsinki: Reports of National Research and Development Centre for Welfare and Health 1997:217.

Pirkanmaa Polytechnic (2002a) Degree programme in social services, Degree programme in nursing and health care. Retrieved 11 June 2002 from the World Wide Web: http://www.piramk.fi/english/degree_programmes/dp.

Pirkanmaa Polytechnic (2002b) Kotihoito 2005 projekti. Retrieved 17 June 2002 from the World Wide Web: http://www.piramk.fi/palveluosasto/hankkeet/Kotihoito2005/index.html

Rajaniemi, J./Sonkin, L. (2002) *Palveluverkostot ikääntyvien tukena. Mix-projekti 1998–2001* (Service networks as support for elderly people. The Mix project 1998–2001). Helsinki: Reports of Kuntokallio, Center for gerontological training and research 2002:1.

Ranta, H. (ed.) (2001) *Sosiaali- ja terveydenhuoltolainsäädäntö 2001* (Statutory social welfare and health care services 2001). Helsinki: Kauppakaari; Talentum Media Oy.

Rintala, T./Elovainio, M./Heikkilä, M. (1997) *Osiensa summa – Tutkimus sosiaali- ja terveydenhuollon yhdistämisen taustoista ja vaikutuksista* (The sum of its parts: Study on the background factors, and the effects of, combining social welfare and health care). Helsinki: Researches of National Research and Development Centre for Welfare and Health 1997:75.

Risikko, P. (2000) 'Työelämän ja koulutuksen yhteistyö – tulevaisuuden edellytys' (Co-operation between working life and education – a precondition of the future), pp. 195-202 in Uusitalo, H./Parpo, A./Hakkarainen, A. (eds.), *Sosiaali- ja terveydenhuollon palvelukatsaus 2000* (Social welfare and health care service review 2000). Helsinki: Reports of National Research and Development Centre for Welfare and Health 2000:250.

Rissanen, S./Laitinen-Junkkari, P./Hirvonen, R./Sinkkonen, S. (1999) 'Vanhusten kotihoidon laatu Kuopiossa 1994 ja 1997 – arviointitutkimus kotipalvelun ja kotisairaanhoidon yhdistämisen vaikutuksista kotihoidon laatuun vanhusasiakkaiden, omaisten ja työntekijöiden arvioimana' (The quality of elderly home care in 1994 and in 1997 – The evaluation study on the effects on the quality of home care after the merging of home help service and home nursing as evaluated by the clients, their relatives and staff involved), *Gerontologia* 13 (2): 71–81.

Ruotsalainen, P. (2000) 'Asiakaslähtöinen palveluketju ja tietoteknologia' (Customer-oriented chain of service and information technology), pp. 7-32 in Nouko-Juvonen, S./Ruotsalainen, P./Kiikkala, I. (eds.), *Hyvinvointivaltion palveluketjut* (The chain of services of welfare state). Helsinki: Kustannusosakeyhtiö Tammi.

Ruotsalainen, P./Nouko-Juvonen, S./Kiikkala, I. (2000) 'Esipuhe' (Preface), pp. 5-6 in Nouko-Juvonen, S./Ruotsalainen, P./Kiikkala, I. (eds.), *Hyvinvointivaltion palveluketjut* (The chain of services of welfare state). Helsinki: Kustannusosakeyhtiö Tammi.

Seiskari, R. (1997) 'Hoitotyö yhdistyneen sosiaali- ja terveystoimen kotihoidossa' (Nursing in home care of the integrated social and health affairs), pp. 149-160 in Parviainen, T./ Pelkonen, M. (eds.), *Yhteisöllisyys – avain parempaan terveyteen* (Communality – the key for better health). Helsinki: Reports of National Research and Development Centre for Welfare and Health 1997:217.

Siltari, T. (1998) 'Espoon kotihoitopalveluiden laadun ja taloudellisuuden arvioinnista' (Some facts concerning the assess the quality and economy of Espoo's home care services), *Vanhustyö* 8: 17-19.

Sinkkonen, S. (ed.) (1995) *Kotihoidon sisältö ja laatu Kuopiossa 1994* (Content and quality of home care in Kuopio in 1994). Kuopio: Kuopio University Publications E, Social Sciences 30.

Sinkkonen, S./Tepponen, M./Paljärvi, S./Rissanen, S. (2001) 'Kotihoidon sisältö ja tapaustutkimukset kotihoidon organisoinnista yhdistetyssä sosiaali- ja terveystoimessa' (Content of home care and case studies on the organisation of home care), *Kunnallistieteellinen aikakauslehti* 29 (3): 177-195.

Sipilä, J. (1997) 'Introduction', pp. 1-8 in Sipilä, J. (ed.), *Social care services: The key to the Scandinavian welfare model*. Aldershot/Brookfield, USA/Hong Kong/Singapore/Sydney: Avebury.

Sipilä, J./Andersson, M./Hammarqvist, S-E./Nordlander, L./Rauhala, P-L./Thomsen, K./ Warming Nielsen, H. (1997) 'A multitude of universal, public services – how and why did four Scandinavian countries get their social care service model?', pp. 27-50 in Sipilä, J. (ed.), *Social care services: The key to the Scandinavian welfare model*. Aldershot/Brookfield USA/Hong Kong/Singapore/Sydney: Avebury.

Suoninen, L. (1996) 'Lammilla ja Tuuloksessa tiedetään vanhuksen onnistuneen kotiutumisen avainsanat' (In Lammi and in Tuulos are known the key words of sucessful discharge), *Sosiaaliturva* 16: 30-33.

Tervala, A. (2002) *Toimialaraportti 2002. Terveyspalvelut* (Report on health services of line of activities 2002). Kauppa- ja teollisuusministeriö; TE-keskus.

The elderly working team of Leppävaara's social and health centre (1994) *Vanhustenhuollon kehittämisohjelma 1994–2000 (2010)* (The development programme for elderly care 1994–2000 [2010]). Espoo: Leppävaara's social and health centre.

Tilastokeskus (2001) Kuntien palkat ammateittain 2001 (Municipal salaries by occupation in 2001). Retrieved 11 June 2002 from the World Wide Web: http://www.tilastokeskus.fi/

University of Tampere (2002) Research programme on ageing of the Academy of Finland 2000–2002. Retrieved 22 August 2002 from the World Wide Web: http://www.uta.fi/laitokset/ tsph/itu/ohjelma.htm

Vaarama, M./Lehto, J. (1996) 'Vanhuspalvelujen rakennemuutos 1988–1994' (The structural change of services for the elderly in 1988–1994), pp. 39-60 in Viialainen, R./Lehto, J. (eds.), *Sosiaali- ja terveyspalveluiden rakennemuutos. Laitoshoidon vähentämisestä avopalvelujen kehittämiseen* (The structural change of social and health care services. From diminishing of the institutional care to development of outpatient services). Jyväskylä: Gummerus Kirjapaino Oy.

Vaarama, M./Hakkarainen, A./Voutilainen, P./Päivärinta, E. (2000) 'Vanhusten palvelut' (Services for the elderly), pp. 75-98 in Uusitalo, H./Parpo, A./Hakkarainen, A. (eds.), *Sosiaali- ja terveydenhuollon palvelukatsaus 2000* (Social welfare and health care service review 2000). Helsinki: Reports of National Research and Development Centre for Welfare and Health 2000:250.

Vaarama, M./Voutilainen, P./Kauppinen, S. (2002) 'Ikääntyneiden palvelut' (Services for the elderly), pp. 76-105 in Heikkilä, M./Parpo, A. (eds), *Sosiaali- ja terveydenhuollon*

221

palvelukatsaus 2002 (Social welfare and health care service review 2002). Helsinki: Reports of National Research and Development Centre for Welfare and Health (STAKES) 2002:268.

Viitala, R (2000) 'Ikääntyvän väestön hyvinvoinnin ja palvelujen kehittäminen' (Development of welfare and services for the ageing population), *Vanhustyö* 1: 5-8.

Working Group Investigating the Significance of Non-Institutional and Institutional Care (2001) *Memorandum (Final Report) of the Working Group Investigating the Significance of Non-Institutional and Institutional Care.* Helsinki: Working Group Memorandum of Ministry of Social Affairs and Health 2001:30.

Unpublished References

Parikka, T./Salonen, P. (2002) E-mail exchanges and telephone discussion on the elderly care in Pirkkala on 19 June 2002.

Prunnila, S (2002) *Tampereen kaupunki palveluiden järjestäjänä* (City of Tampere as a service provider). Unpublished lecture in Hoiva-alan koulutus- ja kehittämisprojekti in Tampere 23.4.2002.

Väänänen-Sainio, R./Lotvonen, S. (2002) *Ennalta ehkäisevät kotikäynnit 75-84 – vuotiaille kotona asuville ikääntyneille Höyhtyän ja Kaukovainion suuralueella. Hankesuunnitelma* (Preventive home visits for 75-84 years old elderly people living at home in regions of Höyhtyä and Kaukovainio. Project plan). Unpublished project plan. City of Oulu, Social and health affairs, Regional elderly work, Oulu.

222

Annex: Project Descriptions

A1 Discharging from Hospital to Home Care

Provider	City of Helsinki, Social Office and Health Office (Heiskanen et al., 2001)
Objectives	• To develop cooperation between hospital and home care concerned with the discharge of elderly patients in the city of Helsinki • To develop elderly patients' discharge towards a more customer-oriented, safer and more flexible process, with the help of a new operations model
Target group	All elderly patients discharged from hospitals in the city of Helsinki
Number of staff involved	All staff involved in the discharge process, follow-up treatment and care in hospital and at home
Methods	• A new operations model was developed by a working group involving nurses doing elderly nursing in home care and hospital • The operations model consists of phases of the discharge process, and the content of every phase covers operations, functions, and instructions on who is in charge of the task in question, and how documentation and flow of information will be checked
Strengths and weaknesses	• The concepts used in the discharge process and home care were determined in order to ensure that everyone participating in the discharge process and elderly care knows the basic issues • A new method – the operations model – was developed, and the development work was done by persons who are actually doing elderly care work • The operations model can be used in different kinds of settings in elderly work • The clear content and instructions of this model help to make practical work easier, more flexible, safer and presumably cheaper, and in that way the model will benefit all providers involved in the discharge process, as well as follow-up treatment and care • As a weakness it could be mentioned that, so far, there has been no evaluation of the operations model in practical use

A2 Development Programmes for Elderly Care in Leppävaara

Provider	City of Espoo, Leppävaara's social and health centre (The elderly working team of Leppävaara's social and health centre, 1994; Lindström, 2000)
Objectives	• The main target of these development programmes was to develop elderly care in Leppävaara • The objective of the first development programme was to estimate the current situation, and to propose change factors which the future may require from the current point of view • Objective of the second development programme was to clarify the most essential problems, challenges and development needs in current elderly care
Target group	All persons aged 65 or older in Leppävaara, the number of this population being 4,371 in the year 2000
Number of staff involved	All staff involved in elderly care in Leppävaara in the year 2000: • Number of physicians: 23 (health centre) • Number of nurses: 22 (health centre) • Number of home care staff: 102
Methods	Two development programmes were drawn up by a multiprofessional team • SWOT analysis was used as a basic instrument when drawing up the development programmes. It included possibilities, strengths, weaknesses and threats of elderly care taking the current situation and the future into account
Strengths and weaknesses	• Two development programmes were prepared by a working group representing employees of both the administrational and practical level • In both programmes the starting situation was thoroughly clarified • Possibilities, strengths, weaknesses and threats of elderly care were clarified with the help of SWOT analysis • The development operations were mainly focused on the weaknesses and threats • The development activities were thoroughly described in both programmes The second programme mentioned that the operations of the first development programme had been evaluated, but it was not explained how the evaluation had been carried out. Anyway, improvement in elderly care has obviously occurred during the first period as could be stated from the following:

- The first development programme has acted as a good framework whenever services have been developed for elderly care
- The challenges stemming from the first development programme have been well responded to, and the operations have been developed and changed in the desired direction

A3 Kuopio Studies

Provider	University of Kuopio (Rissanen et al., 1999)
Objectives	The main purpose of this study was to assess the effects of the merging of home help service and home nursing on the quality of home care with regard to two aspects: • To assess the quality of home care in relation to the quality objectives which were set for the integration • The quality objectives of the organisation were (a) to guarantee the quality of home care and (b) to add ability to recognise clients' problems, and (c) to assess the quality of home care in relation to expectations of elderly clients, their relatives and staff in two different periods (1994 and 1997)
Target group	Elderly people (65 years of age or older) who received home care services in Kuopio, their relatives and the staff directly involved or in interaction with these clients on a regular basis • Sample in 1994: 77 elderly clients and 86 relatives • Sample in 1997: 81 elderly clients and 100 relatives • A part of the subjects were similar in both samples
Number of staff involved	1994: 105; 1997: 104
Methods	Information was based on interviews (elderly clients) and questionnaire forms (relatives and staff) and a part of the data was analysed with factor analysis
Strengths and weaknesses	• The data was collected before and after the merging of home help services and home care, which enabled the assessment of the effects on the quality of home care • It is slightly difficult to estimate which of the effects are consequences of the merging and which resulted from other changes occurring at the same time (e.g. a reduction in resources)

225

- The fact that only part of the subjects participated in both assessments reduces the value of the results to a certain degree
- One of the powerful strengths was that elderly clients, relatives and staff acted as estimators. This gives many-sided information about how the clients and the parties involved in care assessed the quality of home care. Because the assessments of these groups were quite similar, the results could be considered as very reliable

A4 Laatuvanttu Project in Lammi and Tuulos

Provider	Municipalities of Lammi and Tuulos, Hämeen lääninhallitus, National Research and Development Centre for Welfare and Health, Sosiaalikehitys Ltd (Autio, 1996; Suoninen, 1996)
Objectives	• To find out how the timing of discharge from a health centre ward could be optimally planned • To consider ways which could support elderly people's coping at home as well as possible
Target group	Social service and health care personnel
Methods	• Basic information was based on interviews with elderly persons living at home or in service homes, old-age homes or health centre wards • According to the results of the interviews, a working group defined the contributory factors concerning safe living at home and successful discharge from hospital • Discussion between different professionals • Health centre ward visits
Strengths and weaknesses	• During the project, practical means (lists of contributory factors) were found to help elderly discharge persons both in health centre wards and at home as well as over the whole discharge process • Flow of information between different professionals improved • Co-operation between different care providers improved • After the project, the change of patients has increased enormously and these figures really prove that the development project has been successful • The number of long-term beds rapidly decreased, showing that goals were reached, and the fact that there was no queue, at least in 1996, from the central hospital to the health centre ward confirmed the achieved improvements

These, as well as the increase in the change of patients, were notable findings, even if they were not defined as development targets
- Some information, such as the number of interviewed persons and the number of participants, was not contained in these articles

A5 Dementia Research in Kuopio

Provider	University of Kuopio, Brain Research and Rehabilitation Center "Neuron", Kuopio University Hospital, University of Helsinki, University of Oulu, Oulu University Hospital (Eloniemi-Sulkava et al., 2001)
Objectives	• To determine whether community care of demented patients can be prolonged through a 2-year support programme based on nurse case management
Target group	100 demented patients in five Finnish municipalities: Kuopio, Iisalmi, Siilinjärvi, Maaninka and Vehmersalmi
Number of staff involved	One nurse and one study physician
Methods	• Patients in the intervention group and their caregivers were provided with a support programme, in which they received systematic and comprehensive support given by the coordinator for a period of two years • The control group received the usual services provided for geriatric patients in community care by the municipal social and health care system or the private sector • The chi-square test, Kaplan-Meier method and Cox regression analysis were used in the analysis
Strengths and weaknesses	• The study was a randomised trial with intervention and control groups • During the follow-up time there were two endpoints • The intervention was well designed and implemented • It could be proved by the trial that by the help of well-implemented intervention, living at home of dementia patients can be prolonged • As a weakness it could be mentioned that a copy of the original doctoral thesis could not be found, nor therefore be used when analysing this case

227

Providing Integrated Health and Social Care for Older Persons in France – An Old Idea with a Great Future[1]

Michel Frossard †, Nathalie Genin,
Marie-Jo Guisset, Alain Villez

1 Introduction

Published in 1962, *Rapport Laroque* is considered as the first official report establishing guidelines for a policy for the elderly. Its main idea is to consider the older people as real citizens by giving them decent incomes through the pension system and to encourage their integration in the community. The development of domiciliary services is the key point to help older persons to remain in their own home. Already at that time coordination was encouraged as a good means to improve the efficiency of the health and care services.

Since the publication of Pierre Laroque's report in 1962, gerontological coordination has been a recurrent theme of policy for the elderly, although it has never been adopted as a structuring element of local policy targeting that group.

It just seems as if this type of coordination was simply unable to escape from a subtle dialectic between declarations of good intent and confinement to the ghetto of innovatory action.

This absence of meaningful political will was most clearly evident after the adoption of France's devolution laws which, by devolving responsibility for county-level policies in favour of the elderly (residential and home care for the most disadvantaged) to the county councils (*Conseils Généraux*), led to the withdrawal of the state from its leading role in local gerontological policies without, however, inciting the county councils to take on this function to its fullest extent.

This report demonstrates that the organisation of the offer of home and residential care is still far from being structured in integrated networks. The different initiatives taken to coordinate the gerontological interventions collided with the fracture that separates activities of the medical side from those of the social sector.

The successive policies of governing health expenditures and the subsequent implementation of the new "Personalised Autonomy Allowance" (APA) supplied the most determining impulses in this still very widely utopian objective of the gerontological coordination which remains the only way identified to meet the needs of older persons in an adequate way.

2   The Legal, Structural and Financial Framework

2.1   *The Legal and Structural Framework of Help and Care Services and Gerontological Policies*

The separation between health care and social or socio-medical structures that has contributed to organise and finance the entire sector of services for the elderly was considerably strengthened by the devolution laws of 1983.

Two major framework laws mark out the institutions and policies dedicated to the elderly: the law on social and medico-social institutions of 30 June 1975, updated by the law of 02/02/02, and the hospitals law of 1978, updated in 1991 and completed in 1996. However, only those institutions linked to the health care sector have benefited from legal funding guaranteeing the implementation of and a future for evolutive solutions. As far as the social and medico-social sector is concerned, the solutions proposed on residential and home help only offered legal funding for elderly people recognised as being economically needy.

Another factor has contributed very substantially to restructuring the gerontological landscape since 1984: the policy initiated by the public authorities for controls on health expenditures, based on the search for solutions as alternatives to hospitalisation.

Since the elderly were found to be the principal consumers of health services, the forecasts on demographic change and especially the ageing of the population have contributed to promote the re-emergence of debates on care for the very old having lost their independence, thus becoming a key element of decisions concerning the development of gerontological policies.

"Dependence" thus has gradually become the most important factor of old age policy, although it cannot be sustained that older persons in general are facing more important social risks than persons with disabilities below the age of 60.

Currently the planning mechanism operates as follows:

Name of the body	Competent authorities
CORERPA Conférence régionale des retraités et personnes âgées (regional conference of the retired and the elderly)	State Ministries Region D.R.A.S.S. (Regional department of health and social affairs) C.R.O.S.S. (Regional committee on health and social affairs)
CODERPA Comité départemental des retraités et personnes âgées (county-level committee for the retired and the elderly)	County council (Conseil Général) Prefect D.D.A.S.S. (County-level department of health and social affairs) The county-level Gerontological Plan
I.L.C.G. Instance locale de coordination gérontologique (local gerontological coordination body)	District Local politicians Communes and other actors Canton

The local gerontological coordination body is the basis of the whole mechanism, and is the channel for the flow of information concerning the needs of the elderly at local and national levels. Its mission comprises needs analysis, definition of resources and the management of state funding for a defined geographical area. Its legal status varies as it can be affiliated to the municipality (public status) or may have an associative status.

Each body has a local coordinator whose position was funded by the state for a period of 4 years, between 1982 and 1987. His mission was to provide a liaison between the different stakeholders and to encourage the development of a coherent local services and equipment policy.

The implementation of this coordinating mechanism was slowed down by the promulgation of the devolution laws of 1982 and 1983, which transferred a large part of state responsibilities – including social action in favour of older persons – to local authority level, in particular to the county councils (Conseils Généraux). According to the new constitutional law, the latter now have full competence in the areas of housing and home care policies for persons with lower income.

All those mechanisms and bodies still exist but after 20 years we observe quite some differences depending on the local situation – some of them are almost asleep and inactive while others are dynamic. For instance, most of the new active "Centres Locaux d'Information et de Coordination" (CLIC) are former ILCG.

The model ways of working presented in the French report have been chosen to illustrate the diversity of ways to coordinate, through some initiatives in France. Plenty of them exist all over the regions either as ILG or more recently as CLIC. Some local authorities (departments) have really promoted such projects by financial support, hence in those regions coordination is more developed. But mainly ILG or CLIC exist because given the strong will of the local partners involved in such strategies, it is of course better when this will meets the local authority's interests.

2.1.1 A New Generation of Gerontological Coordination: The Gerontological Networks

EXPERIMENTAL PROJECTS FINANCED SINCE 1993 BY THE CNAVTS
Amongst the objectives attributed to these experimental networks, the following should be mentioned: needs assessment, guidance towards suitable solutions, better harmonisation of solutions and the services available. The structuring elements of the networks are the gerontological area, with its local services and residential structures and "consultations" for geriatric regulation, preferably through the hospitals. Besides those elements, there is a local action contract signed by those who are active in the field and a socio-medical diagnosis which identifies the help and care plan best suited to the case.

HEALTH CARE-BASED TREATMENT NETWORKS AND THE SO-CALLED
"SOUBIE" NETWORKS[2]
With the 1996 hospital reform and new directives seeking to control health expenditures, the state organised the promotion of distinct networks in the

health care sector, being careful not to exclude the social services involved in the field. As they were conceived as a general mechanism operating within the health system, these "cure" networks are organised to focus on certain pathologies or specific target groups (AIDS, people without resources, drug addicts, palliative care and treatment for the elderly). This emphasises the point that these networks, up to date, have had little to do with the elderly. However, the primary objectives of the networks are to be noted as they were to improve the quality of services provided, to reduce expenditure on "cure" and to promote networking in the provision of community- and hospital-based treatment by means of a coordinating doctor and by giving the end-user more responsibility through a contractual agreement.

There are two new dimensions to these care networks, *namely the involvement of the end-users* who are required to sign up to a care plan proposed to them. There is also a commitment to be made by the carers, who are required to sign a charter that is specific to the network, containing an ethical dimension and promoting care quality; and the evaluation of practices and user satisfaction.

With respect to the so-called "Soubie" networks mentioned above, it should be noted that these networks offer the possibility for exceptional arrangements, e.g. the funding of time spent by independent practitioners in coordinating health care.

The new law of March 2002 on "the patients' rights and the quality of the health care system" redefined the modes of authorisation and financing of experiments initiated by hospitals and independent health care professionals. It also brings together all initiatives under a single "health networks" umbrella .This charges them with facilitating people's access to health care, promoting interdisciplinary cooperation in treatment and integrating education, prevention, diagnosis and treatment for more effective assessment. In fact this law introduces the unique and official designation of "health networks".

LOCAL INFORMATION AND GERONTOLOGICAL COORDINATION CENTRES
(CLIC – CENTRES LOCAUX D'INFORMATION ET DE COORDINATION)
In order to legally recognize gerontological coordination initiatives that had been developed since the beginning of the 1980s, in June 2000 the Ministry for Employment and Solidarity launched a 5-year programme for the creation of 1,000 so-called "Local Information and Gerontological Coordination Centres" (CLIC – *Centres Locaux d'Information et de Coordination*).

The objective is to set up a geographically-based network with financial support from the state with three levels of competences:

- Level 1 – welcoming, informing, advising and supporting,
- Level 2 – assessing needs, compiling personalised care plans,
- Level 3 – implementing, monitoring and adapting those care plans.

A certification process allows the actions carried out by each CLIC to be qualified for each of these levels. There were 280 CLICs by December 2002, of which 43% were Level 1, 28% Level 2, and 29% Level 3. For the time being, there are only a minority of CLICs involved in an effective capacity in the field of coordination of help and care (Level 3). However, over time, we should see a positive development of this notion of networking. For the time being, we observe that for the second and third levels, the CLICs' mission partially overlaps with that of the socio-medical teams working within the departments on the implementation of the new "personalised independence allowance" (*Allocation Personnalisée d'Autonomie* – APA) which was created in January 2002 (see below). This is a source of confusion for providers and beneficiaries alike.

ILCG AND CLIC

The ILCG as local coordination bodies appear first in 1982. This form of organisation of local partners willing to join their efforts to provide better services is still alive in many places around the country. When CLICs have started to be set up since the year 2000 several ILCG became CLIC. In a way one can say that ILCG is the ancestor of CLIC, but as CLICs are quite new, at the moment the two forms co-exist depending on the places.

2.2   Funding of Help and Care Services for Older Persons in France

2.2.1 Domiciliary Services

Home help services are managed mainly by not-for-profit associations, more seldom by the local authorities themselves or community social action centres (CCAS). In exceptional cases, they may be managed by commercial providers. These services, which come under the heading of "social and medico-social institutions" (law n° 2002-02 of 2 January 2002), provide assistance for daily needs of older and disabled persons in need of care. These services are financed by:

- social funds from the county councils if recipients have low incomes;
- the social action branch of pension funds for all other people, up to a threshold beyond which the cost is entirely at the end-user's expense.

For persons who lost their self-care abilities, a new allowance has replaced the old *Prestation Spécifique Dépendence* ("specific dependence allowance") to contribute to the funding of miscellaneous types of help and support for people with care needs living in the community. The *Allocation Personnalisée à l'Autonomie* (APA – "personalised independence allowance"), introduced by the law of 21 July 2001, funds daily care needs up to a threshold fixed on the basis of the degree of the individual's loss of independence that is assessed by a special tool, called the AGGIR,[3] which categorises beneficiaries into six different groups (see Overview 1).

Overview 1: **Main Features of the "Allocation Personnalisée à l'Autonomie" (APA – "Personalised Independence Allowance")**

Eligibility Criteria	Applicants must have at least 60 years of age, live at home or in a family placement or in a nursing home. The assessed care needs for the essential activities of daily life must be classified in the first four groups of the railing (bars) AGGIR.
	As a universal allowance the access to the APA is not subordinate to criteria of financial resources. The amount paid by APA has no impact neither on the succession nor on donations made to the heirs.
Amount	APA is an allowance paid in cash but earmarked (thus it resembles a voucher) as it is intended to directly pay for help at home (employees of a service or informal carers employed directly by the person) or in institutional care, where it should cover the part of the fee corresponding to the help provided for basic care.
	It should be noted, however, that the APA scheme at home is also to finance other types of support than personal services such as needs-related adaptation of housing, meals on wheels, day centres, etc.
	The amount of the APA at home varies from 474,33 to 1106,77 € according to the degree of dependence (groups 1, 2, 3 and 4 of the railing [bars] AGGIR). A financial contribution is paid when resources of the recipient exceed 948,66 € monthly.
	The financial contribution of the recipient varies between 0 and 80% of the amount of APA.
	The amount of APA paid when institutional care corresponds to the cost of the services (performances) given for help in

235

	daily living activities. The amount is fixed by a dependency rate modulated on three levels: for persons in group 1 and 2 of the railing(bars) AGGIR, for persons in group 3 and 4, and for persons in group 5 and 6. The amount of the APA in institutional care is also modulated if resources of the person exceed 2025 € monthly. APA is paid either directly to the beneficiary or to the nursing home or to the service chosen by the beneficiary.
Management and financing	The county councils are responsible for ensuring the APA's management and a large proportion of its funding. The remainder is provided by a contribution from the "Fonds National d'Autonomie" (the national independence fund) using funding from the national social security system (0.1% of the "Contribution Sociale Généralisée" – CSG – the generalised social contribution on earnings, plus a contribution from the health and social action fund of the social security funds).

By the end of 2002 about 650,000 persons have received APA. The number of older persons needing care is estimated at 800,000 (in levels 1 to 4 of AGGIR) and 1,300,000 persons (in AGGIR levels 1 to 6).

- Domiciliary nursing services are managed generally by associations, more seldom by the local authorities and community centres for social action (CCAS). Their creation is subject to prior authorisation from the Prefect (the state representative at county level). They provide home care which is usually administrated by auxiliary nurses under the supervision of a coordinating nurse. The funding is provided entirely by the national social security health insurance scheme, with no contribution from beneficiaries.
- In 2000, about 60,000 old persons were in care with 1,600 domiciliary nursing services.
- Related services: the provision of meals-on-wheels and needs-related adaptation of housing are provided by the local authority or associations that are contracted in. The cost of these services, which are provided on a discretionary basis in the framework of social assistance schemes, is covered mainly by means-tested user contributions paid to the local authority or pension funds.
- New services: day centres, mobile night guards, temporary residential care and other forms of support to family carers are part of a more recent concept, and the services provided are still at an experimental stage. Day centres and temporary residential centres seek to provide respite to those families who are involved in supporting a dependent

relative, whilst mobile night guard services offer an alternative solution to having permanent assistance at home, for which the cost to beneficiaries is such that only the really very well-off have access to them. It should be noted that there are very few options available for financial support for these services beyond social aid provided by the county for low-income individuals, and, more recently, the APA.

2.2.2 Residential Structures

Sheltered Housing (logement-foyer)
These are groups of accommodation units specifically designed for an exclusive use by older persons. They are offering collective services (restaurant, permanent security), for which use and regularity of use are optional. These structures offer a way of life that is based on independent living, and are therefore – at least in theory– not accessible to people needing care.

Given this dual vocation (both the provision of social housing and social residential housing for the elderly), sheltered housing is subject to the dual supervision of the Ministry of Social Affairs and Solidarity and the Ministry of Housing.

Access is subject to authorisation from the chairman of the county council. Pricing for sheltered housing is subject to the provisions of the law on social and socio-medical institutions (law n° 2002-02 of 2 January 2002). In this respect, if the building is approved for accommodation for persons receiving social support, the cost is fixed by the chairman of the county council, and rents for persons with lower income can be supported by the county-level social assistance department. Sheltered housing can include medical treatment if the average level of dependence of the occupants exceeds a threshold level defined by the regulations.

"Medicalised or Non-medicalised" Retirement Homes, Homes for Older People Needing Care (MAPAD – *Maisons d'Accueil de Personnes Agées Dépendantes*)
These somewhat older concepts are subject to the same regulatory provisions as sheltered housing schemes referred to above,[4] with the difference that they offer complete provision for all of the everyday needs of their residents. In this respect, residents of MAPADs suffer from higher levels of care needs. Since the major reform of residential care for dependent elderly people (*Etablissements d'Hébergement de Personnes Agées Dépendantes* – EHPAD)

pricing is organised in three separate packages:[5] "accommodation" which covers food and lodging; "dependence", covering social care in everyday life and provision for incontinence; and "care" which covers the expenses for medical staff, general medical surveillance and medical equipment. These three packages are administered by separate authorities: the county council for expenses linked to accommodation and dependence, the Prefect (the state representative of decentralised departments: DDASS, DRASS) for health care expenses. The medical bill is entirely covered by the statutory health insurance, while the cost for long-term care (dependency) is paid by the APA, without any financial contribution from beneficiaries up to a limit of 2,025.07 Euro.

This new mechanism, replacing medicalisation with the creation of medical therapy is being put in place very gradually: as of 1 July 2002, it had been implemented in only 700 residential care structures out of the 9,000 potentially affected by this reform. According to the terms of the law, the reform is due to be completed by 31 December 2003. Following this date any establishment not having signed up to "the tripartite agreement" will no longer be authorised to host dependent older persons.

Table 1:   Number of Residential Institutions in France

	Number of institutions	Number of beds, accommodations
Nursing Home	6,322	416,029
Short-term housing		7,366
Sheltered Housing	3,097	156,781
Long-term care services		83,215
Total	11,000	663,381

2.2.3 Innovative Structures

SMALL "LIVING UNITS" (BELOW 25 PLACES)

During the past 15 years, a number of so-called "small units", i.e. residential care homes at reduced scale, were set up. They focus on the enhancement of residents' independence, even for those categorised as dependent, and on their attachment to the local community, through the availability of community care services. The APA – the personalised independence allowance – for this reason was made available to fund also these establishments under the same conditions as home care services.

PAID FAMILY PLACEMENT

Paid care for the older or disabled persons within private houses is subject to fairly recent regulatory recognition; indeed, the law of 10 July 1989 gave chairmen of county councils the responsibility of approving these practices that had hitherto been developed completely beyond the existing regulatory framework. Approval is given on the basis of permanent or temporary accommodation for a maximum of three people in a normal family home. Housing conditions are negotiated within the framework of a case-by-case contract, based on a given model contract defined through the normal regulatory channels.[6] The price of the accommodation is broken up into three parts, and negotiated between the host and the guest: remuneration for the host, a maintenance payment (food, washing and maintaining of the property), and finally, a payment based on the availability of private and shared facilities.

All costs of the stay can be covered by county-level social assistance schemes. Currently, about 5,500 older and disabled persons are accommodated in adult family placement.

239

2.2.4 The Geriatric Sector and Health Care Institutions

These are almost exclusively managed by public hospital structures under the auspices of respective legislation and state control through regional hospitalisation agencies (*Agences Régionales de l'Hospitalisation* – ARH). The ARH director decides on the overall budgetary allocation required for annual funding, through credits made available by health insurance schemes for establishments and services falling within this sector.

People are directed towards health care institutions and services under this scheme upon prescription. The patients concerned more often than not present multiple pathologies requiring technical care and constant medical supervision:

- Short-term geriatric services, providing acute medical care.
- Monitoring and rehabilitation services (non-specialised), providing convalescence care and rehabilitation services required to help patients return to normal living conditions.
- Long-term health care services, providing long-term accommodation in a hospital environment.[7]
- Geronto-psychiatric units offer short-term care for people with a mental illness and those presenting behavioural problems linked to deficiencies in their cognitive functions.

- Day-care hospitals allow diagnosis and treatment activities without having to stay overnight – these services often have a geronto-psychiatric tendency.
- Home hospitalisation services are different from nursing care services on account of the intensity of the care provided and their capacity to offer health care at home.
- Geriatric consultations offer proper external specialised consultations but are today very rare in hospital complexes. They are set up as part of the five-year plan aimed at the development of the geriatric sector, as adopted in 2002 by the Ministry of Social Affairs and Solidarity.

Table 2:   Financing of Different Services (1998)

	Health Insurances (Social Security)	Local Authorities (Départements)	APA (2002)
Housing			
Nursing homes	1.57 billion	930 million	240 million
Long-term care services	1.11 billion		
Home care			
Domiciliary nursing services	530 million*)		
Home help	530 million	300 million	ca. 820 million

Source: Ministry of Social Affairs; *) Social Action branch of pension funds (Social Security).

2.3   A Service Provision that Is very Unevenly Distributed across the Country

In France, we can observe that health care services are characterised by a high degree of disparity over the country. As the poor quality of service in certain institutions and departments is threatening the efficiency of old-age policies that are aiming at keeping the elderly in their own homes as long as possible, the Ministry is trying to redress the balance through specific programmes of service provision development, for instance through the 5-year plan for the creation of additional home-nursing services.

Furthermore, the negligible dispersion of day-care services (still in an experimental stage) and short-term care structures is seen as a major problem.

2.4   The Stakeholders Involved in Providing Services and Their Mode of Cooperation

The services described above include four families of actors helping older persons to remain in their own homes:

*   Home helpers employed by providers (so-called "mandating" associations and social workers) that have been approved by the Ministry of Social Affairs and Employment, operating under the status of "family employment" and recruited directly by those receiving support, since a law was introduced in 1987 facilitating direct employment of informal carers by older people.
*   Residential care structures that are operated by commercial, public and private non-profit providers.
*   The health care institutions, i.e. public and private hospitals which are accredited by the government or part of the public hospital network.
*   Independent health workers, a category which includes doctors, nurses and other paramedical professionals.

241

The relationships between those actors are marked by competitive distortions linked to the status of institutions and staff, and to the way in which funding and payment are organised. These distortions are particularly acute in the home help sector where tensions between the companies which employ home-help staff and the case-by-case recruitment of helpers by the elderly themselves have become more than evident. The battle to secure the lowest possible hourly costs by employing home helpers in order to increase the number of hours financed within the framework of services that are only financed up to a defined ceiling, was particularly visible during the specific dependence scheme experiment (*Prestation Spécifique Dépendence*) which ran from 1997 to 2001.[8] As part of that programme, socio-medical teams organised by the county council and given the task of assessing needs and drawing up care plans, tended to go for case-by-case employment, thus rendering older persons, who were no longer in full control of their intellectual capacities, employers of their personal assistants. It does not seem that the now introduced "APA mechanism", although giving a certain priority to service provision for the most dependent individuals, has been any more successful in reversing this trend.[9]

Tensions have also been felt between home help services and residential institutions; one suspected the other of delaying applications for entry into residential care, thus resulting in newly-arriving residents that had got ever more dependent.

Other distortions have risen in the provision of home nursing services that can be provided either by employed nurses or by independent nurses; the former have to operate within an overall budget financed from the social health insurance scheme, the latter on the basis of individual approvals for the financing of treatment by the same health insurance scheme. The competitive environment in the area of institutional care should also be mentioned, with commercial companies competing with non-profit organisations from the private and public sector. Such commercial structures, absent from the gerontological field 20 years ago, now account for nearly 25% of places, that is to say that their share has almost reached that of private associations providing these services. Recently there has been a drop in demand for residential care possibly due to the demographic dip of the First World War. Paradoxically, some residential homes now have empty beds despite the anticipated increased demand for this type of care. It remains to be seen whether the increase in the number of elderly people[10] forecasted for the next three years will contribute to correct this situation.

3   Coordination, Integrated Health and Care Services, Service Networks for the Elderly: Towards a Typology[11]

The need for better coordination or integrated health and care as an idea is as old as social and health policy targeting the elderly itself. It is the result of a fragmentation of services, structures and funding. There is a very great diversity of practical examples, due to the conjunction of three separate elements: a highly individualised approach to the needs of people on the part of the professionals from each sector, the emergence of a decentralised or local approach, without any pre-defined generalised model to work from, and generally unsuitable regulatory and financial conditions, reflecting the fragmentation of services, requiring highly-developed imagination to get around the obstacles in place.

The experience of France in this field is characterised by a large empirical dimension and a strategy that seeks to allow for considerable room for manoeuvre to the professionals operating in the field. Unfortunately, this does not always come along with financial support! It was only in the 1990s that the *Fondation de France*, and then the Ministry of Social Affairs and Solidarity, started to commission studies and research activity on this subject to define organisational and operational models. The work done to date has contributed to the implementation of coordination models within the framework of experiments financed by the said institutions and through advances made by recent socio-medical policy aimed at the elderly: the specific dependence allowance (*Prestation Spécifique Dépendence*), the personalised independence allowance (*Allocation Personnalisée d'Autonomie*) and the local gerontological information and coordination centres (*Centres Locaux d'Information et de Coordination Gérontologique*). It is noticeable that the literature available on the subject has primarily emerged from these public and private commissions, and that the trend has not been for researchers to seize upon the theme of their own volition. As for the professionals from the sector, they have put little down on paper, with the exception of some often very succinct experiments, emphasising the positive side of the exchange which allows work to be carried out in a coordinated manner when compared to traditional, more fragmented approaches. Nevertheless, these contributions are primarily grey literature, with little to offer from a practical, methodological point of view.

243

In the following, we will elaborate on four points: a clarification of notions and concepts, in particular using a multidimensional typology, a specifically economic approach to address the issues raised by an organisational information chart on coordination, and the conclusions that can be drawn from these theoretical and semantic analyses as a means of understanding the current incentive and assessment mechanisms developed over recent years.

3.1 Concepts and Definitions

The question of networks and coordination has very much to do with that of the principles and operational parameters of collaboration and exchanges between actors within a production system. The economic analysis distinguishes market and hierarchy concepts, the extreme forms between which an intermediary situation exists, called "cooperation". The market is a decentralised organisation, which is based on principles having to do with deriving the greatest possible satisfaction or usefulness by the agents concerned, who must negotiate a balanced trade, an appropriate quantity/price balance and with regulation occurring as a result of market pressures in a competitive environment. At the other end of the scale, the hierarchy is a centralised organisational form characterised by the integration of a diversified set of activities under a single decision-making entity. The vertically integrated company (providing intermediate products right through to final products) and the horizontally integrated company (providing a series of products of the same type) is the current model for this type of entity. Each element is supposed to work towards the same objective, of which there is one, and only one for the whole of the organisation. This is left in the hands of the single decision-making authority. Cooperation is an intermediary form, an association of production units having different objectives and preferring not to invest in complementary activities or not being able to do so, because of the prohibitive cost of the "entry barriers" into the business.

On the basis of these theoretical foundations, we would propose the following definitions:

- *Integrated services* are a set of services made available for a specific population group over a given geographical area, or for the population of a given geographical area, by a single company or organisation, grouped together under a single decision-making authority.

- *Network or coordination* is a voluntary organisation of professional people (which may include voluntary workers) who pool their means and resources to develop information, social and health care, and prevention services designed to resolve complex or urgent problems, which have been identified as priorities over a given geographical area, according to criteria decided in advance on a consultation basis. In the first case, the result will be a stable organisation providing for the complete coverage of health care needs of a given population. In the second, it will be a temporary or permanent collaboration between different organisations working towards a specific objective.

It is worth clarifying a semantic detail at this point, when comparing France and Southern Europe on the one hand, and the Anglo-Saxon world on the other. Coordination and networking in the French sense is a process and organisation of case management. Its operations require a professional to manage individual cases: that individual will be referred to as the "case manager" according to the English language tradition, and *"référant"* in French. It is the coordinating organisation which will refer the individual to the case manager. The coordinator is a professional person who runs the coordination structure.

3.2   *Moving towards a Typology*

Several approaches are possible, and serve to further clarify. Very much along the lines of what we have already described, we turn first of all to the approach adopted in the UK by Davies (1992). Using already quite old studies, the authors propose a case management typology, with the notion of "coordination based on a person" being the equivalent for the French reality. This typology comprises a fundamental level, the state of relations between the members of the network, supplemented by other complementary typologies concerning the content of tasks, the design of the care provided, the leadership or the place of professionals and end-users in the coordination.

The first level distinguishes an institutional integration model for services (Consolidated Direct Service Model) and one without institutional integration, the "Brokerage Model". This in turn is divided up into two possible variants, the "Advocacy Model", in which the case manager "pleads" the case before the services concerned with a view to setting up a care plan within the framework of a network which can be formalised to differing degrees. The second variant is the "Brokerage Agency Model", in which the case manager has the authority and the financial means to allow him/her to get past the professional service framework in the strictest sense, or to go beyond standard norms, meaning that s/he can play a more incentive-driven role than applied in the previous model.

The institutional integration model is the equivalent of that used by the vertically integrated company as, for instance, represented in US private insurance companies and in particular in the US Social Health Maintenance Organisations. There is no profit-making private equivalent in France, but there is embryonic evidence of it in France's "*mutuelles*" (mutual insurance companies), and, more significantly, at municipal level, in *social action centres* in those cases where they provide community care services, meals on wheels and so forth.[12] In France, this model was developed in theoretic literature during the 1980s for a health care application, rather than for sociomedical purposes or services directed at the elderly (Launois, 1985). We can illustrate this by the case of a coordination service presented in Annex A3. The "gerontological coordination" has been created in the 1980s to follow up people at home with health difficulties. Today, older adults are the main persons asking for care plans (90%), but also disabled people or persons that are socially isolated. The coordination is supported by local institutions (so-

245

cial action centres of the city, the department), which translates a strong political involvement and facilitates its funding and functioning. It also enables to secure a wide coverage of professionals. It is now coming back, however, in the form of so-called "*Soubie* networks" (see above) (see Annex A6, "Réseau Gérontologique du pays de Retz" which received the Soubie Agreement in November 2001). The vast majority of French experiments in coordination are close to the advocacy type of the brokerage model (Frossard, 1996), with variants: one-stop shop (*Fondation de France*, 1992) with fixed or variable design, or the "Network head-end" (*à tête de réseau*) model (Groupe de Travail DGS-DAS, 1995; Comte, 1996). The *Brokerage Model* is used in Kent in England, where the case manager has a budget to provide support in the home to about 30 older citizens in need of care; it is currently emerging in France promoted by county councils as part of specific experiments with repect to the specific dependence service (PSD) and in preparation for that tool to being more widely developed.

The typology founded on tasks connected to coordination involves listing a series of functions. It has been systemised in the US (Geron/Chassler, 1995): here we find information, personal assessment, creation of a care plan, and its implementation, monitoring and evaluation and the decision to bring it to a close. Practical coordination can include one or all of these levels, which themselves can be the subject of sequenced implementation over time, which is the main and guiding idea of the CLIC in France with their quality labelling process (the different sequences are presented in the first part of this report). This is why, today, most coordination projects seek to be labelled as a "CLIC" to have their activities recognized by the government and to secure – not least important – subsidies and political support guaranteeing their development. Indeed, most of the projects presented in the Annex have to cope with financial instability. Two of them, the "CLIC de Châlus" (Annex A1) and the "Maison des Aînés" (Annex A5) are recognized as "CLIC", categorized at level 2, i.e. they can give information, advice, and guidance to the older persons and their families. They also carry out needs assessment with a pluridisciplinary approach and propose personalised care plans at home.

We would also suggest superposing another typology over this typology of organisational forms: one concerning the intervention principles of integrated services and networks. The practical observation of experiments we have been able to analyse and our study of respective literature encourage us to propose two approaches: one that we will call *care system* and another one that we would describe as *accompaniment*. Whilst the notions of sector and network are well used today, definitions of them are not so readily available. We would suggest the following:

- A care system describes the trajectory of a person or patient in a network or an integrated ensemble; this trajectory is legitimised either by the state of scientific knowledge or professional experience, or indeed, by regulatory or price approaches.
- A trajectory is the process followed by a person or patient within a mechanism providing services or health care; this journey is characterised by switches from one service to another and by a whole series of aid and health care types.

The sector approach is essentially one adopted by the sponsor looking for efficiency at the best possible cost, on the basis of a standard reference. The *accompaniment approach* is based on the individual design of the health care provision and its financing, rejecting any form of standardisation and notions of imposed references. This distinction sums up quite neatly the challenges faced by assessment today. The question asked of public health evaluators and economists alike is whether or not a generalisation of care system practices should be imposed, and how to evaluate practices used when no universal referencing system is available.

247

Persons responsible for financing coordination are first and foremost interested in the demonstration of pertinence and proof of good cost/efficiency ratios. In the meantime, this issue of the superiority of the coordination approach over a non-coordination approach requires no further proof, and particularly no economic proof (Frossard, 1992).

4   Model Ways of Working

Since Pierre Laroque's report national policies have intended to develop domiciliary help and care provision. The need of coordination to improve the efficiency of the given services was regularly stressed but only a few providers adopted such a perspective. Through 30 years, coordination as a model way of working remained dependent mainly on a voluntary basis. Despite the lack of strong and incentive public financial support, more and more local actors began to coordinate their actions for a better integration of the services they offer.

4.1 Gerontological Coordination, Joint Working

"St-Martin d'Hères Coordination Gérontologique" is one of those initiatives initiated in the 1980s; with a largely medical leaning, the St-Martin d'Hères coordination missions are to set up services to keep people with health problems in their own homes. 90% of the clients are elderly.

- The team assesses the needs of those requiring assistance, sets up and coordinates aid provided, monitoring the support process as it evolves, "respecting the natural environment and the choices of the individuals involved".
- Collective support for the families (the commune has a strong family-based culture).
- An individual case file is opened by the social workers and made available to all the teams (coordination, personal aid, health care, activities). It contains information on the person's identity, health condition, family and social environment, services put in place, resources, living conditions, social coverage, etc.
- After the health and care plan has been implemented, monitoring is carried out through visits to the person's home or interviews in the office, but also via the different services involved in the aid plan, that provide information on the individual's progress (benefits or problems observed).
- Operational meetings (gerontological coordination) with the permanent staff take place once a month.
- The strong points of the project are to have succeeded in grouping all services under a single umbrella, which is known and recognised as the commune's gerontological hub.
- Major institutional support and recognition: direct person-to-person links and applications are processed rapidly. The coordination has led to a raising of the "tolerance threshold" of services and families thanks to teamwork and the elimination of professional isolation that those providing the services sometimes experience in the field. The partners stress that now there is a very strong gerontological culture within the commune, reinforced by this coordination (partnership practices, common tools, support between the various teams, good cohesion). This project shows the importance and quality of an initial assessment in the home by social workers: good communication of clear, enlightened information to the teams.

It is one of the oldest projects of joint working to have been developed and managed with a regular success in spite of difficulties due to a lack of recognition of the work done by certain professionals and recently and increasing work with the introduction of APA.

Another illustration of joint working coordination is the "Réseau Gérontologique du Pays de Retz" (in Brittany). Initiated in 2000 by a geriatric hospital, this project is one of the very few "health care networks" (see 2.11) dedicated to the elderly after the new hospital reform in 1996. Its missions are:

- To reduce the use of hospitalisation and institutionalisation by attempting to prevent a total loss of equilibrium specifically for vulnerable people aged 75 and over (identification by GPs). The GP carries out a medical and social assessment at the person's home, in collaboration with a social worker of the CRAM or the county council;
- To define a medical and social accompaniment plan for a period of one year; depending on the case, the doctor or the social worker will be the coordinator; and
- to develop a common culture thanks to training actions.

In terms of tools and methods the "Réseau gérontologique du pays de Retz"uses AxiAge, a computer programme for old patients designed to measure the degree of vulnerability of the individual + MMS (Mini Mental State) + MNA (Mini Nutritional Assessment) + social evaluation. A summary meeting with the GP, the social worker and a hospital geriatrics representative, results in the drawing up of an accompaniment plan for a period of one year. Also joint training actions involving the different professionals on the theme of vulnerability and tools available are regularly organised.

After two years, success in getting doctors and social workers to work together while they were not used to doing so has become visible. The multidisciplinary assessment has allowed professionals to take a fresh look at certain situations. Nevertheless, partners conclude that the process is very time-consuming for those leading it: two years to put the project together and assemble the professionals around it; the operation of the network relies on the motivation of a small number of people.

4.2   *The Implementation and Evaluation of Coordination*

With this spontaneous organisation of providers of social and health care services, gerontological coordination has received some special attention over recent years from public authorities and those responsible for the regulatory texture. And this has been to such a degree that those operating in the field, having legitimately complained that coordination has no funding behind it and therefore no means to ensure its survival, now fear that their initiatives are going to be "borrowed"; or else, they feel disorientated faced with the multitude of mechanisms that are available now (see section 2). Here, we will defend the position that the given diversity of current incentives has as a consequence that the criteria requiring the respect for diversity must preside over any innovatory social experiment.

We will not be looking at incentives and funding mechanisms here, since this is done in the first part of this report. For the time being, we will refer to the main points in the literature on evaluation.

Evaluation has become a compulsory dimension of private and public projects and project funding in social and health care.[13] The diversity of projects and the way they are organised, funded and implemented cannot be an excuse for fragmented evaluation criteria and measures. The risk is patently there. The work done by ANAES, the National Agency for Evaluation in Health Care, the IMAGE group and CREDIS, the INSERM group from Montpellier and the CPDG today provides a corpus of evaluation methods which allow appropriate tools to be developed to meet the requirements of specifications imposed upon projects by funding organisations.

Without suggesting that the list is exhaustive, the main evaluation items that can be identified from the literature on the subject would include:

- Rate of coverage and targeting
- Cost, productivity, optimal size of the coordination
- Efficiency: costs avoided, user satisfaction, reduction in implementation time for aid plans, effective implementation of aid plans, improvements in quality of life
- Development of professional collective learning
- Respect for freedom of choice
- Readiness to pay on the part of end-users, service providers and administrations.

For more detailed information about those items, or methods and results in general, it could be interesting to have a look at reference works, in particular with the CPDG and the INSERM team in Montpellier, the two major centres for the production and execution of research on the issue of coordination.

250

5   Conclusions

The slow emergence of policies for the elderly further to the publication of Pierre Laroque's report in 1962 has meant that no clear solutions to the delicate question of the respective roles of national solidarity and family solidarity have been found in respect to older persons experiencing declining autonomy and needing assistance in daily activities.

The subtle combination of informal help provided by the person's immediate environment and professional services provided through socialised funding (county-level social assistance and state health insurance schemes) still suffers from the problems of accessibility of existing service provision at local level.

Even though the introduction of the personalised independence allowance (*Allocation Personnalisée à l'Autonomie* – APA) is a sign of progress, in the sense that it recognises the loss of autonomy as being a social risk that needs to be paid for from the social protection system (when compared to the former PSD which was no more than an assistance service reserved to the most dependent and most disadvantaged), French policies have not followed through to the natural conclusion of providing the universal services needed.

Arbitration is still required to decide on the means-testing of APA on the basis of the individual's resources and level of dependence and the issue of compensating families for the financial cost of their own support. The solution that suggests that families should be employed by their own ageing relative cannot be sustained, as it converts family solidarity into a salaried status; an uncomfortable example of catering to the needs of employment policy!!

On the other hand, the *culture of gerontological coordination* should benefit from the introduction of these new mechanisms based on a much more systematic orientation through the formalisation of aid plans drawn up by socio-medical teams. A national evaluation of CLICs is about to be undertaken, at the behest of the Ministry, before the end of 2002. This will allow to better understand methodologies, the strategies of those concerned and the role of the funders, and to assess at last the contribution of these new mechanisms designed to improve the quality of life of older persons living in their own homes.

Substantial progress is expected in the field to see to it that these new orientations are directed towards the promotion of *territorial gerontological*

251

networks, involving all local-level actors and institutions. There is still a long way to go to achieve this objective, in particular with respect to the challenges concerning funding and authority which need to be addressed when attempting to promote such a mechanism.

Notes

1.   This report was written and compiled by Michel Frossard † (Professor of Economic Science; Director of the Multi-disciplinary Gerontology Centre and of the Inter-University Gerontology Laboratory, University of Grenoble), Nathalie Genin (Research Engineer – CPDG, Grenoble), Marie-Jo Guisset (Gerontologist – UNIOPSS, Paris) and Alain Villez (Technical Advisor – UNIOPSS, Paris).
2.   From the name of "Raymond Soubie": first president of the National Committee of Health Care Networks.
3.   AGGIR: *Autonomie Gérontologique Groupe Iso Ressources* (Gerontological Independence, the Group Iso Resources).
4.   Law n° 2002-02 of 2 January 2002 on social and socio-medical institutions.
5.   Law of 24 January 1997; the same law with which the specific dependency allowance (*Prestation Spécifique Dépendence*) was introduced.
6.   The new mechanism introduced by the social modernisation law of 17 January 2002 which substantially reformed the status of families receiving elderly and handicapped people in this way.
7.   In-depth studies are currently being carried out by the Ministry of Social Affairs and Solidarity to assess whether this type of service should be kept within the health sector. In a long-term perspective, it is expected that most long-term care beds will be moved into social and socio-medical care structures. Whilst these new measures are under investigation, the long-term health care services (*Services de Soins Longue Durée*) are the only hospital-based services that charge their patients for their stay, or charge county-level social services when the individual's resources are insufficient to meet the costs.
8.   Reference to the law of 24 January 1997 which fixed the highest amount at about 850 € per month.
9.   Law of 20 July 2001which introcuced the "Allocation Personnalisée d'Autonomie" (APA).
10. The French population is set to experience an acceleration of its ageing due to the arrival of the baby-boomers at retirement age.
11. The elements developed here are the result of work carried out on behalf of the *Fondation de France*, the initiator of the project, the Ministry of Employment and Solidarity, the County Council and the Rhône-Alpes social security health insurance body (*Caisse Régionale d'Assurance-Maladie*). The project was carried out at the multidisciplinary gerontology centre (*Centre Pluridisciplinaire de Gérontologie*) by Michel Frossard in collaboration with Anne Boitard, a research engineer.
12. Also SIPA (integrated services for the elderly – *Services Intégrés pour les Personnes Agées*) services, tested in Montreal, are part of this category. They are based on the American HMO model and the Canadian models developed in Ontario and Alberta.
13. The Fondation de France over the last ten years has promoted a number of coordination projects. It was also the first institution to demand evaluation of the projects that it funded, and was at the root of the development of evaluation methodology (see Frossard et al., 2000).

References

ANAES (2000) *Evaluation des réseaux de santé* (Evaluation of health care networks). Paris: ANAES.

Argoud, D. (1996) 'Reflexions sur quelques expériences de coordination gérontologique' (re-flections on some gerontological coordination experiments), pp. 309-322 in: Aymé, S./ Henrard, J.C./Colvez, A. (eds.), *Handicap et vieillissement. politiques publiques et pratiques sociales* (Handicap and ageing. Public policy and social practices). Montpellier: Les Editions INSERM.

Béjean, S. (1994) *Economie du système de santé. Du marché à l'organisation* (The health care economy. From market to organisation). Paris: Economica.

Colvez, A. (1999) *Evaluation de l'expérience de Lunel, rapport d'évaluation* (evaluation of the Lunel experiment: an evaluation report). Montpellier: INSERM.

Colvez, A./Gay, M. (2001) *Evaluation de cinq expériences de CLIC* (evaluation of 5 CLIC experiments, report to the DGAS). Montpellier: INSERM.

Comte, J.F. (1996) 'La coordination gérontologique: de la théorie à la pratique' (Gerontological coordination: from theory to practice), pp. 302-307 in: Aymé, S./Henrard, J.C./Colvez, A. (eds.), *Handicap et vieillissement. politiques publiques et pratiques sociales* (Handicap and ageing. Public policy and social practices). Montpellier: Les Editions INSERM.

Davies, B. (1992) *Care Management, Equity and Efficiency: The International Experience.* Kent: University of Kent at Canterbury/PSSRU.

Dherbey, B. (1994) 'La coordination des services' (The coordination of services), *Gérontologie et Société* 69 (June): 72-76.

Dherbey, B./Guisset, M.J./Jallaguier, J. (2000) *L'accueil de jour, un maillon du soutien à domicile des personnes fragilisées.* Paris: Fondation de France.

Dherbey, B./Jurdan, C. (2002) 'Les dispositifs de coordination un outil de développement', *Gérontologie et Société* 100: 65-74.

Ennuyer, B. (1996) 'Coordonner ou ordonner? Du rapport Laroque à aujourd'hui' (Coordinate or command? From the Laroque report to the present), pp. 323-332 in: Aymé, S./Henrard, J.C./Colvez, A. (eds.), *Handicap et vieillissement. politiques publiques et pratiques sociales* (Handicap and ageing. Public policy and social practices). Montpellier: Les Editions INSERM.

Fondation de France (1992) *La coordination gérontologique, démarche d'hier, enjeu de demain* (Gerontological coordination: yesterday's practices, tomorrow's challenge). Paris: Fondation de France (Cahier de la Fondation de France, no. 5).

Fournier, P. (2002) 'La collaboration Ville-Hôpital – de la Filière au Réseau gérontologique', *Gérontologie et Société* 100: 131-147.

Fourtane, P.H. (2002) 'Le CLIC de Châlus (Haute-Vienne)', *Gérontologie et Société* 100: 95-110.

Frossard, M. (1992) 'Analyse économique de la coordination' (An economic analysis of coordination), pp. 106-114 in: Fondation de France (ed.), *La coordination gérontologique, démarche d'hier, enjeu de demain* (Gerontological coordination, yesterday's practices, tomorrow's challenge). Paris: Fondation de France (Cahiers de la Fondation de France, no. 5).

Frossard, M. (1996) 'Case Management in France: An Economic Perspective', *The Journal of Case Management* 5 (4): 161-166.

Frossard, M./Boitard A. (1997) 'Evaluation des réseaux de coordination gérontologique: une approche économique' (An evaluation of gerontological coordination networks: an economic approach), *Revue d'Epidémiologie et de Santé Publique* 45: 429-437.

Frossard, M./Boitard, A./Jasso Mosqueda, G. (2000) *L'évaluation des coordinations gérontologiques* (The evaluation of gerontological coordinations). Grenoble: Université Pierre Mendès France/CPDG/Fondation de France.

253

Geron, M.S./Chassler D. (1995) 'Advancing the State of the Art. Establishing Guidelines for Long Term Case Management', *The Journal of Case Management* 4 (1): 9-13.

Groupe de Travail DGS-DAS (1995) *Sur la coordination gérontologique* (On gerontological coordination). Document de travail. Paris: DGS-DAS.

Guinchard-Kunstler, P. (1999) *Vieillir en France. Rapport au premier Ministre* (Ageing in France. Report for the Prime Minister). Paris.

Guisset, M.J./Puijalon, B. (1995) 'La coordination gérontologique' (Gerontological coordination), *Retraite et Société* 8.

IMAGE-CREDES (2001) *L'évaluation des réseaux de soins. Enjeux et recommandations* (Evaluation of health care networks. Challenges and recommendations). Paris: IMAGE-CREDES.

Launois, R. (1985) *Les réseaux coordonnés de soins* (Coordinated health care networks).

Puijalon, B./Guisset, M.J. (2002) 'La Coordination, une longue histoire mouvementée' (Coordination: a long and moved history), *Gérontologie et Société* 100: 13-23.

Villez, A. (1997) *La viabilité économique des petites unités de vie*. Paris: Fondation de France.

Villez, A. (2000) 'Quelle Prestation Dépendance pour demain?', in: *Encyclopédie Protection Sociale, Quelle refondation?* (art.135). Paris: Editions Liaisons/Economica.

Villez, A./Vinsonneau, A. (2001) *L'APA en 23 Questions* (A.P.A. in 23 questions). Paris: UNIOPSS.

Annex: Project Abstracts

The following seven cases present projects that have been chosen in agreement with the monitoring committee of PROCARE France. The initiatives presented illustrate the diversity of the approaches and typologies presented in the report. Certain actions are recent, whilst others are not, clearly illustrating the progressive construction of coordination and network concepts in France over the past 20 years.

A1 CLIC de Chalus (Haute-Vienne)

Project initiators	Association de Coordination des Actions en Faveur des Personnes Agées (ACAFPA – Association for the coordination of actions in favour of the elderly)
	SCAPA: Service coordonné d'aides aux personnes âgées (coordinated services for the elderly)
	An association created in 1982 under the 1901 law on associations, further to the circular of 07/04/82 on medico-social policy in favour of pensioners and the elderly
Institutional partners	In addition to the partners of the association, professionals from the fields include: • Mandatory service for local employment • Relationship support services • Municipality-Hospital network (CHU, Red Cross, Pact'Arim)
Professional partners	• Elected representatives of the canton (county council, mayors) • Directors of centres for the elderly from Châlus and Cars • Representatives of services to help the elderly stay in their homes (ADPA home help, meals on wheels, nursing care) • Chairpersons of pensioners' clubs • Social workers • Members of the medical and paramedical professions • Volunteers and all those taking an interest in issues relating to ageing
Financial partners	• The county council (21%), communes (14%), state (4%), Fondation de France (10%)

Objectives and missions	• Information, advice, guidance for the elderly and their families • Precise assessment of needs (functional disabilities, remaining or potential capacities, existing human and/or technical resources, environment/housing, economic resources, affective, family and social environment, representation of the person's health condition and quality of life, psychological aptitude to accept the help on offer) • Prevention of loss of functional independence linked to age • Aid for help in the home to compensate the elderly's loss of functional independence
Number of staff	• 1 coordinator, a social worker by training • 2 assistants (deputy coordinator + activity leader) • 2 voluntary assistants • 1 referral agent: CIPA • 2 medical referral agents: 1 independent and 1 from hospital
Tools	• coordination meetings: at the request of the family doctor, with the coordinator and the professionals concerned: setting up of a guidance project which is proposed and negotiated with the person and his/her family (respect for freedom of choice) • steering meetings: evaluation of the project/aid plan. The frequency of these meetings depends upon how things develop. Emergency meetings held in case of problems • newsletter on the new aid plan for the elderly, to the family and the professionals involved • creation of summary files of successive evaluations • NB: the professionals are paid to attend the meetings • Evaluation in two stages: 1) Gerontological evaluation audit (BEG) = MMS (Mini Mental State) + MNA (Mini Nutritional Assessment) + unipodal station + GDS (Geriatric Depression Scale) 2) Overall assessment of functional independence: SMAF (Système de mesure de l'Autonomie Fonctionnelle – functional independence measurement system) • home-hospital liaison tool: transfer file specifying that the person is being monitored through the coordination with the BEG, the guidance project and the services adopted + synopsis of social situation + medical report (in an envelope marked "confidential")
Strengths	• initiative rooted in practicality (home help services), started up by local politicians in 1982 that has been able to adapt to the political and social context right through to acquiring the "CLIC-approved" label

	• 20 years of existence and experience • involvement of all local and institutional actors • general assessment of the elderly, using standardised and complementary transversal tools • continuous monitoring of beneficiaries • continuous training for assistants • number of beneficiaries in 2000: 41
Weaknesses	• fall in the number of people following PSD • mandatory service, job insecurity for home helps • accompaniment of people with extensive needs requires the involvement of different aid services and usually at great cost to the individual
Evaluation results; Keywords	Has been externally evaluated Evaluation planned through the CLIC Proximity – shared tools – global evaluation – multi-disciplinarity

A2 *Association Locale de Développement Sanitaire* (ALDS – Local Association for Health Care Development), Canton of Meulan, Yvelines

Project initiators	At the start of the project in 1981: l'Amicale des Médecins du Canton de Meulan (AMCM) Since 1983, ALDS has widened the network to include all the independent health professionals from the canton Since 2001, creation of AML (Association des Médecins Libéraux de l'ALDS – ALDS association of independent doctors) to deal with the strictly medical aspects of coordination
Institutional partners	The ALDS management board is composed of the following representatives: • health professionals • end-users, associations and institutions (hospitals, retirement homes, clinics) • member communes The institutional and financial partners are the Caisse Régionale d'Assurance Maladie (regional social security health insurance fund), Yvelines county council, the Yvelines healthcare and social agency (DASS), member communes, the MSA agricultural social mutual organisation and the Caisse Nationale d'Assurance Vieillesse (national pension scheme)

Objectives and missions	• Keeping elderly and dependent people in their own homes – information, dialogue, advice – medico-social assessment of needs – guidance and provision of resources – evaluation and monitoring of actions • through the introduction of various services: – nursing care in the home (Service de Soins Infirmiers à Domicile, domiciliary nursing service), in 1983 (64 cases processed), to provide quality care – Tele-assistance, created in 1986 – Personal aid services in 1990: mandatory service, i.e. the elderly person is the employer, ALDS deals with administrative management, supervises the assistants and makes the relational link between the family and the person being aided – Gerontological coordination service, in 1997: needs assessment and implementation of aid plans in emergency situations targeting dependent individuals • Promotion of the coordination of care between the municipality and the hospital • Creation of the medico-social unit under the APA umbrella. Involved in 24 different communes, i.e. a geographical area of some 120 km^2
Number of staff	1 supervisor per service and each ALDS service has its own funding and accounting: • the domiciliary nursing service is financed by the Ile de France Caisse Régionale d'Assurance Maladie (regional social security health insurance fund) – 16 employees • the coordination service is funded by Yvelines county council – 2 employees • personal aid services include 2 employees and 60 auxiliaries • the tele-assistance service is funded by members – 1 employee • the association – 2 employees, including a medical coordinator • the APA unit – 3 employees, including one doctor • the association is funded by the member communes and the beneficiaries of the services
Tools	• preparation of a combined medico-social dossier to apply for the aid for dependent individuals and professionals (hospital or at home): draft • multi-disciplinary meetings to coordinate health care provision for the individual (for someone returning home) • setting up of working groups of independent professionals from the health sector on specific subjects (creation of a website) • evaluation questionnaire for patients (quarterly) and health care professionals

258

	• compilation of a directory of independent and hospital health care professionals in the ALDS area
Strengths	• experience in the field of 18 years • the mechanism is entirely integrated into existing structures • very close collaboration with all independent and other professionals has developed at the initiative of the independent sector • 2001: 240 elderly people cared for daily
Weaknesses	• short-term financial stability • still insufficient resources given the demand from dependent people
Evaluation results; Keywords	Has been evaluated by an external body twice (CPDG) Renewal of funding within the framework of a FAQSV fund to improve the quality of care in the community mechanisms in 2002 Independent sector – network – multi-disciplinarity

A3 Coordination Gérontologique, Isère (Gerontological Coordination)

Project initiators	Centre Communal d'Action Sociale de St Martin d'Hères (St Martin d'Hères community social services centre) Began in the 1980s, initially with a largely medical leaning
Institutional partners	• Ville de St Martin d'Hères (St Martin d'Hères municipality) • Isère county council • UNCCAS (national union of community social action centres) • UDASSAD (county-level union of home health and personal care associations) • Pension and health insurance bodies • Direct work in the field with the services of the CCAS (community social action centres): • support: service-providers, mandatory and tele-alarm • domiciliary nursing service (40 places); nurses to administer care + the day centre • catering: meals on wheels and hostel restaurants • entertainment service for pensioners
Professional partners	• Partnership with: • Centre de Prévention des Alpes (CPA prevention centre, Alps): centre for multidisciplinary gerontological audits and evaluations for pensioners • Accommodation structures (EHPAD) • University hospital complex (medical + social services) • Independent health care professionals • Psychologists working for health care structures

	• Associative network: ALMA (Allo Maltraitance – physical abuse help-line); UDIAGE (information and guidance service) • SCAPH 38 (independent counselling experiment for physically handicapped people in the Isère) • Accommodation and integration hostels
Objectives and missions	• Services to keep people with health problems in their own homes. 90% of the people being aided are elderly, but there are others (the sick, the handicapped, the socially isolated, those undergoing re-integration, etc.). The team assesses the needs of those requiring assistance, sets up and coordinates aid provided, monitoring the support process as it evolves, "respecting the natural environment and the choices of the individuals involved" • Collective support for the families (the commune has a strong family-based culture)
Number of staff	2 social workers (80% and 100% working time) 1 part-time geriatric doctor (13 hours per week) 1 psychologist (half-time) 1 secretary (half-time)
Tools	• Gerontological sector meeting of the CCAS (community social action centre) which is more institutional, also held once per month • The CMT (Comité Médical Technique – technical medical committee): departmental meetings between professionals: once per week for the health care services and day centre, and twice per month for the residential hostel, the mandatory service and meals on wheels. For the service providers, the exchange of information occurs on a daily basis
Weaknesses	• The introduction of the APA caused delays in the work in the field. The APA has become a victim of its own success, creating a gap between the amount of allowance paid and the actual nature of the needs • A lack of knowledge and recognition of the work done by certain professionals (those operating in people's homes), very difficult, precarious working conditions for certain categories (home help) • Coordination work requires a major investment, substantial availability and flexibility in terms of actions and time-tabling. It also requires time investment in consultation and support within the team to allow people to step back and better interpret what is going on
Evaluation results; Keywords	No evaluation to date Common gerontological culture – single site – common tools – teamwork

A4 Gerontological Coordination and Local Networks in the Cantons Cysoing, Pont à Marc et Seclin

Project initiators	Association created in 1992 under the 1901 law on associations, comprising: – a hospital doctor – a GP – 2 local politicians
Institutional partners	Agence Régionale d'Hospitalisation (ARH – regional hospitalisation agency) Nord-Pas-de-Calais county council Caisse Régionale d'Assurance Maladie (CRAM – regional social security health insurance scheme) Mutualité Sociale Agricole (MSA – agricultural social mutual organisation) Union Régionale des Secours Miniers (URSSM – regional miners' support union) Elected representatives of the communes in the area and county councillors
Professional partners	Independent doctors / paramedics – Centres de Soins Infirmiers (CSI – nursing care centres) – Service de Soins Infirmiers à Domicile (SSIAD – domiciliary nursing service) Hospitals / home help associations / residential establishments
Objectives and missions	• Inform – assess – direct – coordinate • Set up aid plans in collaboration with the professionals of home help services • Organise hospital discharges • Run training courses for the network and for professionals • Identify prevention actions for end-users
Number of staff	2 employees: – 1 full-time coordinator nurse – 1 full-time secretary
Tools	• Multi-disciplinary committees • The aid plan: a vector of information and communication for the professionals involved • Charter for the members of the network • Workshop training courses to enhance working practices
Strengths	• Multidisciplinarity • Good collaboration with the hospital • Recognition from the professionals of the sector of the actions carried out over more than a decade • Long-standing collaboration with the "Nord" county council and the politicians from the area

Weaknesses	• a large number of network users, but always the same people take on an active role • small and therefore vulnerable structure, few people trained, changes in staff are not easy to cope with • very heavy workload for the administrative staff • insufficiently visible, premises not centrally located
Evaluation results; Keywords	An evaluation of the network was carried out in 2001 by ANAES (National agency for evaluation in health care) Participation in training workshops Annual number of calls Number of aid plans managed Number of professionals involved in the work of the committees Network – multi-disciplinarity – teamwork – recognition – training

A5 *La Maison des Aînés* (The Elders' House), CLIC de Belfort

Project initiators	County council (approved in 2000) The municipality via the CCAS (community social action centre)
Institutional partners	State / Municipality / CRAM (regional social security health insurance scheme) Youth and Sports ministry at local level: equilibrium workshops (experiment being run by the CRAM to give renewed confidence to young people who have fallen by the wayside) + training courses within retirement homes
Professional partners	3 representative associations within the Maison des Aînés: • gerontological conference, comprising professionals from the gerontological sector (medico-social institutions, hospitals, home help services, the centre for improved housing) • Comité Départemental des Retraités et des Personnes Agées (CODERPA – county-level department for pensioners and the elderly) • L'Office des Personnes Agées de Belfort et du Territoire (OPABT – the Belfort area office for the elderly): • confederation of OAPs clubs which are very active in this county • independent doctors and the paramedical professions • independent nurses, social funding sources

	• pension funds, the Institut Universitaire et Technologique (IUT – technology university)
Objectives and missions	• reception and time to listen (by phone and in person) to OAPs and their families thanks to a one-stop-shop system • information, advice and support with a view to making elderly people's everyday lives better, to do with prevention, legal matters, housing, transport, quality of life and comfort, social and cultural life, the provision of services to keep people in their homes and residential care over the county • assessment of needs in the home • creation of a personalised aid plan by those services responsible for keeping people in their homes (using gerontological counsellors in particular, but also via other professionals if asked to become involved) • monitoring and proposals for changes to the aid plan for a referral case (who did the assessment, coordinator of services and person responsible for overseeing changes in the individual's situation) • complementary mission of the gerontological confederation: participation in the definition of a county-wide study group in the form of reflection and discussion (a sort of observatory of the needs and actions to be developed throughout the area
Number of staff	9 sector-based gerontological counsellors (full-time), from different professional horizons (nurses, social workers, social and family sector) 1 person for the tele-alarm (80% working time) 2 secretaries (full-time)
Tools	Meetings currently take place but are in the process of being validated by the CLIC: • The guidance committee, a sort of observatory at county level bringing together institutional partners who tend to be involved with the CLIC. Its mission: – to analyse and organise the network of institutional and professional partners from the gerontological sector – to consider the needs of the elderly in the county – to fix objectives and means of functioning for coordination – to identity difficulties encountered in the coordination of gerontological initiatives • The CLIC bureau, or the Bureau of Directors (county council, establishments), oversees the implementation of guidelines identified by the orientation committee through meetings. It solicits the support of the gerontological confederation which encompasses all those involved: once per month

263

		• The coordination and monitoring unit: this is individual coordination (at least 2 operations in the home). It carries out assessments, defines aid plans, implements and coordinates the different aid services: 2 hours per month
Strengths		• one-stop-shop with good availability (5 days per week) • county coverage, small area (60 km^2), meaning the gerontological professionals involved have better intelligence and partnership work is encouraged, as is the setting up of information relay points • resources made available (9 gerontological counsellors) • setting up of thematic discussion groups • setting up of a training programme for home help assistants (pre-qualification), equivalent to 130 hours of initiation (130 trainees per year) + CAFAD (home help) certificate training
Weaknesses		• small network – everybody knows everybody else, lack of new blood • it takes a great deal of time to enter into a coordination: it was quick for professionals working in the home help field and establishments. On the other hand, we are starting to see the integration of independent doctors, but these are very early days • lack of candidates as home help assistants: poor recognition for this type of work • 101 communes in a small county, meaning lots of dispersion and time required to coordinate actions and negotiate with the local politicians
Evaluation results; Keywords		No evaluation to date. Some are planned within the framework of CLIC One of 20 experimental sites due for evaluation -> evaluation in progress Retired – proximity – one-stop-shop – political will

A6 Réseau Gérontologique du Pays de Retz (Loire Atlantique)

Project initiators	1 hospital doctor (St Nazaire) and GPs Managed by an association operating under the 1901 law on associations, bringing together professionals from the gerontological health sector "Soubie"-approved network, November 2001
Institutional partners	Agence Régionale d'Hospitalisation (ARH – regional hospitalisation network) Caisse Régionale d'Assurance Maladie (CRAM and CPAM – regional social security health insurance scheme) County council Hospital establishments in the area Independent health professionals (doctors, nurses) Hospital doctors
Professional partners	Health care and social establishments for the elderly
Number of staff	A part-time secretary RQ: GPs are paid on the basis of the audits carried out (260 €/year); the social workers are paid by the institution they are affiliated to (CPAM or county council)
Tools	• for the identification of candidates
Weaknesses	• unfavourable context for the launch of the network (GP strike, and they are major actors in the candidate identification process) • "vulnerability" of mobile medical care: doctors are "independent" people who are not easily integrated into a network – political difficulties, in particular with the Allocation Personnalisée Autonomie (APA – personalised independence allowance) • the network enables the actions of the professionals to be coordinated, but because the funding comes from different sources (ARH, CRAM, county council), there is a tendency to compartmentalise it
Evaluation results; Keywords	No evaluation to date, but one is planned and budgeted for in the project Health care network – multi-disciplinarity – proximity – time/motivation

265

A7 *Permanence d'Accueil et d'Orientation Gérontologique* (PAOG – Permanent Gerontological Reception and Orientation Service), Drôme

Project initiators	Crest Hospital and the county council (social services) Created in October 1995 as a CLIC project
Institutional partners	Hospital County council Representatives of the CCAS (community social action centre) Municipalities Caisse Régionale d'Assurance Maladie (CRAM – regional social security health insurance scheme) Mutualité Sociale Agricole (MSA – agricultural social mutual organisation) Union Départementale des Affaires Familiales (UDAF – county family affairs union)
Professional partners	ATMP Directors of retirement homes Crest medico-social centre Mutuelles de la Drôme, home help services Director and departments of Crest Hospital Firms of independent nurses Home help services Domiciliary nursing services Physiotherapists, GPs
Objectives and missions	• reception and information for the elderly and their families • multidisciplinary assessment of needs at the person's home • orientation • creation of a personalised aid plan • coordination of services required by the individual • training and exchanges (project to help the helpers)
Number of staff	1 half-time coordinator 1 secretary
Tools	• 2 open days, "blue week" reaching out to a large number of people • consultation meeting (once per month) with professional partners • gerontological group (twice per month) • coordination meeting with hospital and geriatric services • preparation of an information brochure for the elderly

	Existing files: • welcome form in the geriatric ward (person's ID, medical questionnaire, AGGIR chart) • social file • explanation of the AGGIR chart • liaison report outlining services in place
Weaknesses	• lack of time and means: a half-time coordinator, secretariat and psychologist • heavy workload of independent nurses and lack of space in the domiciliary nursing service SSIAD are problems when it comes to returning people to their own homes
Evaluation results; Keywords	The site has been the subject of a CPDG study Gerontological network – multidisciplinarity

List of Acronyms

AGGIR:	A new French assessment tool
APA:	Personalised independence allowance
ARH:	Regional health state agency
CCAS:	Communal and municipal centres for social welfare and social affairs
CHU:	University hospital centre
CLIC:	Local information and coordination centres
CNAM /CRAM:	National/regional social security insurance company
CNAVTS:	National pension fund for workers (employees)
CNRPA:	Committee for retired and elderly people
CODERPA:	County level committee for retired and elderly people
EHPAD:	New acronym for institutional care structure for vulnerable older persons
ILCG:	Local gerontological coordination body
MSA:	Mutual insurance company for agricultural workers

CHAPTER 7

Providing Integrated Health and Social Care for Older Persons in Germany

Günter Roth, Monika Reichert

1   Introduction

In Germany, social and health care services for the elderly are characterised by marked *fragmentation*.[1] With the growth and differentiation of health and social welfare services for older people in need of care, there have long been complaints of a lack of *transparency*, *coordination*, *efficiency* and *effectiveness* on the part of the strongly specialised subsystems, as regards orientation to quality, results and patients, but also ethical conditions, among other things. These complaints have intensified with the pressing problems affecting financing of the welfare state since the 1980s. The decisive reasons for frequently uncoordinated simultaneous and conflicting projects and for the failure of many models designed to improve coordination and integration of health care and welfare support systems were seen as lying in the subsequent institutional disparities. Such criticism is supported by the recent increase in international comparisons, which show that the German health care sector is extremely expensive, but of at most average quality (WHO, 2000; OECD, 1999), and also by the debate on "competition for locations" and a look at similar debates on reform in other countries.

Corporatist organisation, which has a substantial presence in the German health care system, less so in welfare services, possesses its own strong dynamic and a capacity for persistence, even when set against the increasing efforts to achieve policy reform since the late 1980s. The institutionalised *separation* between the *health care* and *social security systems*, with health, long-term care, pensions and accident insurance and welfare benefits, which has developed in the course of time, has become as firmly established as the gulf between *"outpatient" and "inpatient" care*. In line with the *heterogeneous* organisation of financing and supply, their professional and interest organisations (including doctors, nursing occupations, social work and psychologists) and training courses are also organised *separately*. Here, mention should also be made of the *decentralised* state organisation and the associated antagonism of German federalism and its "interlinked policy trap" ("Politik-verflechtungsfalle"; Scharpf, 1985).

Key features of the way in which health care and welfare services are organised in Germany are the historically based reticence of state organisations *(principle of subsidiarity)* and the high level of "self-management" of implementation. This means that *charitable associations*, most of which are denominational or ideological ("weltanschaulich") in nature, feature relatively strongly among suppliers of welfare and health care services, including inpatient health care, although the number of *private commercial* suppliers and outpatient care have also been increasing in recent times. Another striking feature of outpatient health care is the prominent part played by *licensed medical practitioners* in private practice with the associations of panel doctors ("Kassenärztliche Vereinigungen", KV), who are at the same time responsible for important state-authorised control functions.

Given the aim of the research project PROCARE (defining new concepts of an integrated health and social care for older persons in need of care by comparing and evaluating different national modes of care delivery) this report will first give an overview on the very complex legal and structural framework of health and social care provision for elderly people in Germany, including numerous regulations of financing, stakeholders etc. In this sector there are also descriptions of the main aspects of the process of care provision (Who provides what and on which basis?). As part of the fragmented system of the German health and social care system there exists also a longstanding and broad discussion about improvements in coordination and "integrated care provision" with numerous model projects, which is the theme of section 3. In this section, first the state of research and some definitions of terms of "integrated care" will be outlined, then the longstanding and broad discussion of concepts and models of improvements, before five concrete model ways of working with "integrated social and health care for older people" will be described. Finally, conclusions will be made concern-

270

ing the lessons learned from the situation regarding "providing integrated health and social care for older persons in need of care in Germany".

2 Legal and Structural Framework and the General Discourse on Integrated Care Provision

2.1 Structure of Provision (Regulations, Institutions, Stakeholders)

In Germany, *health, accident, care and pensions insurance* on the one hand and *public social welfare* schemes on the other are, in particular, involved in the provision of social and health care services for the elderly.[2] All areas are covered by federal legislation, supplemented by regulations at the regional level ("Länder"). As a general rule, the federal legislation requires a high level of consensus between the Federal State and the Länder, which in some cases restrains fundamental changes. One reason for this being is that the composition of the majority in the Federal Council (Bundesrat) is often the opposite of that in the Federal Parliament (Bundestag). In the area of social security, the ensuring and organisation of provision are largely left to be "self-managed" by funds and supplier associations (e.g. medical associations or hospitals), which conclude framework agreements and detailed regulations for contract drafting, financing and organisation at the regional level (Bäcker et al., 2000: 51 ff.).

2.1.1 Health Insurance

In Germany, *health care* provision is dominated by *panel doctors* (acting as small businessmen) and their associations (KV). The latter are not only responsible for outpatient provision on the basis of contracts with funds, but they also influence and coordinate other services and systems. For example, a referral by a doctor who is licensed by the association of registered doctors is required for inpatient treatment at the health insurance fund's expense and, conversely, other suppliers, such as hospitals, are largely prohibited from providing outpatient treatment. The 23 regionally (at the "Länder" level) structured associations of registered doctors, whose members are panel doctors (compulsorily if they settle accounts with social health

271

insurance), are, together with the federal and regional associations, subject to medical self-management, and only to *legal* supervision by the competent regional authorities and the Federal Minister of Health. The medical associations are responsible for ensuring provision (in which they have to work with the funds), and they conclude group contracts with the funds covering services, appraisals and remuneration. The association of registered doctors then settles up with the panel doctors. It also monitors their activities and is responsible for planning of requirements (in respect of doctors, large-scale equipment, etc.) in conjunction with the funds. On the other hand, the Länder are responsible for planning of hospital requirements and provision (investment costs), which again results in financial problems for incentives and coordination problems.

In 2000, the associations of doctors and of suppliers (e.g. charitable associations, hospital groups) were faced with 420 independent (traditionally based on corporate or professional groups, "Stände") *health insurance funds* (STABU, 2001: 468), whose self-management function is exercised by a management committee composed of equal numbers of employee and employer representatives. While the scope of the statutory health insurance funds' services is extensively laid down by legislation, in recent years there has been an increase in the funds' management authority and in competition among them (Bäcker et al., 2000: 54).

In Germany, *benefits in kind* are to the fore in public health care services, i.e. medical and dental treatment, hospital care and pharmaceutical supply, which account for approx. 85% of overall expenditure. Policy holders are not involved in the financial processing, and simply identify themselves with their insurance card on admission to provision. Hence there is a potential for patient data to be exchanged and for coordination of provision to be optimised. This has often been discussed, but is impeded both by fear of restricting freedom and the right to self-determination and by various organisational interests.

A number of reasons for the lack of efficiency and effectiveness in health care provision, i.e. for "inappropriate and over- and under-provision", are due to this corporatist structure. In this context, particular importance is attached to a variety of *coordination problems*, especially between the outpatient and inpatient sectors (SVRKAG, 2002). The problems include the mixing of commercial concerns with professional responsibilities and the obligation in respect of or assumption of the public interest, in the context of a monopolistic self-management of the providers. The suppliers thus determine the instance and scope of service and influence framework conditions and budgets. Here, the well-known problems of excessive demands resulting from "moral hazard" intensify the overall difficulties (Mager, 1996; Rothgang, 1997: 97-126).

Nevertheless, there have been many – often rather half-hearted – *reforms* in the health insurance field since the mid-1980s. For instance, with the 1992 Law on the structure of health care (Federal Law Gazette Part I, 1992: 2266 ff.) the right of policy-holders to a free choice of funds and *competition between funds* was introduced as from 1996. To date, however, this has largely been established *without* the relevant competition among suppliers and according to prevailing opinion, without equal conditions for competition,[3] so that funds have above all sought to "take the pick of the bunch", i.e. they have competed for rich young contributors, and there is still a great deal of scope for increases in efficiency (SVRKAG, 2002). Moreover, health reform resulted in the introduction and expansion of the patients' own contributions, limitations in services provided, as well as various attempts with legal limitation and control of sectorial *budgets*. In addition to such reactive measures of *curbing cost expansion* (Eberle, 1998; Meyer, 2002), which are usually successful only in the short term, the recently introduced billing of expenses according to diagnosis-related groups (DRGs) in hospitals (see below, 2.2) and the regulations passed with the health reform law 2000 (Federal Law Gazette part I 1999: 2626 ff.) for "integrated care" (§§ 140 ff. Code of Social Law V) offer innovations which could have a more structural impact.

This report is concerned primarily with the regulation for "*integrated care*" according to § 140a-h Code of Social Law V, whereby for the first time the outlined cartel of standardised services that are provided based on the group contract on the health insurance side is broken down experimentally. Thereby competition on the side of the providers and the health insurance companies is intensified in this sector and the integration of the forms of care is pursued (Korenke, 2001: 268 f.). Accordingly, health insurance companies can conclude contracts for "integrated care" directly with selected cross-sector provider networks (physicians in private practice, hospitals, outpatient care and rehabilitation services, etc.), mostly without participation of the associations of panel doctors (KV).[4] This is connected to expectations of increasing efficiency through increased competition, on the one hand, and the integration of care systems (e.g. outpatient and inpatient care), on the other hand – repeated examinations, unnecessary referrals, selective

273

treatment strategies, revolving door effects, etc., which involved in particular multi-morbid older persons, should thus be avoided (Schulz-Nieswandt, 2000). The *opponents* of the regulation (e.g. the KV, Weber, 2001) stress that the reform increases the negotiation power of the health insurance companies one-sidedly, whereby these are primarily interested in curbing cost expansion, so that, with reference to the USA and the health maintenance organisations (HMOs), the result would be ruinous competition and decline in services. Moreover, reference is also made to the familiar weaknesses of a market economy organisation of health care services and advantages of corporatist control (e.g. low transaction costs, similarity of care) (Weber, 2001). Dangers are also seen in the fact that risk selection and information deficits of the clients could become more intense.

Here, too, the *implementation* of the regulation that was begun hesitantly is still not settled. The main obstacle is seen in the fact that there continue to be different financial regulations and sectorial budgets in the outpatient and inpatient sector (Gerlinger, 2002: 25). Further, it is still unresolved how the relationship between old forms of regular care and new integrated care will look like in detail, and whether panel doctor companies will succeed in bringing their interests to bear on the implementation in order to circumvent the intention of the legislature (Korenke, 2001). A further question is the extent to which the health insurance companies will be able to limit the free selection of physicians by patients participating in integrated care (which is not provided for in the law) and the extent to which it will be possible to interest patients in participating in integrated care. Given the shortage of quality assurance and quality transparency of medical care, the free selection of physicians will be an essential criterion for those involved.

Along with the attempts to integrate or strengthen *competition* in the German corporatist health system, *quality assurance* was considerably expanded beginning with the health reform law of 1989 up till the health care reform of 2000. This has run into problems of acceptance and implementation until now, however, especially with physicians in private practice, among other reasons because of the related increase in complexity and amount of work as well as the lack of incentives and sanctions (Weber, 2001: 256; SVRKAG, 2002: 254). Such defence strategies applied by the physicians in private practice are also reported from numerous *model projects* trying to improve integration or coordination of health and social care, because such projects are often viewed as a "luxury" and as additional burden in addition to the actual (because economically and medically necessary) work

(Kühn, 2001: 22). The new regulation for integrated care also offers, at least theoretically, improved options because it provides health insurance funds with a means of selecting providers also based on qualitative factors and, to this end, to conduct an pro-active comparative information policy (also from the side of the providers). The latter has not been available hitherto even in rudimentary form, because clients have hardly any access to information on the performance of health care service providers.

2.1.2 Long-term Care Insurance

With the enactment of the *long-term care insurance* ("Pflegeversicherung"; in the following: LTCI) in 1994[5] the social security system – in spite of increasing criticism – was further developed in a "path-dependent" way. First, to provide coverage for those in need of long-term care, which was handled previously via social welfare systems (means-tested for the poor), recourse was taken to the "proven solution" of social insurance and, second, a new branch was created. An integration in other systems providing social security (e.g. health insurance) was not considered in spite of numerous references to additional coordination problems, in particular with health insurance and social welfare systems. Furthermore, the criticised outpatient-inpatient dichotomy was unfortunately maintained. During the political decision-making process, aspects of political enforcement, and, paradoxically, reform goals which were to be realised more easily in a new partial system, played a major role (Haug/Rothgang, 1996). On the one hand, the separatist and corporatist system of social security was continued with the LTCI, thus aggravating the problems. On the other hand, a number of essential *reforms* were introduced within the system that must be evaluated partly as experimental field or pioneering achievement in particular in terms of a *market* oriented restructuring of the health system, or even of the entire welfare state. The following aspects can be emphasised as the main *innovations* of the LTCI (Rothgang, 1997; 2000)

1. Introduction of direct *competition* between long-term care providers for customers,
2. *Transfer* of the responsibility for securing care provision to LTCI agencies set up within the health insurance agencies (i.e. not, as in health care, with the providers),[6]
3. Introduction of a "*gatekeeper*" in the form of a medical service of health insurance agencies (MDK) for needs assessment (i.e. to avoid excessive claims, but also to control quality).

275

4.   The legally established *maximum budget* for monetary and benefits in kind (per capita lump sums based on the level of needs and the selected form of service to be provided), which generally offer only *partial* coverage for each case and service type (the health insurance companies' principle of demand coverage was thus not accepted [Rothgang, 1996]), and

5.   last not least, the expanded *legal* instruments, i.e. not only those controlled by self-administration, in order to limit costs (Roth/Rothgang, 1999) and to regulate quality (Roth, 2001; 2002).

According to § 14 Code of Social Law XI, a person in need of care is defined as someone who, due to a physical or mental illness or handicap, requires long-term (expected to be more than half a year) specific forms of assistance (personal hygiene, feeding, mobility and housekeeping). Three levels are defined, depending on the extent of assistance required. Among the *sectorial* services, for the entitled person may choose between a *cash benefit* (attendance allowance) for self-procured informal care and assistance (based on levels: € 205, 410 and 665), and a *benefit in kind* for home care services (up to € 384, 921 and 1,432, in hardship cases up to € 1,918); both kinds of service can also be combined. For care provided in short-term care facilities and in nursing homes, the benefits in kind are much higher: up to € 1,023; 1,279 and 1,432; and in hardship cases up to € 1,688.

Finally there are some vague programmatic regulations for improving the *coordination* of participants (e.g. §§ 8, 12 Code of Social Law XI; cf. Eifert et al., 1999a and b), which have still not taken on a very concrete form. Especially interesting here is also the newly introduced § 8a[7] which allows to create "models" up to a budget overall of € 5 Mio. per year with personal budgets, which means that care provision is given beside the strong frontiers of type of care, i.e. ambulatory or stationary care. Moreover, there exist individual initiatives for improving the care infrastructure due to the "Planning and Promotion of the Care Infrastructure" on the regional level ("Länder") based on § 9 Code of Social Law XI. This also holds true for the general structural conditions which are relevant for "integrated care". Among the regional regulations, those of *North Rhine-Westphalia* deserve special mention. In order to create a more effective coordination of long-term care, this state provided guidelines for setting up neutral consultation offices and *Long-Term-Care conferences* on the local level, as well as for contractual agreements to improve the transition from hospitals to rehabilitation or nursing facilities (Eifert et al., 1999a and b). Similar regulations are found in their initial stages in other regions (Eifert et al., 1999b). Meanwhile, the ambitious goals in North Rhine-Westphalia have encountered considerable implementation problems on the regional and local level, e.g. with implementing binding agreements for organising a seamless transition from hospitals to follow-up care. Apparently, the "smoothing out" or "avoidance" of heterogeneous incentives of institutional macrostructures on the regional micro-level can only partially succeed (Eifert et al., 1999a; Wingenfeld, 1999), an aspect which will be further pursued based on the numerous model experiments shown below (cf. 3). At the same time the legal mistake of allocating costs to various providers and for having refrained from a "monistic" form of financing, must also be considered.

Overall, the regulations of the LTCI Act can be characterised as a *barrier*, rather than an opportunity, to the integration of social and health care services for older persons. The LTCI Act reinforces the *separation* between medical, nursing and rehabilitative care, in-house and inpatient care, layperson and professional care, and preventative, rehabilitative and curative care. This leads to the even more severe "interface problem" which has been discussed for years, especially because of the standardised and limited budgets that are oriented to the narrowly delimited services and to the sector-based, individual service systems, so that necessarily a large number of cost units come into play (Rothgang, 1997; Schmidt, 2002).

277

2.1.3 Services for the Handicapped and Social Welfare Services

Further services for older persons in need of long-term care and for physically or mentally handicapped persons will be provided as part of book IX of the Code of Social Law for the *rehabilitation and participation of handicapped persons* produced in 2001 (Federal Law Gazette I: 1046, 1047, changed on 23 July 2002, Federal Law Gazette I: 2850). Existing lack of clarity is supposed to be limited by this time by regulations that are presented in summary form for multiple social services areas. No fewer than 29 laws concerning services for the handicapped are listed in an information brochure of the responsible Federal Ministry of Labour.[8] Services planned for the handicapped (thus not only, but partly also for older persons) are medical rehabilitation, services for participating in working life and life in the community (§ 5 Code of Social Law IX). The statutory health insurance companies are responsible for rehabilitation, but also the statutory pension insurance (insurance body), statutory accident insurance (Employer's Liability Insurance Association) and social compensation (pension and integration offices; "Versorgungs- und Integrationsämter").[9] In addition, the law mentions the (responsible subordinate) public welfare providers for the first time (§ 6 Code of Social Law IX). For the *coordination* of the still largely unconnected rehabilitation services, *"combined service units"* should be set up according to § 23 par. 1 Code of Social Law IX in all districts and district-free cities as integrative centres for the handicapped where comprehensive consultation could be ensured and all rehabilitation services of the providers could be coordinated quickly.

Finally, various reform efforts have also been surfacing in recent years in the area of *social welfare systems ("Sozialhilfe")*, which serve as a residual network of means-tested social support for individual assistance. Reactive cost-curbing measures also predominated the reforms of the Federal Social Assistance Act (BSHG). Here, financing, organisation and services are primarily under local government; in several regions the states also participate to varying degrees. Traditionally, government-supported charitable or voluntary non-profit organisations (*"Freie Wohlfahrtspflege"*) are playing a dominant role as providers of social services and facilities, while private commercial providers hardly existed prior to the enactment of the LTCI. Those and other simultaneous reforms as part of a *new public management* resulted mostly from financing problems, they had similar goals and a major impact on social services for older persons. Instead of subsequent reimbursements or lump-sum financing of facilities, which had been the general standard until 1994 and had not provided any incentives at all for providers to economise or to increase their output, services and prices were hence supposed to be arranged prospectively by contract and under circumstances of increased competition (Roth/Rothgang, 1999). These reforms, but above all the "boom" of newly-established private providers that started to mushroom following the introduction of the LTCI, resulted overall in a steep *reduction* in *locally provided* social services for older persons. Among the services that were completely eliminated in many regions were the "complementary services" (housekeeping, meals-on-wheels, family nursing, etc.) and those of the so-called "open care of the elderly" (cultural and social programmes for seniors, meeting places, etc.), thus service areas that were not covered by the LTCI. Thus, the LTCI and the "explosion" of private health and long-term care services was used above all by local authorities (partly also by regional authorities) to achieve savings and to re-balance their precarious financial situation, i.e. to retreat from locally supported provision of basic-level supply (*"kommunale Daseinsvorsorge"*; see 2.2).

278

2.2   *Financing*

Regulations for financing are a *basic prerequisite* for improving the coordination or integration of health and social services for older persons. Connected
to this are essential incentives for participant activities, whereby the complicated separate structures in Germany have numerous negative effects.

Total *health expenditures* in Germany for the year 1999 were € 211 milliards or 10.9% of the entire gross domestic product (STABU, 2001: 460;
Deutscher Bundestag, 2002: 394 f.).[10] Of the total expenditures in 1999, more
than half, or € 118.5 milliards, came from the *statutory health insurance* companies and 7% was from the LTCI ; 11% was financed by *private budgets* and
governmental budgets covered 8%.[11] The latter item includes the aid for long-
term care financed by taxes, the net expenditures of which in 1999 amounted
to € 2.3 milliards.

The lion's share of health expenditures is financed by *social insurance*.
This is financed primarily by contributions, *one half each* by the *insured* and
the *employer*, which are assessed based on a percentage of the gross income
up to a maximum limit. The amount of the percentage in *statutory health
insurance* is determined by the health insurance companies themselves, and
in early 2002 it was on average 14% (in 1970 it was still 8.2%), whereby variations of several percentage points occur between the health insurance companies; since the effect of the recently expanded risk structure adjustment,
however, this variation has noticeably decreased. The contributions are assessed independently of risk, and family members are also insured (solidarity
principle).[12]

The contributions to the *LTCI* were legally set at 1.7% of the gross income of employees. Further, *investments* of both hospitals and care facilities
are financed in part by *taxes*. In addition, attention should be drawn to mostly
regionally funded public subsidies (financed through taxes) for various social services and private non-profit organisations for which, however, no
statistics or coherent reports exist due to their generally local, very heterogeneous organisation and financing.

2.2.1 Health Care Services

Among the *expenditures* of the statutory health insurance companies, those
for treatments in hospitals dominated and made up 32.4% in 1999; other
important items were medical and dental treatment (22.1%) and expenditures for medication (24.2%). It should be noted in this connection that about

10% of the insured were responsible for approximately 80% of the costs (Winkelhake et al., 2002). Further, health costs and long-term care needs increase, as is well known, in particular in advanced age, as multi-morbidity, chronic degenerative illnesses and dementia occur more frequently (STABU, 2001: 432; BMG, 2001).[13] Also in view of this situation, efforts to increase efficiency and effectiveness of the health system, i.e. to avoid "insufficient, excessive, and incorrect care" must begin especially with these groups (SVRKAG, 2002).

Invoicing between statutory health care agencies and *physicians in private practice* is generally based on federal legal guidelines as part of the independent administrative agencies based on about 2,500 *individual performances* (fee for services) with uniform assessment standards and points systems (Bäcker et al., 2000: 76 ff.).[14] In connection with a higher value given to technologically expensive services, this creates incentives for excessive specialisation and increases in referrals, dominance of partial analyses instead of integrative results orientation, and overall insufficient effectiveness and efficiency (Schulenburg, 1992). With the Health Care Structure Act of 1992 and the first and second statutory health insurance revision act, therefore, *budgeting* of the total compensation package agreed upon by social health insurance and health insurance companies and of the expenditures for medication and remedies was introduced along with concurrent introduction of liability of contracted physicians for exceeding budgets. This noticeably put a restraint on the trend to quantity expansion (Gerlinger, 2002: 12 f.). In addition to the reforms, a lump-sum compensation for each visit was introduced along with the continued compensation for individual services. Consulting services and personal conversations with medical personnel were upgraded and technical services were *downgraded*. Further, a change of course was attempted by assigning lump-sum compensation to family doctors treating the handicapped, demented, or the terminally ill (Bäcker et al., 2000: 79). A negative consequence of flat-rate budgets, however, is the minimisation (rationing) of services, thus an inadequate provision of care for older persons, especially when budgetary limitations threaten to be reached or exceeded (Gerlinger, 2002: 13).

Moreover, the effects which the 2000 health care reform, above all the regulation for integrated care and disease management programmes, will also have on the financing of services of physicians in private practice who are supposed to get integrated into networks of various providers, is still unclear. In general, however, there is a lever for continuing to break up encrusted and separated financing and incentive structures towards an integration of outpatient *and* inpatient services using *combined* fees (case-based or per capita lump sums) (Deutscher Bundestag, 2002: 442). The harmonisation of the financing regulations in outpatient and inpatient areas is a necessary precondition to succeed with integration approaches, as otherwise basic incentives for integration are lacking and contrary forces continue to exist (Gerlinger, 2002: 20).

With the above-mentioned regulation of the 2000 health care reform for financing *hospitals* via DRGs (based on models in the U.S. and Australia), fees are no longer determined by the traditional, retrospective method based on actual demonstrated expenses that have been incurred, i.e. through per capita daily lump sums, but rather on *prospectively* determined diagnosis and case group-related *lump sums*, independently of the actual duration of stay and costs per case. As a result, backers anticipate an increase in competition, shorter stays and savings. Critics, on the other hand, expect intensified "raisin picking", primarily economically oriented and deficient treatment, rationing, premature discharges with frequently uncertain follow-up care and thus above all further "revolving door effects", in particular for older persons (Sell, 2000; Schulz-Nieswandt, 2000). It seems to be indisputable that the reform, also in view of American experiences, will involve considerably higher demands on the cooperation and outpatient care because patients will be released "quicker and sicker" from the hospital (cf. below 2.3). However, concrete consequences cannot yet be reported as implementation has just begun.

Medication and other aids are distributed in the outpatient area based on prescriptions by physicians in private practice via commercial drugstores; since the above-mentioned health care reforms, certain indications of "minor" illnesses (e.g. common colds) are excluded and increasingly co-payments by patients are being introduced to reduce public spending (Bäcker et al., 2000: 80 f.).[15] Still, the number of medications authorised by the law governing the manufacture and prescription of drugs in Germany remains very high and includes 145,000 preparations (Bäcker et al., 2000: 81). Hospital studies assume that about 22% of prescribed expenditures are for medications of doubtful usefulness (Bäcker et al., 2000: 83). Based on the strong position and advertising activity of pharmaceutical manufacturers, supply-induced increases in demand and thus inappropriate care services can also be assumed in this area. Moreover, deficient qualifications and routines of physicians in private practice, but also cultural aspects or expectations of patients who assess the "success" of treatment based on a specific output such as the prescribed medication, must also be considered as causes.

2.2.2 Home Care Services and Institutional Care

By tradition, community care services and nursing homes in Germany were part and parcel of the residual welfare systems, and thus financed by public (regional or local)[16] budgets and means-tested user contributions. One of the main objectives of the LTCI was thus to shift long-term care costs from local government. Hence, long-term care outside the hospitals is now financed primarily by the LTCI. As the scheme was conceived as a *contribution* to partly cover costs that are due to long-term care needs, however, the tradition of user co-payments and means-tested social welfare contributions has remained as a general feature of long-term care service financing in Germany. With the introduction of the LTCI public budgets for long-term care were about doubled (cf. Rothgang, 1997; Roth/Rothgang, 2001). Total expenditures in 2001 of LCTI made up a total of € 16.87 milliards (www. bmgesundheit.de) while the social welfare systems that until 1995 had covered most costs of long-term care had in 1999 € 2.3 milliards net expenditures on this budget line.

Costs in *nursing homes* are broken down into long-term care costs, investment costs, and costs for board and lodging.[17] Accordingly, the LTCI covers primarily long-term care costs by means of lump-sums according to the three (four) defined levels of long-term care needs. If these budgets are exceeded, which for institutional care is more likely than for community care, the client has to pay from his own financial resources. If these do not suffice, s/he has to apply for means-tested support of the local social welfare office. Prior to the enactment of the LTCI, investment costs for old-age and nursing homes were traditionally subsidised by the regions (Schölkopf, 1999a) and the remainder was paid privately or by social welfare. Since 1995, the regions were supposed to ensure – according to political agreements between the federal government and the regions and based on state legislation (§ 9 Code of Social Law XI) – that at least half of the savings incurred by the local social welfare systems were reinvested to support investment costs for long-term care facilities. Despite considerable savings in social welfare budgets, regions and local authorities, however, did not heed this agreement, so that with this cost item considerable gaps continue to exist (Roth/ Rothgang, 2001). In addition, even with support of investment costs all regions retained more or less the outpatient and inpatient dichotomy and refrained from creating any *cross-sectoral* service and need-oriented support apart from the type of provision (Eifert et al., 1999a and b). In the end, costs for board and lodging in nursing homes remain to be paid by the residents (or by the social welfare system) as well as do costs for further social or health-related services and aids that are not covered, e.g. for housekeeping, by the LTCI. Unfortunately, in recent years it was especially here in the local sector that considerable savings and cuts were made by local authorities in reaction to the LTCI.[18] Overall the result was that even today a significant number of those in need of long-term care remain dependent on social welfare.[19]

The financing of health and social services for older persons in need of care in Germany is thus to a considerable extent separatist, which results in incentives for the various cost units or policies to shift costs and benefits from one area to another (Rothgang, 1997). A problem connected to the *lack of integration* is seen, for instance, in the *rehabilitation* of persons in need of care, which represents an important objective of the LTCI, but which is due to this disintegration, among other reasons (e.g. qualification deficits of medical professionals), realised to a minor degree only (Deutscher Bundesag, 2002: 570). Rehabilitation is not covered by the LTCI, although it would profit from successful rehabilitation processes, but remains a primary responsibility of pension and health insurances. However, health insurance has no economic incentive for implementing *rehabilitation* – quite on the contrary, in a successful rehabilitation case it would indirectly relieve other insurance agencies from costs. The latter is due to income adjustments which are regulated differently: While a simple adjustment of expenses takes place with LTCI agencies, meaning that extra expenses can be externalised, a risk structure adjustment takes place, occurs with health insurance agencies and this initiates competition. This means that "a patient who is insufficiently supported and treated, who 'wastes away' and only generates costs that can be passed on to other health insurance companies via the expense adjustment of the long-term care insurance, is in any case better for an insurance agency that is oriented to competitive advantages *vis-à-vis* other agencies than a patient who has been supported in rehabilitation at the expense of the statutory health insurance and whose treatment costs remain with the agency itself" (Rothgang, 1997: 161).

Among the outlined general structural conditions, the LTCI generates also a "classic" product orientation, i.e. *adopting* performance-oriented serv-

283

ices in the *quickest manner* instead of an "activating" and "understanding" long-term care that is oriented to the maintenance and recovery of self-care.[20] Prevention and above all interaction with, as well as the support of, self-care is less often rewarded than the *adoption* of long-term care in traditional, encrusted and often outdated structures.[21] Integration could, to that extent, only succeed with person- and needs-oriented overall budgets that are supported *independently* of existing care structures (cf. Schmidt, 2002). In this connection according to the supplement law for long-term care benefits or services "Pflegeleistungs-Ergänzungsgesetz" from 20.12.2001 (Federal Law Gazette I No 70, p. 3728, 3733) and here the new paragraph 3 of § 8 SGB XI the long-term care insurance companies could promote model projects up to € 5 millions per year, especially for personal budgets and new forms of housing for persons in need of long-term care.

The system of price negotiations and reimbursements between long-term care services and facilities as well as statutory health insurance agencies underwent reform in recent years, but not in an integrative direction. In community care, reimbursement is handled mostly (80%) through service-packages systems and until now with fixed point systems that are usually consistent on the regional level – partially differentiated by associations,[22] to a lesser extent (11%) via fee for individual services or according to time spent (7%); in addition, there are combinations of reimbursements by service systems and time spent (8%) (Schneekloth/Müller, 2000: 117). For the providers of community care, similar to the outpatient health care services, generally incentives are created to expand the services offered and to reduce the amount of time spent on individual services (Schulenburg, 1992). In the institutional sector, traditional per diem rates are still paid based on the level of care. However, while prior to the enactment of the LTCI the *subsequent* complete cost recovery through the social welfare systems was dominant, a limitation of costs was the primary goal of *prospectively* agreed-upon compensation, guidelines for highest increase rates, introduction of profitability checks, and an extensive standardisation of services and their costs (Roth/Rothgang, 1999). As ever, costs and "prices" are usually determined administratively in collective negotiations between provider associations and purchasers, and not as a result of market mechanisms. Persons in need of long-term care and their relatives and representatives generally do not participate in the collective negotiations.

2.3   Process of Care Provision

2.3.1 Demand and Provision of Care

As a starting point for the long-term care of older persons it should be observed that *self-help* and family-based or informal long-term care today still rank far above professional care both as a general expectation and in their empirical quantitative significance.[23] Currently, care of older persons in Germany as in other industrial nations is still performed predominantly free of charge by female family members at home (cf. Jacobzone, 1999: 12). Out of a total of 1.9 million persons entitled to LTCI provisions in 2001, almost 70% were cared for in their own homes; 50% received attendance allowance for informal assistance they arranged for themselves, i.e. a lump-sum cash benefit to be used at their own preferences, 29.7% institutional care, 8.4% professional community care, and 10.5% a combination of community care and attendance allowance; the rest is assigned to respite care, day or night care services and short-term care. From the about 1.3 million persons cared for at home, 55% were assessed in level I, 35% in level II and 10% in level III. The percentage of those seriously in need of care at level III who were cared for at home has decreased in recent years. The demand for long-term care can be attributed to a considerable degree to the loss of mental abilities or "gerontopsychiatric" problems. This holds true, e.g. for 63% of those at level III, 47% of those at level II and 40% of those at level I (Schneekloth/Müller, 2000: 48).

  The number of personnel in *outpatient geriatrics and home care services* has expanded enormously since the 1980s, in particular since home care services were financed by the social health insurance in the late 1980s and since the LTCI came into effect in 1995, where annual growth rates in home care services were noted up to 10% which, however, by late 1999 had markedly declined (Schölkopf, 1999a and b; Roth, 2000a and b; Fretschner et al., 2001; Roth, 2003). In late 1999 there was a total of 184,000 persons employed in about 11,000 community care service agencies with care contracts according to LTCI (STABU, 2001: 477). The services provided and the demand for health and social care services, when compared with the leading European countries, the northern European welfare states and the Netherlands, where around 10-20% of the elderly population take advantage of such services, are still rather underdeveloped.[24] Beyond this, it is unclear how many facilities and personnel are available in other local social services and facilities (e.g. housekeeping services, geriatric meeting centres, etc.). However, mention was already made of the tendency to dismantle the local public funding of these services in reaction to the LTCI.[25]

Finally, the 8,800 *nursing homes* with a total of 645,000 beds (1999) and 441,000 employees (a quota of provision with about 5,5% of the elderly in the age of 65 and more) as well as the 2,200 hospitals with 565,000 beds and 1.1 million employees (including 111,000 physicians and 416,000 nursing personnel) should also be mentioned (STABU, 2001). But the number of beds in hospitals has fallen from 618,000 (1994) to 565,000 (1999), or only just 80% of the capacity of 1980. The number of beds per 1,000 inhabitants has decreased from 6.91 (1990) to 5,98 (1999). The average stay of patients in hospitals in 1999 was 10.5 days and just 60% of the value of 1980; in 1994, it was still 12.7 days (STABU, 2001).

It seems certain that *in the future* both the need and the demand for outpatient health and social services for older persons will continue to grow for reasons of demography alone. While the accuracy of individual prognoses remains uncertain (Fretschner et al., 2001; Blinkert/Klie, 2000, 2001; Rothgang, 2001; Jacobzone, 1999) social and cultural changes such as the rise in number of gainfully employed women, the transformation of family structures, the increase in persons living alone and the "modernisation" of societal relationships in general, will call for additional efforts to extend the supply structures. In Germany, the number of persons receiving home care as a percentage of all persons entitled to the benefits of the LTCI has decreased sharply in recent years and the share of those cared for by professionals showed a strong increase (www.bmgsbund.de). The demands for coordination and integration of different types of services increase accordingly.

2.3.2 Public vs. Private Services and Regional Variations of Care Provision

As already mentioned, ideologically ("*weltanschaulich*") oriented *charitable private non-profit organisations* traditionally hold a strong position in the area of health and social services for older persons. Their predominance was broken, however, by the health care reforms and above all by the introduction of the LTCI, but also by reforms in the framework of new public management approaches. While *private* commercial providers of outpatient care services from the mid- to late 1980s did not yet exist, in late 1999 they provided already 51% of all home care services (number of facilities) in Germany. Charitable private non-profit organisations provided only 47%, and public (local) providers with a share of 2% had almost disappeared (STABU, 2001: 476). Consideration must also be given to the fact that private commercial providers had on average significantly fewer personnel than did charitable private non-profit organisations, so that the latter continue to provide the largest share of home care for older persons (Roth, 2000b; 2003; Schneekloth/Müller, 2000). Similar, though not as apparent developments can be observed in the institutional sector (STABU, 2001: 448). Due to the competition initiated and intensified by the reforms mentioned, problems arise, however, in terms of the coordination and integration of social and health care services, e.g. when information is merely shared with competitors. Even greater problems result when coordinating bodies are set up, which is discussed in more detail below (section 3).

Finally, the provision of health care and social services in Germany is *regionally* and *locally* very different, which is in particular the result of the fact that government responsibility for a long time was primarily on the regional and local level. First of all, the demand and the provision of community care services in rural regions is generally somewhat less pronounced than in urban areas, where a better coverage can be assumed (cf. Roth, 2000b; Roth, 2003). However, according to data from North Rhine-Westphalia, a "catch up" process of provision structures between rural and urban regions can be observed, so that traditional differences disappear with processes of an ongoing "suburbanisation" (Roth, 2000b). The predominance of specific organisations and provider associations is also regionally very diverse. For example, there are several regions in North Rhine-Westphalia in which charitable private non-profit organisations still provide around 70% of community care services. On the other hand, also in some regions private commercial providers retain a market share of 70-80% (Eifert et al., 1999a: 185 f.).

287

2.3.3 Boundaries of Care Provision and of Professions

Until today, and in sharp contrast to the German care reality, representatives of the mainstay of informal care – if existing at all – have not taken an *active* part in professional and institutional discussions. Therefore, integration models should start in particular with the connection between professional and lay care and the empowerment of users. The domination of institutions was the hallmark of German provision of long-term care for older persons which was traditionally oriented to the clinic and nursing home and did not produce outpatient nursing, social and health services in great numbers until the mid 1970s – apart from physicians in private practice. The contact between professionals and next-of-kin often was and remains to be seriously deficient. In spite of increasing customer surveys persons in need of care and their relatives are still considered mainly to be "troublemakers" rather than "king customers" (Roth, 2001). Empirical surveys also show that the selection of services is marked to a considerable degree by randomness and that the consultation and determination of need on the part of the long-term care services is often seriously deficient, so that inappropriate care of those in need cannot be excluded.[26] This results from frequently discussed problems of the transition between various care facilities and branches, for example in the case of the quick and minimally coordinated discharge from hospital (see 3.). In this connection a general trend in the inpatient sector which is important for outpatient care should be mentioned: the elimination of hospital beds and the concurrent increase in case numbers, and the shortening of the length of stays for patients (Schaeffer/Ewers, 2001).

288   Mention should also be made that social law provides many more incentives to reward and control professional services as a substitute for informal care, rather than to its pro-active support and preventive measures. It must also be taken into consideration that, from the perspective of potential users, professional care services just represent a "second choice" and that generally, especially with older persons, there is inhibition against, or even rejection of, social-political institutions and professional care (Pöhlmann/Hofer, 1997; Giese/Wiegel, 2000), so that they are used only if there are no other options (Brandenburg/Zimprich, 1995; Blinkert/Klie, 1999; Runde/Giese, 1999; Gräßel, 1998a; Kliebsch et al., 2000; Schneekloth/Müller, 2000). In this context, finally, the temporal, physical and mental burden placed on informal carers should be considered (Halsig, 1995; Adler et al., 1996; Gräßel, 1998a; 2000; Schacke/Zank, 1998; Wilz et al., 1999; Schneekloth/Müller, 2000), so that, e.g., nursing courses or other professional programmes that are thought to provide relief, in reality imply additional efforts for family carers.

The lack of integration of health and social services is worsened, as we have shown, by institutional disparities, various interests of associations and federations, and also by conflicting interests, roles, cultures and actual qualifications of *professional groups* (esp. between nurses and physicians) (Döhner/Schick, 1996; Garms-Homolová, 1996a). Time and again nursing sciences criticise the lack of willingness to cooperate with care personnel, above all on the side of family doctors and medical specialists (Schaeffer, 1999: 244 f.). Nursing personnel, with generalised training in social skills and nursing and whose special expertise remains somewhat unclear, stands against the technologically highly specialised physician often working from a limited point of view.[27] In the nursing professions in Germany there are many basic qualification and quality deficiencies, regardless of formal professional degrees (Flügel 1996; Kühnert/Schnabel, 1996; Kühnert, 1999). Thus, 69% of the nursing personnel in outpatient care have completed training as specialist, but specialised methods such as geriatric assessment or a systematic care planning and quality assurance are at the same time mostly unknown or are not used (Roth, 2001). With considerable variations between the qualification profiles of outpatient nursing services, nurses dominate among the personnel with an average of 52%, followed by geriatric nurses with 17%, nursing assistants and geriatric assistants with 10% and others with 5% (esp. social-pedagogical and domestic service training), and 16% of personnel have no professional training (Schneekloth/Müller, 2000: 111, 237).

289

Long-term care has not yet been established as a profession with specialised technical knowledge, academic research etc. and corresponding societal recognition (see: Voges, 2002), in spite of professionals' efforts to obtain independence or self-reliance, an emancipation process, in particular *vis-à-vis* the physician-dominated hierarchy. Corresponding to the differing status of professionalisation, societal recognition and professional positions is the fact that *incomes* of the professional groups in the field of social and health care are also very diverse – though, data on this issue are very unsatisfactory.[28] Differences in status and hierarchy that are increasingly challenged by the nursing professions, undoubtfully complicate the cooperation between physicians and nursing professions. In this perspective, training and access possibilities to care professions, which are differently regulated from region to region, also represent a problem. This affects in particular nursing and geriatric nursing as well as pediatric nursing, which in spite of largely uniform curricula is organised in separate degree programmes, whereby the efforts for integrative approaches (Menke/Oelke, 1999; Richter, 2001) have failed for the time being.[29]

3   Model Ways of Working

3.1   State of Research and Definition of Terms

In Germany, debates about coordination, networking and integration of health and welfare services for elderly people are mainly based on Anglo-Saxon models of *"Care* und *Case Management"*, which are combined with integrating Health Maintenance or Managed Care Organisations (Wendt, 1993; Schweikart, 1999; Engel/Engels, 2000a, b.; Haubrock et al., 2000; Kühn, 2001). The following proposal was made to distinguish between these *terms* (Schweikart, 1999: 81; Ewers/Schaeffer, 2000: 8). The term *"case management"* denotes the coordination or integration of help in favour of the individual case (as a case, i.e. not necessarily as a person) and of his/her immediate personal environment. Conversely, the term *"care management"* denotes the coordination of help and networks of service providers at the level of the general public in a care region. Both concepts, which have elicited wide-spread discussion without producing any final definition of the terms (Kühn, 2001: 46), aim to *improve* the efficiency and effectiveness of care provision systems by means of coordinating and integrating management. It should be of utmost importance to promote and enhance the patient's or client's independence, and his/her ability to engage in self-help. As regards the levels of integration, a distinction can be made between *vertical* (care provision by primary care physicians, specialists as well as in the inpatient and outpatient settings) and *horizontal* levels (medical, nursing, welfare services, etc.) (Haubrock et al., 2000: 83).

To date, there is a paucity of German, but a plethora of American, data available on care und case management and on the myriad model projects for coordination and integration of health and welfare services for elderly people. On the whole, these results tend to be *non-standardised* and un-satisfactory (Green, 1989; Challis/Traske, 1997; Eng et al., 1997; Miller et al., 1998; Foley, 1999). Nonetheless, American research in particular has given rise in Germany to informative discussions about health and welfare services for elderly people. Although the need for research into care management is stressed time and again – in view of the lack of coordination of professional care systems and their intrinsic rationales, which is constantly lamented in the literature – there are only isolated reports of satisfied patients and on the whole mostly disappointing empirical findings. For example, as a result of managed care systems, readmission of patients to hospital after discharge or admission to a nursing home were not less common compared with control groups; indeed, the opposite trend was noted. Likewise, mortality rates, functional capacities, self-care abilities as well as the patients' activities appeared to have shown little improvement; nor was there any reduction in the amount of medication taken or in the costs incurred (Foley, 1999: 6; Green, 1989). Furthermore, managed care apparently confers more benefits on younger patient groups than on the elderly, for whom even particularly restrictive and negative effects were observed. Contrasting to these findings, Eng et al. (1997; see also Schnelle et al., 1999) draw markedly more positive conclusions. They concluded that the rate of admissions to institutions had been reduced by the scientifically accompanied managed-care programme and that costs were also reduced, while high levels of client satisfaction could be recorded, too.

Overall, a comprehensive review of the empirical literature available on evaluation of managed care organisations in the USA attests to the tremendous importance of financing systems (single-service reimbursement or prospective flat-rate fees), indicating that the performance capability of managed care organisations compared with individual medical practices is superior especially if the prevailing conditions could be neutralised (Robinson/Steiner, 1998; cf. Kühn, 2001: 72). Döhner et al. (2002: 18 f.) quote other factors and numerous international studies on geriatric-gerontological case- and care-management measures. The following issues were reported as important factors for success: having a decent amount of time and creating trust between the parties concerned, the enormous importance of interpersonal relationships for the successful outcome of procedures, the relevance of the intensity, duration and continuity of procedures and finally the ability of positive and negative consequences of greater activation and mobilisation of the clients concerned. An interim summary highlights the problem whereby care or case management is always linked to economic distribution issues and to different sets of vested interests, so that e.g. the independence and role of the case manager as an advocate and protector of patients' interests is accorded just as much importance as is the objectivity of long-term orientated evaluation. Most probably, it will be difficult to implement all these aims, when set against the background of the special theoretical difficulties encountered in evaluating health and welfare services, financial restrictions and also in light of the American experiences, where the main goal of managed care was to reduce costs (Kühn, 2001: 38). Likewise, it should be borne in mind that with case management, gatekeeping and cost reductions, specialisation advantages may be forfeited with the risk of insufficient care provision, for instance if, as mostly intended in Germany, the position of the general practitioner is strengthened (Emanuel/Dubler, 1995; cf. Kühn 2001: 42).

Thus, for evaluation purposes there is an urgent need for *process- and outcome*-orientated measurements which should be conducted in large representative settings (with control groups as well as combined longitudinal and cross-sectional analyses), so that the numerous potential influences can be controlled. In Germany, research into care and nursing is comparatively underdeveloped. Accordingly, while the numerous model experiments for coordination and integration of health and welfare services are regularly "evaluated", there is an inevitable preponderance of the model character (subject to extremely unfavourable framework conditions or to a "hostile environment") with small case numbers, and the qualitative interpretative character of action or concomitant research. Furthermore, initiators, submitting entities, sponsors and researchers are often entwined in complex sets of interests and fall prey to the political influence of associations, so that failure of model projects rarely tends to be noted. In Germany, this has hardly ever served to furnish proof of the reliability and validity, representativeness and objectivity of methods and instruments used in research into integrated care provision concepts; nor has it been able to provide a differentiated proof of effects.

3.2 Models of Integrated Care in Germany

In Germany, a plethora of model projects were initiated over the past few years aimed at coordination and integration of the highly fragmented care provision systems. In 1999, the Federal Ministry for Family Affairs, Senior Citizens, Women and Youth (BMFSFJ) launched the model programme "*Futuristic Help Structures for the Elderly*". Following the call for the expression of interest, more than 400 project proposals were made, of which 28% were focused on improving coordination, networking and integration of care systems (BMFSFJ, 2000: 7f.). Furthermore, there are reports of more than 400 physicians' networks and a number of integrated treatment systems (physicians-hospital integration) engaged in discussion of integrated care in the health care sector (§ 140 Book V of the German Code of Social Law – SGB V) (Deutscher Bundestag, 2002: 450; Döhner/Schick, 1996; BMFSFJ, 2000; Ewers/Schaeffer, 2000; Haubrock et al., 2000; Tophoven, 2001).

292

An initial, frequently encountered, approach to overcoming the fragmentation of health and welfare services for elderly people focuses on improvement of the *transition* from the hospital to subsequent care or rehabilitation institutions or other forms of outpatient care (Domscheit/Wingenfeld, 1996; Wingenfeld, 1999). The much-criticised discharge is facing more stringent requirements, set against the background of short and possibly more frequent hospital stays and of the decline in "misallocation" of hospital beds to patients in need of care[30] in the wake of the introduction of the LTCI. It is not unusual that a patient is discharged from hospital at short notice – thus often with increasing care needs or facing care needs for the first time – right before the weekend without having organised adequate provision for domestic care or for rehabilitation and without adequate coordination with the familial self-help facilities, the outpatient or welfare service, general practitioners, department of social welfare, etc. This means that there is a risk of avoidable admissions to nursing homes or imminent readmission to hospital due to inadequate treatment and care (Döhner et al., 2002: 21 f.). Often, in particular the persons concerned and their relatives, and also the nursing services and physicians, have not been given vital information on further treatment,[31] on the available services (nor on prices)[32] or on how to apply for different welfare benefits. In brief, this "wandering about" by patients and the choice of the forms of care provision and of care processes, which to a large extent is governed by pure chance, are an often-described result of fragmented care provision structures (Ewers/Schaeffer, 2000; Giese/Wiegel, 2000; Meier-Baumgartner/Dapp, 2002; SVRKAG, 2002; Schmidt, 2002; Döhner et al., 2002). In order to improve the discharge from hospital, a variety of documents called *"Discharge or Forms or Instruments"* have been compiled at a regional level, with the aim of standardising and improving the exchange of information between hospitals, outpatient nursing services and licensed medical practitioners as well as other parties concerned (Domscheit/Wingenfeld, 1996; Wingenfeld, 1999; Hüning et al., 2000; Krause, 2000; DVSK, 1999; Courté-Wienecke et al., 2000; Hillers, 2000). Critics, however, have stated that merely improving the discharge itself and introducing forms or information channels were too little to achieve a lasting improvement of the health status and to promote the independence of older persons in need of care (Döhner et al., 2002: 20).

Furthermore, special *centres*, *organisational units* (e.g. hospital social services) or *multidisciplinary geriatric teams* were set up, composed either of hospital personnel or of staff from different organisations. Their much-discussed approach is to reinforce the integrating role of the *general practitioner*,

293

who should act as a "navigator" or gatekeeper in care provision, but often also in collaboration with geriatric multidisciplinary teams or centres (SVRKAG, 1995; Döhner/Schick, 1996; Förster/Nottenkämper, 1996; Döhner, 1998; Kauss et al., 1998; Meier-Baumgartner/Dapp, 2002; Döhner et al., 2002). One central problem that has emerged so far derives from the fact that physicians are not receptive to the model endeavours to improve coordination or integration. This is often due to lack of financial incentives and legal obligations, inadequate qualifications and poor understanding of the problem involved, but also due to conflicts of interest. This reticence is revealed for example by the frequent complaints about physicians' poor participation in such model projects (Garms-Homolová, 1996a: 41; Döhner/Schick, 1996; Garms-Homolová/Schaeffer, 1998; Döhner et al., 2002).

Other projects are developing integrated care and organisational concepts of joint working by means of *health care centres* or multidisciplinary *service provider networks* with a comprehensive range of services being offered as *a package,* e.g. outpatient surgery, outpatient rehabilitation, nursing, domiciliary services, etc. (Haubrock et al., 2000: 107f.). It thus seems premature to have closed down the much greater integrated care provided by the *polyclinics* in the former German Democratic Republic after the reunification of Germany (Deutscher Bundestag, 2002: 455). While these models are being ascribed more importance, especially as a result of the aforementioned regulations governing "integrated care" within the framework of the Health Reform in 2000, little progress has been made yet in implementing them. Underpinning this approach, new integrated *forms of living and care* such as "supervised living" ("sheltered housing"), are being offered. However, there is hardly any statistical information available on these, despite the success scored by these forms of care over the past few years. This once again reflects the magnitude of institutional disparities between outpatient and inpatient settings. This disparity is also expressed in the legal issues questioning whether such establishments are to be considered as institutions, thus coming within the purview of the Home Act and home supervision, and receive other forms of reimbursement, sponsorship, etc. (BMFSFJ, 2001: 250 f.). In principle, however, such forms of living and care are reported to enjoy a high level of acceptance among elderly people (BMFSFJ, 2001: 249), because they combine self-determination with care and the advantages of institutional services; however, at this juncture, attention must also be drawn to the possibilities (of which little use has been made to date) for adapting housing conditions or for collective housing for the elderly (BMFSFJ, 2001: 246, 252 ff.). Here, too, the problem is that investment costs' promotion of the regions (*"Länder"*) generally is targeted on *either* outpatient *or* inpatient sectors, while these mixed concepts of living and care are less supported. Here, too, a per-person care budget tailored to the actual need and independent of the form of care would provide an integrative solution (cf. Schmidt, 2002: 305).

Models devised on a broader scale for integration of care provision focus as far as possible on efforts such as the creation of independent advisory, initial-contact and brokerage centres, the organisation of coordinating care conferences, round tables, working groups, etc. (Heinemann-Knoch et al., 1995; Eifert et al., 1999a, b; Schweikart, 1999; Rosendahl, 1999; Wendt, 2000). The first mentioned institutions are supposed to provide advisory and information services, also for the general public, either in an individual case or in general as regards issues relating to care needs and to available care services. *"Care conferences"* or other coordination committees primarily serve to promote the flow of information and coordination between the different organisations, institutions or associations. In a broader sense these also discharge socio-political tasks such as the planning of care services at the regional level, acting as advocate for clients' social welfare, etc. However, in general individual cases are not dealt with here, but rather procedures are to be agreed at a regional or local level, the activities of the different parties coordinated and overall the care structures improved (cf. Rosendahl, 1999).

Finally, other concepts are directly aimed at providing coordinating support to *lay caregivers* and self-help, such as e.g. by organising care courses or interacting with relatives (cf. Prümmer, 1997; Bauer-Söllner, 1997; Plück/ Giersberg, 1998; Schild-Woestmeyer/Dietz, 1998; Ward-Griffin/McKeever, 2000). Another link is the proactive provision of advice to elderly people (possibly before they actually need care) on social policy programmes and services. These are meant to have a preventive or proactive effect.[33] In this connection, it should be underlined that such concepts to reinforce the *self-determination, self-confidence and self-preservation* of elderly people within their social networks are of paramount importance for health promotion and prevention. However, empirical findings show major deficits due to non-existent, poorly developed or – as a result of cost-cutting efforts at the local level – even declining services of that kind (see 2.2).

3.3 Selected Models

Projects selected from the variety of model projects for the integration of health and social care services for elderly people living at home in Germany will be presented below. *These* projects are – whenever possible – founded upon a *comprehensive, scientifically based* concept and follow different strategies from among the basic approaches to model projects shown above (e.g. horizontal and vertical integration, care and case management). Furthermore, they are characterised *by linking* different suppliers or associations thus overcoming competition. In addition, we tried to find models that pursue an integrated action not only by developing "soft skills" such as team building processes or striving for coordination, but also by means of "hard" incentives (e.g. common budgets, legal obligations). In the same way not only soft, *qualitative* but also hard, *quantitative* methods (outcome measures, multidimensional assessment with valid and reliable instruments, baseline-follow-up design, control groups, large numbers of cases) should be applied in the evaluation. Finally, selected models should be characterised by the successful or highly probable transition of the model project into mainstream care provision with a potential impact on national policies. It should be said in advance, however, that current model projects in Germany, although numerous, rarely meet all these criteria, so that, to some extent, markedly lower expectations have to be accepted.[34]

The first two model projects described below have already *been evaluated* and published their results. In both cases efforts are being made to continue the projects. The remaining three projects are taken from the BMFSFJ (2000) model programme mentioned above, for which no results from evaluation studies are as yet available. As mentioned above, out of the 400 proposals submitted in this federal government programme, 20 model projects were selected, at least six of which are of interest to PROCARE and three of which were first selected here. It can be assumed that, due to the effect on the public achieved with the programme published by the federal government, and the high number of project proposals submitted, a discriminating pre-selection for quality has already been made. As the model projects run from 2000 to 2003 we want to show the *aims* and *concepts* of the projects as of to date. In addition, initial interim results are available from the accompanying scientific research (BMFSFJ, 2000; Klaes, 2002). According to these, out of 72 individual measures 38% have been implemented, 13% have not yet been initiated, and 25% have been initiated, with limitations however. In this connection it should be mentioned that integration and case management measures clearly lag behind, generally due to the familiar problems such as, for instance, lack of willingness to cooperate on the part of independent practitioners, competition, lack of qualifications, differences in culture and institutional structures[35] (Klaes, 2002: 25 f.; Potthoff, 2002: 27 ff.; Törne, 2002: 38).

3.3.1 Outpatient Geriatric Team Project (Projekt Ambulantes, Geriatrisches Team – PAGT), Hamburg

PAGT was promoted as the model plan by the BMFSFJ and the "Johanna and Fritz Buch Memorial Foundation" between late 1992 and late 1996 in Hamburg and carried out with accompanying research at the University of Hamburg (Döhner, 1998; Döhner et al., 2002). Currently efforts are being made, however, to re-apply and continue the model.[36] Its *aim* was to improve the quality of life of the elderly and their relatives by stabilising or establishing a social network, preventing or at least delaying disease becoming chronic, preventing or delaying the need for care, preventing or reducing clinically unnecessary admissions to hospital, reducing periods spent in hospital, avoiding an unintended transfer to a nursing home and, if possible, returning the person to his/her own home and reducing the mortality rate. In order to put this into practice a *combined approach* of *care and case management* was chosen, for which three teams were formed in two model regions with one or two general practitioners, one person to attend to the patient (case manager) and a regional coordinator (care manager). The latter was a member of all teams. Further representatives, e.g. of the nursing service were included in the teams as necessary. The teams were to autonomously develop means of coordination without numerous guidelines. Various instruments were used for *evaluation*. At the beginning the patient underwent a short screening by the doctor (following Barber/Wallis), in order to determine high-risk patients. Afterwards a geriatric assessment was performed at two moments in time (baseline, follow-up), complemented by intensive interviews with patients. Furthermore analyses were undertaken using interviews, group discussions, patient records and other sources.

Overall 446 patients were screened, 131 of which (28%) were identified as high-risk patients.[37] 89 patients (68% of high-risk patients) were included in the accompanying research, as some could or would not take part. Accordingly, after informed consent was obtained, a home visit with a multidimensional assessment was carried out as a basis of an initial situation analysis and a respective care plan. Thereupon the patient caretakers took over their work, progress was discussed in monthly team sessions, plans were modified as necessary etc. The assessment showed that their need for help (according to self-assessments) and current demands were not covered, especially with respect to assistance in structuring free time, physical therapy and mobility/transport (Döhner et al., 2002: 109). Deficiencies became also apparent in the missing adaptation of sanitary installations to the requirements of elderly people (Döhner et al., 2002: 101).

After having got acquainted, roles and duties had been assigned, the team entered into a routine phase, during which occurring conflicts were settled – with the help of the coordinator's moderation some work processes were modified (Döhner et al., 2002: 129). Interviews showed that the expectations of staff with respect to qualification, a higher degree of work satisfaction and confidence in dealing with patient and coordination problems were satisfied. Medical doctors, for example, acquired a deeper insight in problems such as incontinence, which are too rarely discovered and receive too little attention. Furthermore, new ideas and improvements in care services were developed, e.g. in relation to a lack of coordination and planning of activities (see Döhner et al., 2002: 137 f.). This is exactly where major problems in community care services occur as, on average, at least four different professionals are caring for one person in need of care (Roth, 2001). In two of the three practices moreover, case discussions with representatives of community care services took place after the project was concluded. Nonetheless there are obviously critical findings on cooperation. For instance, reference is made to the duration of, and importance of forming relationships of trust and to the respective personal prerequisites (Döhner et al., 2002: 137). Thus it was underlined once more that permanent functional coordination and integration needs institutional standardisation, formalised work routines and a set of incentives in order to overcome defensive behaviours due to competition or fears of control.[38] What was strongly emphasised by the project was the need for an outreaching consultation of clients and coordinated care. However, especially with personal consultation it was noticed that resistances on the side of the clients had to be overcome (Döhner et al., 2002: 110-120).

A final assessment could be performed in approx. 50% of the 89 patients (the others had died or moved) (Döhner et al., 2002: 179). A comparison of the two measurements (N=43) demonstrated significant deteriorations

298

in ADL scores and in mental and emotional health as a result of the problems of very advanced age. All other areas remained without significant
change. In addition the patient's subjective experience also showed a significant reduction in satisfaction with the availability of social support
(Döhner et al., 2002: 181 f.). It must be taken into account, however, that
generally decreasing health potentials in the clients studied had led to a significant increase of needs, which eclipsed the expansion in supply that could
be realised during the project. This meant that initial expectations of the
model project in relation to improvements in patients' quality of life could
not, however, be fulfilled (Döhner et al., 2002: 199). Nevertheless success was
reported such as the preventive effect of housing adaptations and the priority of care at home, even with persons in terminal care. Due to the *low number
of cases* and the lack of a *control group,* these results, like others reported on
the basis of individual cases, including achievements like the avoidance of
hospital admission, and nursing homes and the shortening of hospital stay
(Döhner et al., 2002: 189-200), are hardly worth assessing. Finally the project
confirms that, should such approaches be successfully transferred to mainstream care, economic incentives and legal regulations, e.g. concerning the
process of screening or assessment, and coordinating procedures, such as
case and care management, are indeed indispensable. Still, these kinds of
basic institutional innovations have not yet been put into effect by Federal
Law. For this reason it is hardly surprising that, in the case of the PAGT model
project, acceptance into routine care has not been successful because financial support was not realised (Döhner, 2002: 218).

3.3.2 Geriatric Network (Geriatrisches Netzwerk) Hamburg

The fundamental assumption behind the work of the Geriatric Network
(Geriatrisches Netzwerk) model project, which is likewise supported by
BMFSFJ, is that geriatric assessment reduces mortality, and can extend the
period in which elderly patients live independently in their own homes. In
particular the problem of "hidden morbidity" was to be addressed (Meier-
Baumgartner/Dapp, 2002: 19, 22). To this end intervention should be preventative and take place within outpatient health provisions (family doctor) and also through home visits (by a social education worker from the
advice centre) before either hospital care or rehabilitation or admission to a
nursing home become necessary. The attempt to achieve this was done by
handing on the geriatric screening as proposed by Lachs (cf. Meier-Baum-

299

gartner/Dapp, 2002) from the geriatric hospital to family doctors. The screening was applied and tested as a filter instrument for frequently occurring problem areas among older people. In the case of a positive geriatric screening, the use of various other assessment procedures (Meier-Baumgartner/Dapp, 2002: 46-98) and of social advice in the geriatric hospital was tested. The resultant coordination and cooperation, responsibility for geriatric matters and further evolution were observed and documented, as were the clients (process, independence, quality of life) and their relatives (burden).

12 family doctors out of 20 were arbitrarily chosen in the region and took part in the 24-month model study (1997-1999), together with a total of 156 female patients (42 of whom participated in the dementia subproject). Also in this case it is planned to conduct a similar follow-up project.[39] Alongside, regular coordination meetings were held in the geriatric hospital, to present key issues and examples of patient cases. A regular exchange of information was organised by means of doctors' letters. A total of 5 screenings were conducted at intervals of 6 months, at times t1-t5, a minimum of 2 social advice sessions, 5 assessments as appropriate, 3 standardised questionnaires to patients, dealing with quality of life and ability to cope independently, and to relatives, dealing with quality of life and the burdens on them. In addition at t1 and t5 family doctors were questioned on the subject of the geriatric patient, the organisation of the practice, geriatric expertise, and any recommendations of the geriatric hospital carried out (compliance). Contacts with patients were quantified and recorded, and measures taken in the coordination and advice centre (t1-t5) and in the subprojects (t1-t5) (Meier-Baumgartner/Dapp, 2002: 50 ff.) were recorded together with time taken. Finally, in the geriatric hospital, regular consultations and case conferences were held.

A total of 133 patients, average 79.4 years, remained until t5 (Meier-Baumgartner/Dapp, 2002: 95, 100). At the beginning and at the end of the project, 80% of the geriatric patients were living at home without an assessment (negative screens). Of those in the dementia subproject 69% were living at home at the beginning of the project, and only 53% remained there at the end. The proportion of those living in care homes rose from 0 to 6% in the first group, and from 9 to 19% in the second group (Meier-Baumgartner/Dapp, 2002: 100). In all groups, but most markedly in the group with dementia, a decline in the ability to cope independently (Barthel index, ADL and IADL) was observed, ranging from mild to severe. Nevertheless, the quality of life of the geriatric patients remained at a relatively constant high level. However, the information provided by the patients themselves was contradictory and must therefore be interpreted with caution (Meier-Baumgartner/Dapp, 2002: 102 f.). When the screening of family doctors was compared, t1 showed abnormalities in the memory category for more than 55% of patients, and t5 for only 45% of patients. This is interpreted as a result of improved clarification within the assessment. Further significant improvements were apparent in sight, and still more in hearing, where figures of $30\%_{t1}$ and more than $20\%_{t5}$ were found, and in social support ($28\%_{t1}$, $19\%_{t5}$). An *increase* in abnormalities on screening was found in the IADL, in activities ($20\%_{t1}$, $35\%_{t5}$) and multiple prescription drug use ($26\%_{t1}$, $35\%_{t5}$), the average number of drugs taken being 3.9-5.4. In addition, on average 5_{t1}-7_{t5} diagnoses were given, with a consultation frequency of 31 doctor-patient contacts during the 24 months (Meier-Baumgartner/Dapp, 2002: 104-113). The questionnaire on social circumstances showed a relatively constant high average value and a small but significantly *increasing* proportion of patients below critical values ($10\%_{t1}$-$16\%_{t5}$). Time expended on social advice was on average 4 hours per patient in 24 months (Meier-Baumgartner/ Dapp, 2002: 122-125).

301

Among those assigned following screening to the dementia subgroup, mild to severe dementia was confirmed in approximately half on geriatric assessment. In the other half only slight cognitive disorders were found. Status remained stable in 65% of the total group between measurements. In 35% an increase in the disorder was found, with particular increases in the groups with moderate or severe dementia (Meier-Baumgartner/Dapp, 2002: 136 f.). Out of those initially assessed as having only slight cognitive limitations, 15% developed dementia. This was judged a positive outcome in comparison to other research results, where the figure is 25%. It is ascribed to the effect of the intensive attendance associated with the project (Meier-Baumgartner/Dapp, 2002: 157). The categorisation made by the family doctors was predominantly confirmed by the assessment; nevertheless at t1, dementia had been categorised as simply mild forgetfulness in 29% of cases, and at t5 the figure was as high as 36%. The reverse occurred to a small degree, with some false positives (ibid.: 138).

Overall, geriatric screening (modified as proposed by Lachs) is claimed to have proved its worth, it could be incorporated into practice without difficulty, met with a high level of acceptance, and was in most cases also used by doctors for patients who were not participating in the model project (Meier-Baumgartner/Dapp, 2002: 152). On the other hand, the value of the assessment tool was judged to be slight by the family doctors, because it was felt to provide few new insights, although the modules measuring cognitive abilities were judged to be enlightening. Similarly the recommendations of the geriatric hospital were only in part put into practice by the family doctors as a result of the assessment, although 80% of them judged these positively. The work of the social advice centre, on the other hand, was judged overwhelmingly positive by the family doctors, because it was found to be supportive in view of the lack of time for organisation and social needs, stated to be a pressing problem (ibid.: 155). The problem of lacking financial incentives for advice in the scale of physicians' charges was reported once more. Also this project was carried out without a *control group* for reasons of cost, thus, real effectiveness could once more not be proven. Therefore the project indicates the significance of the surrounding financial and institutional conditions for the project's permeation into mainstream provision. This effect must also be judged to be limited in the case of the present project, although it should ensure a greater significant expansion in knowledge and use of geriatric screening.

3.3.3 Praxisnetz Nürnberg Nord e.V., HomeCare Nürnberg[40]

This is a regional association in the city of Nuremberg (Bavaria) consisting since 1998 of about 140 physicians in private practice (see in relation to this and below: Kamm-Kohl/Schnetz, 2000: 43 ff.). The idea is to build a comprehensive, integrated care system with the provision of services particularly for older persons in need of care. This involves linking the available provisions and services in the health system and assistance for the elderly, by interdisciplinary quality management and the use and development of state-of-the-art information and communication technologies. A coordination point serves to communicate appropriate, quality-controlled information and assistance to stabilise the quality of life in the home for those in need of assistance. This will also involve the use of economic restructuring at the interfaces of medical, rehabilitation, care and daily need provision, building on the above-mentioned regulations according to § 140 SGB V relating to integrated provision. This project has a particular significance in mapping the way forward, since no such agreements have come to fruition in Germany up till to date, despite the start given by legal regulations. Cost savings are expected, resulting in particular from the optimisation of provision (geriatric advice, with consequent reduction in the length of hospital stays and avoidance of inpatient admissions).

Modules to link and improve medical provision (primary practice, the background service of medical specialists, combined patient health passport and referral letter, quality conferencing and network conferencing) have already been put in place. A set of agreements has been made in Bavaria for the realisation of the medical programme, involving the Bavarian Association of Panel Doctors, the Regional Association of Company Sickness Funds in Bavaria, and the AOK Bavaria. The Federal Association of the AOK has commissioned a scientific study. The project based on this, the "Virtual Home for the Elderly", has as its focus a call centre which deals with all enquiries and provision of services via a single telephone number. This call centre is in process of development, with 2 full-time and specialist staff. In the first instance a market analysis was carried out there, and a data bank constructed as a basis for counselling. In addition to advice and the provision of services, it is planned to carry out assessment (e.g. using the Resident Assessment Instrument, RAI)[41] and Case Management. This is to enable a neutral point of coordination, independent of any providers of services. The advice centre and data bank of service providers and network of participating doctors have already been set up; no information is available as yet about the point reached in establishing the case management as still no evaluation has been published.

303

3.3.4 The Association Structure for Geronto-psychiatric Services in Brandenburg

The Alzheimer Gesellschaft Brandenburg e.V. (Brandenburg Alzheimer Society) and the Fachhochschule (University for Applied Science) Lausitz in Cottbus are the bodies behind the project to develop an association structure for geronto-psychiatric services, in a rural region (Oberspreewald-Lausitz) and a city constituting its own administrative district (Cottbus) (see for the following Neumann, 2000: 146-154). The project design focuses on persons suffering from dementia as the largest group of geronto-psychiatric patients, and on their relatives as carers who often experience an excessive burden and insufficient information, and aims to improve the provision of information, advice, treatment and care. It also intends to benefit the totality of persons suffering from geronto-psychiatric problems, since there has been a lack of information hitherto among medical doctors and professionals concerning the differentiation of clinical assessments of geronto-psychiatric conditions, options for diagnosis and possible remedies ("therapeutic nihilism"), as well as the value of the work done by relatives. A social worker or social education worker was appointed for each region as coordinator for a period of three years, together with a part-time (half-time) project manager. Their task is to promote cooperation between providers by means of newly-established committees, to advice and help in individual cases, and to fill any gaps in provision with services of appropriate quality. To this end, Advice and Case Management for persons with dementia, their relatives and geronto-psychiatric associations is to be established.

The first task is seen as the collection and documentation of individual requirements for assistance, using assessment instruments and the method of case management. Additional areas of activity for case management are given as information about diagnosis, options for the provision of relief and care, advice on questions to do with medical matters, treatment, rehabilitation and legal matters, support in carrying out legal requirements, and the coordination of services. The tasks of the geronto-psychiatric associations are as follows: to contact all providers of relevant services in the region, to organise, prepare, conduct and evaluate association conferences, to supervise the contractually agreed implementation of tasks, to organise monthly case conferences, to produce a handbook of provisions for all partners, to organise and evaluate further training courses as required, and finally to care for public relations. The associations are also being required to develop common quality standards for advice, attendance and care provided to dementia sufferers, to analyse gaps in provision and to develop innovative ways of care. In addition, the project manager has the task to analyse regional features in provision, to develop plans and standards for comprehensive provision for persons suffering from dementia and for carers' respite; further tasks are policy advice, to accompany, direct and evaluate the subprojects, to develop plans for further training, and transfer project results. Finally, this project also aims to disseminate results into mainstream provision by means of a proportionate financing of the association partners, by public sponsorship and by compensation for services rendered on the part of statutory funding bodies and users.

3.3.5 Wiesbaden Geriatric Rehabilitation Network

The aim of the project, which is sponsored by the City of Wiesbaden (Hesse), is to keep the elderly independent and to reduce or remove their need for care (on this and following points see: Haas/Weber, 2000; Weber, 2002). To this end, cooperation is to be improved with a view to geriatric rehabilitation; in particular, the elderly have guaranteed access to this from their own homes. Opportunities for geriatric rehabilitation at home should also arise when medical practitioners in private practice, therapists, geriatric rehabilitation centres and mobile services for the elderly and advisory centres for independent living of the elderly (already available through local authorities)[42] collaborate with the LTCI agencies, and also with the hospital welfare services and the hospitals themselves. Moreover, these measures for geriatric and psycho-geriatric rehabilitation are to be initiated and accompanied by the case management provided by the advisory centre for independent living of the elderly. Although considerable contacts between the advisory centres for independent living of the elderly and the various stakeholders of health services had already been established, practical experience has shown that this is not systematic enough (Weber, 2002: 54). At present, the transition from an acute hospital to inpatient and daily geriatric rehabilitation is subject to qualified monitoring and control by consultant geriatricians from specialist geriatric hospitals. Comparable structures are to be developed and tested for the outpatient and domestic sector.

First, a city project office was set up, an assessment commissioned and a project advisory council installed, with representatives of the various associations. To systemise the flow of information, "standardised selection" was developed as a survey tool to ascertain the personal and domestic situation of the elderly. This tool is used by staff members of the advisory centres or care services[43] and gathers personal and residential data about the elderly. It also keeps information on the objectives from the users' and the professional points of view, points out risk factors and indicates where assistance is already being given. If necessary, a consultation with a geriatrician is recommended. The selected target group are people over 70 years of age who suffer from multiple diseases that limit their function. In particular, the criteria are: change in lifestyle or health problems in the past six months, e.g. need for domestic help or application for provisions from the LTCI; a fall in the past few months; several inpatient stays during the past six months; or application for admission to a nursing home. If at least one of these criteria is fulfilled, the "standardised selection" is applied. This is drawn up in an agreement between the older person and the family doctor. Together with the geriatric consultation and the diagnoses from treatment given so far, this provides an important basis for decisions on how to improve the patient's future care. The project has received broad-based support from the KV (Association of Panel Doctors) Hesse, by their own account, and aroused much interest at the first meeting with family doctors, 60 of whom attended. The prospects for its successful and lasting implementation therefore seem promising (Weber, 2002: 57 f.)

4   Conclusions

Although there have been many and various model projects in Germany to interlink and integrate health and welfare services, specialists have generally been critical, because "in present circumstances such cooperative quality assurance and quality development initiatives tend to be interminable efforts, and prove to be non-viable outside the model context, because the structures which provide the impulse are lacking" (Schmidt, 2002: 294). Garms-Homolová (1996: 41) came to a similar conclusion: "Many attempted solutions have not been followed up, because only some of the "trial conditions" have been manipulated, leaving the true reasons for the inadequate cooperation untouched. Thus, it is now apparent that the establishment of more and more networks and transitional functions has in most cases been less successful than was hoped. The reason is the lack of change in doctors' economic interests and in their resistance to innovation, and especially in the gaps in both doctors' and caregivers' qualifications (not just in their knowledge)". Other projects also report a dismissive attitude and an indifference to cooperation in model projects to integrate health and social services. Döhner (1998: 196) remarks in this connection: "Perhaps there is no project in outpatient geriatric care without its share of complaints about the inadequate integration of the family doctor and poor communication between the various professional groups and institutions." Although the model project initiated by Döhner, the "Outpatient Geriatric Team Project (PAGT)" in Hamburg, was described as successful for all parties concerned, her general assessment of the project reads quite pessimistic (1998: 202) "It has not yet been possible for the PAGT to move from the model stage to the mainstream provision of care. This is not due to the results, which everybody considered very good. Nor was there any lack of commitment by those involved. The many discussions with potential financing authorities (Döhner/Schick, 1996) failed ultimately because responsibility was shunted around in the well-known fashion. Our fragmented system of financing authorities is a decisive obstacle to patient-oriented care, particularly for the elderly, but also for younger persons suffering from chronic illness."

To this extent, reforms to integrate health and social services must be founded on the integration of *financing systems* and the overcoming of *institutional barriers,* especially between outpatient and inpatient care, between health and social services, and between professional and informal care. Therefore, the *fossilised* and *fragmented corporatist structure* of the German health and social service systems would need to be broken down piece by piece, as the regulations of § 140 SGB (Social Welfare Code V) are now attempting to do. Here, outpatient centres (once common in the former East Germany) or health centres could be drawn upon as examples. *Individual budgets* oriented towards objective total personal need rather than the care systems, as hitherto, would provide a fundamental push in this direction. These individual needs could be assessed by a multi-professional team (including informal carers or voluntary representatives) and comprehensive care management. People who need care and their relatives could then, in discussion and agreement with care managers, choose the type of care, processes and suppliers largely by themselves and from one market; always, however, accompanied and coordinated by care managers, who must be as *independent* as possible. This pre-supposes a scientifically-based care management, constantly offering comparative quality criteria and comprehensive information about prices and performance of suppliers and forms of payment. Such approaches have not yet been developed in Germany, as already explained, and it seems that their way is still blocked by many insuperable obstacles and unsolved problems.

    Another special problem lies in the well-known organisational problems of health and welfare systems. Special attention must be paid to the fundamental *assessment problem* and the asymmetrical distribution of information between suppliers and demanders (Akerlof, 1970; Arrow, 1991). Moreover, the quality of personal care services derives from simultaneous production and consumption (*"uno actu"*), its existence necessarily arising from personal relationships and trust. The customer can hardly be said to be sovereign, and problems such as "moral hazard" and external influences come into play (see also Breyer / Zweifel, 1992), making it particularly difficult to control in the sense of "for the good of the whole". This is in fact exceedingly complex. There is, for example, still a tension between *generalists* and *specialists*, which should not be simply glossed over by demanding a "holistic" approach while sacrificing the specialist view. A particular problem with "integrated" control is the organisation of prevention or rehabilitation, which in fact aims to make professional services *redundant*, and thus also targets potential economic sources. For example, there is as yet very

307

little economic advantage for care professionals or doctors to encourage a client towards self-help or recovery, as this would entail a reduction in future income. Another difficult problem is *competition* between suppliers. It is almost impossible, for example, to persuade them to cooperate and coordinate, because this would entail a reduction in their own budgets and consequently disputes about distribution (Kühn, 2001). This is another reason why any stimulus towards prevention and coordination should, for the subjects, first take the form of *self-participation* and *rewards*, and secondly a set of rules, rewards and sanctions (e.g. based on benchmarks) for professional suppliers and case managers. Such systems, however, have scarcely been developed, and, like the multifarious projects to improve coordination and cooperation and the integration of care systems, are far from being adequately evaluated.

Notes

1   Cf. inter alia Döhner/Schick, 1996; Garms-Homolová, 1996a and b; Schulz-Nieswandt, 1998; 2000; Schaeffer, 1998, 1999, 2000; SVRKAG, 2002; Ewers/Schaeffer, 2000, Haubrock et al., 2000; Kühn, 2001; Deutscher Bundestag, 2002; Schmidt, 2002.

2   Just under 10% of the German population are covered by private health insurance, including civil servants. In principle, people can take out private insurance from the compulsory insurance limit of an income of 3.450 € per month, 41.400 € per year (http://www.bmgsbund.de/).

3   To prevent competition from being distorted by a more favourable structure as regards members' health risks, in 1994 equalisation of risk structures was established, under which funds with more favourable risk structures were obliged to make equalisation payments to those with poorer structures. However, the risk structure was not adequately brought into line with morbidity, and this is the aim of the Law of 10 December 2002 reforming the equalisation of risk structures in statutory health insurance (Federal Law Gazette I No. 66: 3465 ff.), for example by means of risk pools and disease management programmes.

4   The regulation follows reforms of the second Statutory Health Insurance Reform Law (Federal Law Gazette 1997, part I: 1520), but goes beyond the structural agreements according to § 73a and model projects according to §§ 63 ff. Code of Social Law and the "networked practices".

5   The "Social Coverage of Long-term Care Insurance Act of 26 May 1994 (Federal Law Gazette I, p. 1014, 2797) went into force by stages. Services for in-home long-term care can be received as of 4/1/95 and services for inpatient care as of 7/1/96.

6   The LTCI Act differentiates, somewhat unclearly, between the care for which the long-term care insurance companies are responsible according to §§ 12 and 69 and the care-providing structure for which the regions ("Länder") are responsible in terms of plan-

ning and support according to § 9; in addition, there are also the local authorities and care facilities mentioned in the vaguely worded § 8, which assigns the task of "working closely together" to the participants and nominates "society's overall" responsibility.

7   With a supplement law to the LTCI "Pflegeleistungsergänzungsgesetz" of 12/14/01 (Federal Law Gazette I, p. 3728).

8   http://www.bma.de/download/broschueren/a712.pdf, 8/14/2002.

9   The latter organisations are in the tradition of social compensation for war veterans and other victims of the Second World War.

10   In 1960, health expenditures in Germany still made up 4.8% of the GNP (Schmidt, 1999: 232).

11   Just as much was apportioned to the private health and long-term care insurance; 2% each was distributed to the pension and accident insurance and private organisations, 4% was borne by employers (STABU, 2001: 460).

12   This principle is restricted, however, by the assessment limit and the possibility of persons of higher incomes acquiring private insurance.

13   Thus, 78% of long-term care recipients in 2001 were 65 years old and above, and also the number of illnesses and health expenditures increase dramatically with age, esp. beginning with age 70; while the average number of illnesses for those aged 20-30 is 1.04, this number increases for those aged 70-80 to 3.4 (Deutscher Bundestag, 2002: 398 ff.; www.bmgesundheit.de).

14   For private physicians, prices are determined by governmental fee schedules. It was already mentioned that patients – except for defined co-payments – are not included in the invoicing procedure between physicians and statutory health insurance companies, thus hampering potential effects to increase efficiency and effectiveness of medical care.

15   In 1999, just under 10% of the expenditures of the statutory health insurance for medication was financed through private co-payments (Deutscher Bundestag, 2002: 452).

16   The most important part of social welfare expenditures is financed by local authorities. However, as most tax revenues are collected on the national level and re-distributed between the regions, it is not possible to give an exact figure for the distribution of social welfare expenditures between the governmental levels (cf. Roth, 1998).

17   In addition, costs of health care and rehabilitation must be considered that are partly the responsibility of the health insurance company or the entities responsible for rehabilitation, and in part privately or through social welfare systems (Rothgang, 1997).

18   The decline in expenditures of "complementary services" in North Rhine-Westphalia between 1994 and 1998 amounted on average to 65% of the initial value, and the decline in expenditures for care of the elderly (communicative, social and cultural programmes such as meeting places) was an average of 25% (Eifert et al., 1999a).

19   As a result of the LTCI, social welfare systems witnessed a decline of clients with long-term care needs, in particular in the community care sector with 67% and in the institutional sector with a decline of 40% between 1994 and 1998; net expenditures for long-term care in social welfare systems were thus reduced by 65% or € 4.3 milliards (Roth/ Rothgang, 2001: 303).

20   Cf. Wingenfeld/Schnabel 2002 for institutional care; to a similar extent this also applies to community care (cf. Schmidt, 2002; Schaeffer, 1999; Ewers/Schaeffer, 2000).

21   Thus, Schmidt (2002: 324), for example, refers in this context to the fact that family members in nursing homes are still considered visitors, not "co-producers".

22   In each service package various types of performance are combined (e.g. in morning and evening care: dressing and undressing, partial or complete washing, oral/dental

care, combing) and assessed via a point system. Due to different areas of overlapping packages between the states, however, a comparison is very difficult. Nevertheless, non-profit organisations in several regions, e.g. in North Rhine-Westphalia achieve higher values per points than private commercial providers (cf. Eifert et al., 1999b; Gerste/ Rehbein, 1998).

23 The desire to be cared for by family members at home is expressed in Germany by 78% of those in need of long-term care and relatives (Schneekloth/Müller, 2000: 63). For the EU: Walker/Maltby, 1997: 105; for the OECD: Kalisch et al., 1998. This desire also results from the fact that the quality of professional long-term care in Germany is often judged to be rather problematic (Roth, 2001; 2002).

24 It is difficult to make a comparison of these data and correspondingly the data of OECD should be evaluated with care. For instance, OECD indicates for Germany in 1999 a quota of 9.6% of those 65 and older using community care services, while the German Federal Statistical Office only reports a quota of 3.1% (12/15/1999, which corresponds to the value of the OECD for 1995 (cf. Hennessy, 1995; Pacolet et al., 1998; OECD 1999; Jacobzone, 1999; Schölkopf, 1999a-c).

25 In addition to nursing services, in late 2000 outpatient care (not only) for older persons had a total of 128,000 physicians and 60,000 dentists (STABU, 2001: 444). For 13.3 million persons aged 65 and older (STABU, 2001) this equals 0.96% physicians per capita which compared to the 1990 figure means a growth of 39%. Other health care personnel cannot be assigned exactly to the target group of older persons and the outpatient area; such personnel includes non-medical practitioners, masseurs, physical therapists, nurses aides etc. from a total of 1.76 million personnel in April 2000, to which another 53,000 pharmacists can be added.

26 Recommendations from acquaintances and family doctors play a more significant role than do service and quality characteristics or prices. The initial consultation by nursing services, according to nursing personnel surveyed (sample throughout Germany, N=533), is less than 30 minutes at 13% of the agencies, and takes longer than one hour at only 15% of them. Only 50% of the nursing personnel affirm the total support of persons in need of care when selecting the suitable care and transition; correspondingly, one third confirmed inappropriate care of those in need for their nursing agency (Roth, 2001).

27 The American Institute of Medicine estimates that each year 98,000 deaths in hospitals occur due to medical errors, which based on the well-founded assumption of similar deficiencies for Germany would mean a number between 25-30,000 (Kühn, 2001: 15). In particular in the area of medication errors, the information problem plays the major role in non-integrated institutions (Kohn et al., 1999, according to Kühn ibid.). It is also assumed, for example, that the usefulness of around half of the medical procedures used in Germany has not been proven (Deutscher Bundestag, 2002: 407 f.). Reference is also made to the lack of willingness on the part of physicians in private practice to participate in continuing medical education programmes, with a surplus of demand for improving in economic skills, i.e. relative to invoicing systems (Kühn, 2001: 21).

28 Thus, physicians in private practice earned in 1996 on average € 8,650 / month in taxable income (Baecker et al., 2000: 79). According to the micro-census (1999), nurses had about € 1,200 net income per month, geriatric nurses only € 1,016 and all physicians combined significantly more than € 2,600 (based on the upwards open-ended top class, which includes most physicians, their actual average income is largely undetermined).

29 The statute on professions in geriatric nursing (AltPflG) as an initially uniform regulation was supposed to become effective on 1 August 2001 (Federal Law Gazette no. 50 of

November 24, 2000). However, by order of the Federal Constitutional Court of 22 May 2001 (ref. no. 2BvQ 48/00), the statute was temporarily annulled, meanwhile accepted by the decision of 10/24/02.

30   Based on insufficient or financially tenable outpatient and inpatient nursing services prior to the LTCI act going into effect, a large number of older persons were stationed in hospitals despite the fact that they had no need for acute medical treatment (cf. Klar, 1989).

31   Insufficient medical care of older patients and "hidden morbidity" is reported internationally (Meier-Baumgartner/Dapp, 2002: 22). According to the findings of the German Society for Nutrition (Deutsche Gesellschaft für Ernährung) about half of the seniors show (often unrecognised) symptoms of malnutrition upon admission to a clinic or nursing home (www.dge.de), cf. also above, 2.3.

32   Thus, overviews with prices and services, which the long-term care insurance companies must publish in accordance with § 7 par. 3 SGB XI were familiar to the long-term care insurance companies in only one third of the researched areas of North Rhine-Westphalia even three years after having gone into effect (Eifert et al.. 1999b).

33   Weber, 1998; similar things are reported from Denmark as being quite successful (Daatland, 1999: 419). Reference is also made to the consulting and controls based on § 37 SGB XI, which must be called regularly at professional nursing services by patients in need of care who have been provided for informally (with attendance allowance).

34   Overall it is striking that projects from the sphere of clinical medicine are very differently endowed in relation to methodical considerations compared to those that originate from social work and social education as well as the nursing profession.

311

35   Also included is the problem that some sickness funds either have no regional organisation or that these regional offices are not given sufficient authority. The latter is concentrated at the Land or federal level (see Eifert et al., 1999b; Rosendahl, 1999).

36   Berlin Prize for Health awarded by the General Local Health Insurance (Allgemeine Ortskrankenkasse, AOK) and the Berlin Physicians Association 2000 (Health and Society 5/2001: 11).

37   Risk factors were first and foremost advanced age (in patients in the accompanying research Æ 84 years), health problems, depression, living alone (66% of the high-risk cases in the accompanying research) and lack of help in emergencies (Döhner et al., 2002: 69-93, 101).

38   These findings correspond to experiences in similar coordination projects (see Kauss et al., 1998; Rosendahl, 1999; Engel/Engels, 2000).

39   Berlin Health Prize of the AOK (Allgemeine Ortskrankenkasse) health insurance fund and the Berlin Physicians Council (Ärztekammer Berlin) (Gesundheit und Gesellschaft Sonderheft [Health and Society Special edition] 5/2001).

40   First Prize, Berlin Health Prize of the AOK and the Berlin Physicians Council (Gesundheit und Gesellschaft Sonderheft 5/2001).

41   This extensively tested, valid and reliable instrument was developed in the USA, in the first instance for the inpatient sector, and imposed overall by means of regulatory reforms (Hawes et al., 1997 a and b; Phillips et al., 1997a-c). There are translations into 14 languages and initial international comparisons (Carpenter et al., 1999), and an adaptation for home use (Garms-Homolová, 1998).

42   These arose from a model experiment in one part of the city in 1983, which gave rise to across-the-board advisory centres (Weber, 2002: 53). This underlines the seriousness of the city's endeavours and the prospects that the project sketched here will endure.

43   It remains to be seen whether the tool used here is tested, reliable and valid.

References

Adler, C./Gunzelmann, T./Machold, C./Schumacher, J./Wilz, G. (1996) 'Belastungserleben pflegender Angehöriger von Demenzpatienten', *Zeitschrift für Gerontologie und Geriatrie*, 29 (2): 143-149.

Akerlof, G. A. (1970) 'The Market for 'Lemons': Quality Uncertainty and the Market Mechanism', *Quarterly Journal of Economics* 84: 488-500.

Arrow, K. J. (1991) 'The Economics of Agency', S. 37-51 in: Pratt, J.W./Zeckhauser R.J. (Ed.), *Principals and Agents: The Structure of Business*. Boston.

Bäcker, G./Bispinck, R./Hofemann, K./Naegele, G. (2000) *Sozialpolitik und soziale Lage in Deutschland*. Wiesbaden: Westdeutscher Verlag.

Bauer-Söllner, B. (1997) 'Stützung häuslicher Pflege statt Überforderung der Pflegenden', S. 151-174 in: Blosser-Reisen, L., *Altern: Integration sozialer und gesundheitlicher Hilfen*. Huber, Bern; Göttingen; Toronto; Seattle.

Blinkert, B./Klie, Th. (1999) *Pflege im sozialen Wandel: eine Untersuchung über die Situation häuslich versorgter Pflegebedürftiger* (Eine Untersuchung im Auftrag des Sozialministeriums Baden-Württemberg; FIFAS, Freiburger Institut für Angewandte Sozialwissenschaft e.V.). Hannover: Vincentz.

Blinkert, B./Klie, Th. (2000) 'Plfegekulturelle Orientierungen und soziale Milieus: Ergebnisse einer Untersuchung über die sozialstrukturelle Verankerung von Solidarität', *Sozialer Fortschritt* 10/2000: 237-245.

Blinkert, B./Klie, Th. (2001) Zukünftige Entwicklungen des Verhältnisses von professioneller und häuslicher Pflege bei differierenden Arrangements und privaten Ressourcen bis zum Jahr 2050. Expertise im Auftrag der Enquete-Kommission Demographischer Wandel des Deutschen Bundestags. Berlin.

BMFSFJ (Bundesministerium für Familie, Senioren, Frauen und Jugend) (Hg.) (2000) *Altenhilfestrukturen der Zukunft*, Auftaktveranstaltung zum Modellprogramm des BMFSFJ am 9./10. März 2000 in Bonn, Berlin, BMFSFJ.

BMFSFJ (Bundesministerium für Familie, Senioren, Frauen und Jugend) (2001) *Dritter Bericht zur Lage der älteren Generation* (BT-Drs. 14/5130 v. 19.1.2001). Berlin: Selbstverlag.

BMG (Bundesministerium für Gesundheit) (Hg.) (2001) *Zweiter Bericht über die Entwicklung der Pflegeversicherung*. Bonn.

Brandenburg, H./Zimprich, D. (1995) 'Lebenssituationen im Alter und die Nutzung der sozialen Dienste — ein empirischer Beitrag aus der Studie "Möglichkeiten und Grenzen der selbständigen Lebensführung im Alter" ', *Zeitschrift für Gerontopsychologie und -psychiatrie*, 8 (4): 237-246.

Brenzel, G. (2000) 'Medizin und Pflege. Wege zu effektiver Kooperation im Team - eine Herausforderung', *Der Onkologe* 6 (6): 540-544.

Breyer, F./Zweifel, P. (1992) *Gesundheitsökonomie*. Berlin: Springer.

Carpenter, G.I./Hirdes, J.P./Ribbe, M.W./Ikegami, N./Challis, D./Steel, K./Bernabei, R./Fries, B. (1999) 'Targeting and quality of nursing home care. A five nation study', *Aging*, 11 (2): 83-89.

Challis, D./Traske, K. (1997) 'Community care', S. 97-116 in: Mayer, Peter P./Dickinson, Edward J./Sandler, Martin (Hg.) *Quality care for elderly people*. London u.a.: Chapman & Hall Medical.

Claus, I. (1995) 'Betreute Überleitung', Heilberufe 47 (11): 12-15.

Courté-Wienecke, S./Wenng, S./Herkert, B./Satzinger, W. (2000) 'Der Patienten-Begleitbogen. Projekt zur besseren Kommunikation zwischen ambulanter und stationärer Versorgung', *Forum Sozialstation* 24 (107): 14-17.

Daatland, Svein Olav (1999) 'Similarities and Contrasts in Scandinavian Care Policies', S. 408-424 in: Naegele, Gerhard/Schütz, Rudolf-M. (Hg.), *Sozialgerontologie und Sozialpolitik für ältere Menschen*. Opladen: Westdeutscher Verlag.

Deutscher Bundestag (Hg.) (2002) Enquête-Kommission – Demographischer Wandel. Herausforderungen unserer älter werdenden Gesellschaft an den Einzelnen und die Politik. Berlin: Deutscher Bundestag, Referat Öffentlichkeitsarbeit.

Döhner, H. (1998) 'Care- und Case-Management durch das Modell PAGT in Hamburg', S. 195-202 in: Schmidt-Ohlemann, Matthias/Zippel, Christian/Blumenthal, Wolfgang/Fichtner, Hans Joachim (Hg.) *Ambulante wohnortsnahe Rehabilitation*. Ulm: Univ.-Verlag.

Döhner, H./Schick, B. (Hg.) (1996) *Gesundheit durch Kooperation. Die Rolle der Hausarztpraxis in der geriatrischen Versorgung*. Hamburg: Lit.

Döhner, H./Bleich, Ch./Kofahl, Ch./Lauterberg, J. (2002) *Case Management für ältere Hausarztpatientinnen und -patienten und ihre Angehörigen: Projekt Ambulantes Geriatrisches Team (PAGT)* (Schriftenreihe des Bundesministeriums für Familie, Senioren, Frauen und Jugend, BMFSFJ, Bd. 206). Stuttgart: Kohlhammer.

Domscheit, St./Wingenfeld, K. (1996) *Pflegeüberleitung in Nordrhein-Westfalen – Konzeptionelle Entwicklungen, Problemfelder und Anforderungen*. Bielefeld: Institut für Pflegewissenschaft an der Universität Bielefeld.

DVSK (Deutsche Vereinigung für den Krankenhaussozialdienst) (1999) 'Die koordinierte Entlassung von pflege- und hilfsbedürftigen Patienten. Ein Projekt des Krankenhauses München-Neuperlach mit einer Drittmittelfinanzierung der Else-Fresenius-Kröner Stiftung', *Forum Krankenhaussozialarbeit*, 1: 16-31.

Eberle, G. (1998) 'Die Entwicklung der GKV zum heutigen Stand', Sozialer Fortschritt 3/1998: 53-58.

Eifert, B./Krämer, K./Roth, G. (1999a) Die Auswirkungen des Gesetzes zur Umsetzung des Pflege-Versicherungsgesetzes (Landespflegegesetz Nordrhein-Westfalen – PfG NW). Untersuchung im Auftrag des Ministeriums für Arbeit, Soziales, Stadtentwicklung, Kultur und Sport des Landes Nordrhein-Westfalen (MASSKS). LT-Drs. 13/11 vom 06.06.2000, Düsseldorf.

Eifert, B./Krämer, K./Roth, G./Rothgang, H. (1999b) 'Die Umsetzung der Pflegeversicherung in den Bundesländern im Vergleich' (Bericht über eine Fachtagung der Forschungsgesellschaft für Gerontologie e.V., Dortmund, und des Zentrums für Sozialpolitik der Universität Bremen am 10.und 11. Dezember 1998 in Köln), *NDV* 8/1999: 259-266.

Eng, C./Pedulla, J./Eleazer, P./McCann, R./Fox, N. (1997) 'Program of all-inclusive care for the elderly (PACE): an innovative model of integrated geriatric care and financing', *Journal of the American Geriatrics Society*, 45 (2): 223-232.

Engel, H./Engels, D. (2000a) *Case Management in Various National Elderly Assistance Systems* (hrsgg. v. Bundesministerium für Familie, Senioren, Frauen und Jugend; Schriftenreihe Bd. 189.2). Stuttgart u.a.: Kohlhammer.

Engel, H./Engels, D. (2000b) *Experiences in Case Management from Nine Countries - Collected Material* (hrsgg. v. Bundesministerium für Familie, Senioren, Frauen und Jugend; Schriftenreihe Bd. 189.4). Stuttgart: Kohlhammer.

Ewers, M./Schaeffer, D. (Hg.) (2000) *Case Management in Theorie und Praxis*. Bern, Göttingen: Huber.

Flügel, K. (1996) 'Pflegeforschung in der Altenpflege. Eine Literaturstudie auf der Grundlage von zwei wissenschaftlichen Fachzeitschriften', *Zeitschrift für Gerontologie und Geriatrie*, 29 (6): 397-403.

Foley, Lisa A. (1999) Care management: Policy considerations for original medicare, in: http://research.aarp.org/health/ib38_care_1.html.

313

Förster, H./Nottenkämper, B. (1996) 'Sozialvisite als Instrument der ambulant-stationären Verzahnung bei Pflegebedürftigkeit', Medizinische Klinik 11/1996: 723-724.

Fretschner, R./Hilbert, J./Rohleder, Chr./Roth, G./Wismar, M./Wörz, M./Erbrich, M. (2001) *Gesundheitswesen und Arbeitsmarkt in Nordrhein-Westfalen* (Hg. Ministerium für Frauen, Jugend, Familie und Gesundheit des Landes Nordrhein-Westfalen), Selbstverlag, Düsseldorf.

Garms-Homolová, V. (1996a) 'Kooperation zwischen Ärztinnen / Ärzten und Pflege in der ambulanten Versorgung - Erfahrungen und Probleme', S. 39-48 in: Döhner, H./Schick, B. (Hg.), *Gesundheit durch Kooperation. Die Rolle der Hausarztpraxis in der geriatrischen Versorgung.* Hamburg: Lit.

Garms-Homolová, V. (1996b) 'Miteinander lernen. Perspektiven der Kooperation zwischen Ärzten / Ärztinnen und ambulanten Pflegediensten', *Häusliche Pflege* 2/1996: 106-108.

Garms-Homolová, V./Schaeffer, D. (Hg.) (1998) *Medizin und Pflege. Kooperation in der ambulanten Versorgung.* Wiebaden: Ullstein-Medical.

Garms-Homolová, V. (1998) 'Qualitätsmessung in der ambulanten Pflege. Erste Erfahrungen mit dem RAI HC-System in Deutschland und Österreich', *Pflegen ambulant* 2: 18-20.

Gerlinger, Th. (2002) Zwischen Korporatismus und Wettbewerb: Gesundheitspolitische Steuerung im Wandel (Working Papers - Veröffentlichungsreihe der Arbeitsgruppe Public Health, P02-204), Wissenschaftszentrum Berlin für Sozialforschung, Berlin.

Gerste, B./Rehbein, I. (1998) *Der Pflegemarkt in Deutschland. Ein statistischer Überblick* (Wissenschaftliches Institut der AOK). Bonn: WidO.

Giese, R./Wiegel, D. (2000) 'Die häusliche Pflege und die Wirksamkeit von SGB XI - Gesetzliche Qualitätssicherung aus der Perspektive der Pflegehaushalte', *Zeitschrift für Sozialreform*, 46 (12): 1023-1047.

Gräßel, E. (1998a) *Belastung und gesundheitliche Situation der Pflegenden.* Egelsbach: Verlag Dr. Markus Hänsel-Hohenhausen.

Gräßel, E. (2000) 'Warum pflegen Angehörige? Ein Pflegemodell für die häusliche Pflege im höheren Lebensalter', *Zeitschrift für Gerontopsychologie und -psychiatrie*, 13 (2): 85-94.

Green, J. H. (1989) 'Long-Term Home Care Research', *Nursing & Health Care*, 10 (3): 139-144.

Haas, B./Weber, J. (2000) 'Wiesbadener Netzwerk für geriatrische Rehabilitation', S. 81-88 in: BMFSFJ (Bundesministerium für Familie, Senioren, Frauen und Jugend) (Hg.), *Altenhilfestrukturen der Zukunft*, BMFSFJ (Bundesministerium für Familie, Senioren, Frauen und Jugend), Berlin.

Halsig, N. (1995) 'Hauptpflegepersonen in der Familie: Eine Analyse ihrer situativen Bedingungen, Belastungen und Hilfsmöglichkeiten', *Zeitschrift für Gerontopsychologie und -psychiatrie*, 8 (4): 247-262.

Haubrock, M./Hagmann, H./Nerlinger, Th. (2000) *Managed Care.* Bern; Göttingen; Toronto; Seattle: Huber.

Haug, K./Rothgang, H. (1996) Die gesetzliche Absicherung des Pflegefallrisikos. Eine Untersuchung der Konsensbildungsprozesse und Wirkungen der Pflegeversicherung (Forschungsbericht der Universität Bremen), Bremen.

Hawes, C./Mor, Vincent/Ph., Charles D./Fries, B.E./Morris, J.N./Steele-Friedlob, E./Greene, A. M./Nennstiel, M. (1997a) 'The OBRA-87 Nursing Home Regulations and Implementation of the Resident Assessment Instrument: Effects on Process Quality', *Journal of the American Geriatrics Society* (JAGS) 45/1997: 977-985.

Hawes, C./Morris, J.N./Phillips, C.D./Fries, B.E./Murphy, K./Mur, V. (1997b) 'Development of the nursing home Resident Assessment Instrument in the USA', *Age and Ageing*: 19-25.

Heinemann-Knoch, M./Korte, E./Voß, M. (1995) Seniorenberatung: Kein psychosozialer Luxus sondern notwendige Aufgabe der Altenhilfe (Bericht über die Modellprojekte zur Erprobung von stadtteil- und gemeindenahen Beratungs- und Vermittlungsstellen für alte Menschen und deren Angehörige in Nordrhein-Westfalen), Institut für Gerontologische Forschung e.V., Köln.

Hennessy, Patrick (1995) *Social Protection for Dependent Elderly People: Perspectives from a Review of OECD Countries* (Labour Market and Social Policy, Occasional Papers No. 16). Paris: OECD.

Hillers, U. (2000) 'Vertrag über den nahtlosen Übergang von der Krankenhausbehandlung zur Pflege', *Forum Krankenhaussozialarbeit*, Nr. 2: 34-37.

Hüning, W./Mört, M./König, S. (2000) 'Nahtlos pflegen. Überleitungsmodell in Borken stellt transparentes Verbundsystem von stationären, teilstationären und ambulanten Hilfen sicher', Häusliche Pflege 9 (7): 18-23.

Jacobzone, Stephane (1999) *Ageing and Care for Frail Elderly Persons: An Overview of International Perspectives* (OECD, Labour Market and Social Policy, Occasional Papers No. 38). Paris: OECD.

Kalisch, David W./Aman, Tetsuya/Buchele, Libbie A. (1998) *Social and Health Policies in OECD Countries: A Survey of Current Programmes and Recent Developments*. Paris: OECD.

Kamm-Kohl, V./Schnetz, D. (2000) 'Virtuelles Altenheim/CareNet Nürnberg, Praxisnetz Nürnberg Nord', S. 43-55 in: BMFSFJ (Bundesministerium für Familie, Senioren, Frauen und Jugend) (Hg.), *Altenhilfestrukturen der Zukunft*, BMFSFJ (Bundesministerium für Familie, Senioren, Frauen und Jugend), Berlin.

Kauss, Th./Kühnert, S./Naegele, G./Schmidt, W./Schnabel, E. (1998) *Vernetzung in der ambulanten geriatrischen Versorgung – die Schlüsselstellung des Hausarztes*. Münster: LIT.

Klaes, L. (2002) 'Wissenschaftliche Begleitung und übergreifende Ergebnisse zum Modellprogramm', *Forum Altenhilfe* Sonderheft 2002, 2: 19-26.

Klar, R. (1989) Umfang von Fehlbelegungen in Akutkrankenhäusern, Forschungsbericht Infratest Sozialforschugn i.A. v. Bundesministerium für Arbeit und Sozialordnung, Bonn.

Kliebsch, U./Fleischle, B./Busch, S./Huchler, U./Pfaff, A./Brenner, H. (2000) 'Utilization of Benefits for Home Long-term care in the German Statutory Long-term care in Insurance', *Zeitschrift für Gesundheitswissenschaften*, 8 (1): 78-91.

Korenke, Th. (2001) 'Innovativer Wettbewerb infolge integrierter Versorgung in der Krankenversicherung?', *Sozialer Fortschritt* 50 (11): 268-277.

Krause, B. (2000) 'Aus dem Krankenhaus in die häusliche Pflege. Wie ein reibungsloser Übergang organisiert werden kann', *Häusliche Pflege* 9 (12): 42-45.

Kühn, H. (2001) Integration der medizinischen Versorgung in regionaler Perspektive - Dimensionen und Leitbild eines politisch-ökonomischen, sozialen und kulturellen Prozesses (Working Papers - Veröffentlichungsreihe der Arbeitsgruppe Public Health P01-202), Wissenschaftszentrum Berlin, Berlin.

Kühnert, S. (1999) 'Strategien zur Qualifizierung und Qualitätssicherung in der Altenpflege', S. 249-261 in: Zimber, Andreas/Weyerer, Siegfried (Hg.), *Arbeitsbelastung in der Altenpflege*. Göttingen: Verlag für angewandte Psychologie.

Kühnert, S./Schnabel, E. (1996) 'Gegenwärtige Personalsituation und Qualifizierungs-erfordernisse in der Pflege', *Zeitschrift für Gerontologie und Geriatrie*, 29 (6): 411-417.

Mager, H.-C. (1996) 'Pflegeversicherung und Moral Hazard', *Sozialer Fortschritt* 10/1996: 242-249.

Meier-Baumgartner, H./Dapp, U. (2002) Geriatrisches Netzwerk: Kooperationsmodell zwischen niedergelassenen Ärzten und Geriatrischer Klinik mit Koordinierungs- und

315

Beratungsstelle (Schriftenreihe des Bundesministeriums für Familie, Senioren, Frauen und Jugend, Bd. 204), unter Mitarbeit von Tom Krause, Kohlhammer, Stuttgart.

Menke, M./Oelke U. (1999) 'Gemeinsame Grundausbildung in der Alten-, Kinderkranken- und Krankenpflege', S. 193-205 in: Schmidt, Roland/Entzian, H./Giercke K./Klie Th. (Hg.), *Die Versorgung pflegebedürftiger Menschen in der Kommune*. Frankfurt/M.: Mabuse.

Meyer, D. (2002) 'Gedanken zur Krise des Gesundheitswesens', *Sozialer Fortschritt* 51 (7/8): 172-177.

Miller, E.A./Weissert, W.G./Chernew, M. (1998) 'Managed care for elderly people. A compendium of findings', *American Journal of Medical Quality*, 13 (3): 127-140.

Moser, R./Won Soon Y. (1985) 'Zusammenarbeit von Sozialstation und Krankenhaus. Ein Erfahrungsbericht aus dem Landkreis Göppingen/Württemberg', *Deutsche Krankenhauspflegezeitschrift* 38 (11): 693-697, 702-703.

Neumann, E.-M. (2000) 'Entwicklung einer gerontopsychiatrischen Verbundstruktur in einer ländlichen Region und einer kreisfreien Stadt', S. 146-154 in: BMFSFJ (Bundesministerium für Familie, Senioren, Frauen und Jugend) (Hg.), *Altenhilfestrukturen der Zukunft*. BMFSFJ Berlin: Bundesministerium für Familie, Senioren, Frauen und Jugend.

OECD (Organisation for Economic Cooperation and Development) (Hg.) (1999) *A caring world. The new social policy agenda*. Paris: OECD.

Pacolet, J./Bouten, R./Lanoye, H./Versieck, K. (1998) Sozialschutz bei Pflegebedürftigkeit im Alter in den 15 EU-Mitgliedstaaten und in Norwegen, Europäische Kommission, Reihe: Beschäftigung und soziale Angelegenheiten, Luxemburg.

Phillips, C.D./Hawes, C./Mor, V./Fries, B.E./Morris, J.N. (1997a) 'Geriatric assessment in nursing homes in the united states: Impact of a national program', *Generations* 21 (4): 15-20.

Phillips, C.D./Morris, J.N./Hawes, C./Fries, E.F./Mor, V./Nennstiel, M./Iannacchione, V. (1997b) 'Association of the Resident Assessment Istrument (RAI) with changes in function, cognition, psychosocial status', *Journal of American Geriatrics Society* (JAGS) 45 (8): 986-993.

Phillips, C.D./Zimmerman, D./Bernabei, R./Jonsson, P.V. (1997c) 'Using the Resident Assessment Instrument for quality enhancement in nursing homes', *Age and Ageing*: 77-81.

Plück, St./Giersberg, A. (1998) 'Pflegepersonen zu Hause schulen. Qualität systematisch beeinflussen', *Forum Sozialstation* 4: 40.

Pöhlmann, K./Hofer, J. (1997) 'Ältere Menschen mit Hilfe- und Pflegebedarf: Instrumentelle Unterstützung durch Hauptpflegepersonen und professionelle Hilfsdienste', *Zeitschrift für Gerontologie und Geriatrie*, 30 (5): 381-388.

Potthoff, P. (2002) 'Zwischenergebnisse des Modellprogramms: Ergebnisse des ersten Monitorings', *Forum Altenhilfe* Sonderheft 2002, 2. Jg.: 27-32.

Prümmer, M. (1997) "Die trinken doch nur Kaffee" - Angehörigenarbeit ist durch Vorurteile belastet. Dabei ist sie ein wichtiger Aspekt der internen Qualitätssicherung, *Altenpflege* 6: 36-39.

Richter, E. (2001) 'Schlüsselfrage Ausbildung. Drei Berufe - eine Profession? Zersplittert in Alten-, Kinderkranken und Krankenpflege schwelt schon lange die Diskussion um eine gemeinsame Ausbildung für alle Pflegeberufe. Im Gerangel um Zuständigkeiten kämpft die Pflege um Qualität, um Kompetenz und ihre Zukunft', *Gesundheit und Gesellschaft* 4 (12): 28-30.

Rosendahl, B. (1999) *Kommunalisierung und korporative Vernetzung in der Implementation der Pflegeversicherung. Wirkungsanalyse regionaler Pflegekonferenzen in Nordrhein-Westfalen*. Münster: Lit.

Roth, G. (1998) 'Veränderungen der institutionellen Finanzverflechtung durch das Pflege-Versicherungsgesetz und Landespflegegesetz Nordrhein-Westfalen. Eine erste systematische Betrachtung', *Sozialer Fortschritt* 2/1998: 37-45.

Roth, G. (2000a) 'Fünf Jahre Pflegeversicherung in Deutschland: Funktionsweise und Wirkungen', Sozialer Fortschritt 8/2000: 184-192.

Roth, G. (2000b) 'Fünf Jahre Pflegeversicherung: Die Entwicklung der Pflegeinfrastruktur - Eine kommunal- und regionalpolitische Analyse', Zeitschrift für Sozialreform, 46 (11): 964-987.

Roth, G. (2001) Qualitätsmängel und Regelungsdefizite der Qualitätssicherung in der ambulanten Pflege — Nationale und internationale Befunde (Forschungsbericht, gefördert durch das Bundesministerium für Familie, Senioren, Frauen und Jugend), Forschungsgesellschaft für Gerontologie e.V., Institut für Gerontologie an der Universität Dortmund, Dortmund.

Roth, G. (2002) Qualität in Pflegeheimen (Expertise im Auftrag des Bundesministeriums für Familie, Senioren, Frauen und Jugend, BMFSFJ), Forschungsgesellschaft für Gerontologie e.V., Institut für Gerontologie an der Universität Dortmund, Dortmund.

Roth, G. (2003) 'Die Entwicklung der Pflegeinfrastruktur in den Bundesländern im Vergleich', Sozialer Fortschritt 3/2003: 73-79.

Roth, G./Rothgang, H. (1999) 'Die Auswirkungen des Pflege-Versicherungsgesetzes auf die Entwicklung der Heimentgelte', *Zeitschrift für Gesundheitswissenschaften*, 7 (4): 307-336.

Roth, G./Rothgang, H. (2001) 'Sozialhilfe und Pflegebedürftigkeit: Analyse der Zielerreichung und Zielverfehlung der Gesetzlichen Pflegeversicherung nach fünf Jahren', *Zeitschrift für Gerontologie und Geriatrie*, 34: 292-305.

Rothgang, H. (1996) 'Vom Bedarfs- zum Budgetprinzip? Die Einführung der Pflegeversicherung und ihre Folgen für die gesetzliche Krankenversicherung', S. 930-946 in: Clausen, Lars (Hg.), *Gesellschaften im Umbruch*. Beiträge des 27. Kongreß der Deutschen Gesellschaft für Soziologie, Band 1. Frankfurt am Main: Campus.

Rothgang, H. (1997) *Ziele und Wirkungen der Pflegeversicherung: Eine ökonomische Analyse*. Frankfurt am Main: Campus.

Rothgang, Heinz (2000) 'Die Pflegeversicherung: Kernstück der Altenpflegepolitik der letzten drei Dekaden, S. 59-86 in: Schulz-Nieswandt, Frank/Schewe, Gisela (Hg.), *Sozialpolitische Trends in Deutschland in den letzten drei Dekaden*. Eve-Elisabeth Schewe zum 70. Geburtstag. Berlin: Duncker & Humblot.

Rothgang, Heinz (2001) Finanzwirtschaftliche und strukturelle Entwicklungen in der Pflegeversicherung bis 2040 und mögliche alternative Konzepte. Endbericht zu einer Expertise für die Enquete-Kommission "Demographischer Wandel" des Deutschen Bundestags. Universität Bremen: Zentrum für Sozialpolitik.

Runde, P./Giese, R. (1999) 'Wirkungen des Pflegeversicherungsgesetzes (SGB XI) auf die Pflegeübernahme und die Pflegeorganisation', *Vierteljahresschrift für Sozialrecht* 4+5/1999: 339-362.

Schacke, C./Zank, S. (1998) 'Zur familiären Pflege demenzkranker Menschen: Die differentielle Bedeutung spezifischer Belastungsdimensionen für das Wohlbefinden der Pflegenden und die Stabilität der häuslichen Pflegesituation', *Zeitschrift für Gerontologie und Geriatrie*, 31 (5): 355-361.

Schaeffer, D. (1998) 'Innerprofessionelle Sicht der Kooperation. Die Perspektive der Pflege', S. 83-102 in: Garms-Homolová, V./Schaeffer, D. (Hg.), *Medizin und Pflege. Kooperation in der ambulanten Versorgung*. Wiesbaden: Ullstein Medical.

Schaeffer, D. (1999) 'Care Management - Pflegewissenschaftliche Überlegungen zu einem aktuellen Thema', *Zeitschrift für Gesundheitswissenschaften*, 7 (3): 233-251.

317

Schaeffer, D. (2000) 'Bruchstellen chronisch kranker Menschen. Die Entlassung aus dem Krankenhaus', S. 11-35 in: Seidl, E./Stankova, M./Walter, I. (Hg.), *Autonomie im Alter*. Wien/München/Bern: Wilhelm Maudrich.

Schaeffer, Doris/Ewers, Michael (2001) 'Ambulantisierung – Konsequenzen für die Pflege', *Gesellschaft u. Gesundheit Wissenschaft* 1/2001: 13-20.

Scharpf, F.W. (1985) 'Die Politikverflechtungsfalle. Europäische Integration und deutscher Föderalismus im Vergleich', *Politische Vierteljahresschrift* 26 (4): 323-356.

Schild-Woestmeyer, K./Dietz, B. (1998) 'Schulungen auf Erfolgskurs. In Münster wird das Angebot an Pflegekursen koordiniert', Forum Sozialstation 12/1998: 40-43.

Schmidt, R. (1999) 'Kooperative und berufsgruppenübergreifende Qualitätssicherung', *Evangelische Impulse* 21 (2): 39-41.

Schmidt, R. (2002) 'Impulse zur sektoren- und systemübergreifenden Qualitätsentwicklung', S. 289-328 in: Klie, Th./Buhl, A./Entzian, H./Schmidt, R. (Hg.), *Das Pflegewesen und die Pflegebedürftigen: Analysen zu Wirkungen der Pflegeversicherung und ihrem Reformbedarf* (Beiträge zur sozialen Gerontologie und Altenarbeit, hrsgg. v. Fachbereich IV der Deutschen Gesellschaft für Gerontologie und Geriatrie (DGGG). Frankfurt a.M.: Mabuse.

Schneekloth, U./Müller, U. (2000) Wirkungen der Pflegeversicherung. Forschungsprojekt im Auftrag des Bundesministeriums für Gesundheit, durchgeführt von I+G Gesundheitsforschung, München und Infratest Burke Sozialforschung. München, Nomos, Baden-Baden.

Schnelle, John F./Ouslander, Joseph G./Buchanan, Joan/Zellman, Gail/Farley, Donna/Hirsch, Susan H./Reuben, David B. (1999) 'Objective and subjective measures of the Quality of managed care in nursing homes', *Medical Care*, 37 (4): 375-383.

Schölkopf, M. (1999a) Altenpflegepolitik in der Bundesrepublik Deutschland: Zwischen Bedarfsdeckung und Marginalisierung. Eine Analyse der Expansion der Pflegedienste im Bundesländervergleich. Diss. Universität Konstanz, erscheint bei Leske + Budrich, Opladen.

Schölkopf, M. (1999b) 'Altenpflegepolitik - an der Peripherie des Sozialstaats? Die Expansion der Pflegedienste zwischen Wohlfahrtsverbänden, Ministerialbürokratie und Parteien', *Politische Vierteljahresschrift*, 40 (2): 246-278.

Schölkopf, M. (1999c) 'Altenpflegepolitik in Europa: Ein Vergleich sozialpolitischer Strategien zur Unterstützung pflegebedürftiger Senioren', *Sozialer Fortschritt*, 11: 282-291.

Schulenburg, J.-M. Graf v.d. (1992) 'Preisbildung im Gesundheitswesen', S. 111-134 in: Andersen, Hanfried H.(Hg.), *Basiswissen Gesundheitsökonomie*. Berlin: Edition Sigma.

Schulz-Nieswandt, F. (1998) 'Zur Zukunft des Gesundheitswesens', *Zeitschrift für Gerontologie und Geriatrie*, 31: 382-386.

Schulz-Nieswandt, F. (2000) '§140 SGB Va ff. und DRGs im Krankenhaus-sektor - Möglichkeiten und Gefahren einer integrierten Versorgung für ältere und alte Menschen', *Sozialer Fortschritt* 49 (5): 115-118.

Schweikart, R. (1999) 'Care Management', S. 76-120 in: Göpfert-Divivier, Werner/Robitzsch, Monika/Schweikart, Rudolf (Hg.), *"Qualitätsmanagement" und "Care Management" in der ambulanten Pflege* (hrsgg. vom Bundesministerium für Familie, Senioren, Frauen und Jugend). Stuttgart, Berlin, Köln: Kohlhammer.

Sell, St. (2000) 'Einführung eines durchgängig (fall)pauschalierenden Vergütungssystems für Krankenhausleistungen auf DRG-Basis. Ein Literaturübersicht', *Sozialer Fortschritt* 49 (5): 103-115.

STABU (Statistisches Bundesamt/DESTATIS) (2001) *Statistisches Jahrbuch der Bundesrepublik Deutschland*. Stuttgart: Metzler-Poeschl.

SVRKAG (Sachverständigenrat für die Konzertierte Aktion im Gesundheitswesen) (1995) *Gesundheitsversorgung und Krankenversicherung 2000: Mehr Ergebnisorientierung, mehr Qualität und mehr Wirtschaftlichkeit*. Baden-Baden: Nomos.

SVRKAG (Sachverständigenrat für die Konzertierte Aktion im Gesundheitswesen) (2002) *Bedarfsgerechtigkeit und Wirtschaftlichkeit* (Bd. III): Über-, Unter- und Fehlversorgung. Baden-Baden: Nomos.

Tophoven, C. (2001) 'Disease Management und Integrierte Versorgung Zur Reichweite zweier gesundheitspolitischer Konzepte', *Arbeit und Sozialpolitik*, 55 (11/12): 30-38.

Törne, I. v. (2002) 'Ergebnisse der Modellprojekte. Handlungsebene: Strukturentwicklung, Kooperation und Vernetzung', *Forum Altenhilfe* Sonderheft 2002, 2: 35-40.

Voges, W. (2002) *Pflege alter Menschen als Beruf – Soziologie eines Tätigkeitsfeldes*. Wiesbaden: Westdeutscher Verlag.

Walker, A./Maltby, T. (1997) *Ageing Europe*. Buckingham, Philadelphia: Open University Press.

Ward-Griffin, C./McKeever, P. (2000) 'Relationship between nurses and family caregivers: Partners in care?', *Advances in Nursing Science*, 22 (3): 89-103.

Weber, J. (1998) 'Qualitätssicherung in der häuslichen Pflege durch aufsuchende Beratungsdienste im Stadtteil', *Archiv für Wissenschaft und Praxis der sozialen Arbeit*, 29 (4) und 30 (1): 365-384.

Weber, J. (2002) 'Case Management im Wiesbadener Netzwerk für geriatrische Rehabilitation', *Forum Altenhilfe* Sonderheft 2002, 2: 52-58.

Weber, M. (2001) 'Wettbewerb im Gesundheitswesen – oder: Warum können und dürfen Einkaufsmodelle der Kassen nicht Realität werden?', *Sozialer Fortschritt* 50 (11): 254-260.

Wendt, W.R. (1993) *Ambulante sozialpflegerische Dienste in Kooperation*. Freiburg i.Br.: Lambertus.

Wendt, W. R. (2000) 'Report on the Evaluation of Case Management in the Elderly Assistance in Baden-Württemberg', S. 10-33 in: Engel, H./Engel, D. (Hg.), *Experiences in Case Management from Nine Countries – Collected Material* (hrsgg. v. Bundesministerium für Familie, Senioren, Frauen und Jugend; Schriftenreihe Bd. 189.4). Stuttgart: Kohlhammer.

WHO (2000) *World Health Report 2000*, in: World Health Report 2000 (http://www.who.int/whr/2000/en/report.htm [February 2002]).hh.

Wilz, G./Adler,C./Gunzelmann, T./Brähler, E. (1999) 'Auswirkungen chronischer Belastungen auf die physische und psychische Befindlichkeit – Eine Prozeßanalyse bei pflegenden Angehörigen von Demenzkranken', *Zeitschrift für Gerontologie und Geriatrie*, 32 (4): 255-265.

Wingenfeld, K. (1999) Konzepte und Maßnahmen zur Sicherstellung des Übergangs von der Krankenhaus- oder Rehabilitationsbehandlung zur Betreuung durch Pflegeeinrichtungen (Teilstudie im Rahmen des Projektes "Evaluation des Landespflegegesetzes Nordrhein-Westfalen" im Auftrag des Ministeriums für Arbeit, Soziales, Stadtentwicklung, Kultur und Sport des Landes Nordrhein-Westfalen), Eigenverlag, Düsseldorf.

Wingenfeld, K./Schnabel, E. (2002) Pflegebedarf und Leistungsstruktur in vollstationären Pflegeeinrichtungen (Eine Untersuchung im Auftrag des Landespfegeausschusses Nordrhein-Westfalen), Eigenverlag, Düsseldorf.

Winkelhake, O./Miegel, U./Thormeier, K. (2002) 'Die personelle Verteilung von Leistungsausgaben in der Gesetzlichen Krankenversicherung 1998 und 1999 – Konsequenzen für die Weiterentwicklung des deutschen Gesundheitssystems', *Sozialer Fortschritt* 51 (3): 58-61.

319

Annex: Selected Model Ways of Working

A1: Outpatient Geriatric Team Project (Projekt Ambulantes, Geriatrisches Team – PAGT), Hamburg

Name	Outpatient Geriatric Team Project (Projekt Ambulantes, Geriatrisches Team – PAGT), Hamburg
Provider	University of Hamburg, Institute for Medical Sociology (Evaluation), Association for Social Sciences and Health (Practical Work)
Objectives	• To improve quality of life of the elderly and their relatives by stabilising or establishing a social network, especially to strengthen their independence, self-determination and choice of support, aid or care services, • preventing or at least delaying disease becoming chronic, preventing or delaying the need for care, preventing or reducing clinically unnecessary admissions to hospital, reducing periods spent in hospital, avoiding an unintended transfer to a nursing home and, if possible, returning the person to his/her own home and reducing the mortality rate, • to guarantee continuity, good cooperation and coordination of service provision especially with informal carers also including social and psychological support and • to help patients and their families to find the correct organisation for their needs.
Target group	Patients 65 years and older which are under medical treatment of general practitioners, with a high risk of dependency, hospitalisation or institutionalisation, i.e. dementia or precarious social factors (determined after a multidimensional Screening), Total: N=466; 131 of which (28%) were identified as high-risk patients. 89 patients (68% of high-risk patients) were included in the accompanying research, as some could or would not take part, N=43 took part in final assessments (N=46 "drop outs", N=29 died).
Number of staff involved	2 teams in 2 model regions with 3 general practitioners (with a small honorarium), 1 care manager for coordination and scientific evaluation (30 hours), 2 case managers for advice and attendance of patients; scientific staff: 1 full-time, 1 student as helper, 1 secretary (28 hours a week) for 4 years.

Methods	Short screening by the doctor (following Barber/Wallis) at beginning, to determine high-risk patients; then geriatric assessment was performed at two moments in time (baseline, follow-up), complemented by intensive interviews with patients with measurements of life quality; furthermore interviews, group discussions, analyses of patient records etc. have been used.
Strengths and weaknesses	*Strengths* • The need for an outreaching consultation of clients and coordinated care. However, resistances on the side of the clients had to be overcome. • Discovery of uncovered need for help (according to self-assessments) and current demands, especially with respect to assistance in structuring free time, physical therapy and mobility/transport. Deficiencies became also apparent in the missing adaptation of sanitary installations to the requirements of elderly people. • Success was reported such as the preventive effect of housing adaptations and the priority of care at home, even with persons in terminal care. • The expectations of staff with respect to qualification, a higher degree of work satisfaction and confidence in dealing with patient and coordination problems were satisfied. Medical doctors acquired a deeper insight in problems such as incontinence, which are too rarely discovered and receive too little attention. New ideas and improvements in care services were developed, e.g. in relation to a lack of coordination and planning of activities. *Weaknesses* • Initial expectations of the model project in relation to improvements in patients' quality of life could not, however, be fulfilled. • Due to the *low number of cases* and the lack of a *control group,* the results, including achievements like the avoidance of hospital and nursing home admission, and the shortening of hospital stay, are hardly worth assessing. • The duration of, and importance of forming relationships of trust and the respective personal prerequisites. But it was underlined once more that permanent functional coordination and integration would need institutional standardisation, formalised work routines and a set of incentives in order to overcome defensive behaviours due to competition or fears of control. • Finally the project confirms that, should such approaches be successfully transferred to mainstream care, economic incentives and legal regulations, e.g. concerning the

321

	process of screening or assessment, and coordinating procedures, such as case and care management, are indeed indispensable.
Results of evaluation/keywords	Underlining the need for an outreaching consultation of clients and coordinated care; discovery of uncovered needs; support for preventive effects of housing adaptations; improvement in inter-professional coordination through multi-professional case management; deeper insight through multidimensional assessment and multi-professional case management for medical doctors in problems, i.e. for incontinence, which are too rarely discovered and receive too little attention; new ideas and improvements in care services, e.g. in relation to a lack of coordination and planning of activities, i.e. patient care planning.

A2: Geriatric Network (Geriatrisches Netzwerk) Hamburg

Name	Geriatric Network (Geriatrisches Netzwerk) Hamburg
Provider	12 General Practitioners, 1 geriatric hospital ("Albertinen-Haus, Hamburg") within a memory clinic, an advisory board and a coordination centre
Objectives	• To extend the period in which elderly patients live independently in their own homes by transfer and use of geriatric assessment in the outpatient health provision through family doctors, in particular the problem of "hidden morbidity" was to be addressed. • To this end intervention should be preventative and take place within outpatient health provisions (family doctor) and also through home visits (by a social education worker from the advice centre) before either hospital care or rehabilitation or admission to a nursing home become necessary.
Target group	12 family doctors out of 20 were arbitrarily chosen in the region and took part in the 24-month model study (1997-1999), together with a total of 156 female patients (42 of whom participated in the dementia subproject) and a total of 133 patients, average 79.4 years, remained until t5; From those without an assessment (negative screens), 80% of the geriatric patients were living at home.
Number of staff involved	12 family doctors, 1 social pedagogue in an advisory board; 1 physician in an assessment unit, 1 neurology and 1 neuropsychiatry therapist (in the memory clinic), 1 secretary; scientific staff: 1 for coordination, 1 assistant for data procession, 2 advisors (chief of the clinic and chief of memory clinic)

Methods	Geriatric screening as proposed by Lachs (1990) as transfer from the geriatric hospital to family doctors. In the case of a positive geriatric screening, other assessment procedures and social advice in the geriatric hospital were tested. The resultant coordination and cooperation, responsibility for geriatric matters and further evolution were observed and documented, as were the clients (process, independence, quality of life) and their relatives (burden). Alongside, regular coordination meetings were held in the geriatric hospital, to present key issues and examples of patient cases. A regular exchange of information was organised by means of doctors' letters. A total of 5 screenings were conducted at intervals of 6 months, at times t1-t5, a minimum of 2 social advice sessions, 5 assessments as appropriate, 3 standardised questionnaires to patients, dealing with quality of life and ability to cope independently, and to relatives, dealing with quality of life and the burdens on them. In addition at t1 and t5 family doctors were questioned on the subject of the geriatric patient, the organisation of the practice, geriatric expertise, and any recommendations of the geriatric hospital carried out (compliance). Contacts with patients were quantified and recorded, and measures taken in the coordination and advice centre (t1-t5) and in the subprojects (t1-t5) were recorded together with time taken. Finally, in the geriatric hospital, regular consultations and case conferences were held.
Strengths and weaknesses	*Strengths* • When the screening of family doctors was compared, t1 showed abnormalities in the memory category for more than 55% of patients, and t5 for only 45% of patients. This is interpreted as a result of improved clarification within the assessment. Further significant improvements were apparent in sight, and still more in hearing and in social support. • Overall, geriatric screening (modified as proposed by Lachs) is claimed to have proved its worth, it could be incorporated into practice without difficulty, met with a high level of acceptance, and was in most cases also used by doctors for patients who were not participating in the model project. • The work of the social advice centre was judged overwhelmingly positive by the family doctors, because it was found to be supportive in view of the lack of time for organisation and social needs, stated to be a pressing problem.

323

Weaknesses
- The value of the assessment tool was judged to be slight by the family doctors, because it was felt to provide few new insights, although the modules measuring cognitive abilities were judged to be enlightening.
- Similarly the recommendations of the geriatric hospital were only in part put into practice by the family doctors as a result of the assessment, although 80% of them judged these positively.
- The problem of lacking financial incentives for advice in the scale of physicians' charges was reported once more. Therefore the project indicates the significance of the surrounding financial and institutional conditions for the project's permeation into mainstream provision. This effect must also be judged to be limited in the case of the present project, although it should ensure a greater significant expansion in knowledge and use of geriatric screening.
- Also this project was carried out without a *control group* for reasons of cost, thus, real effectiveness could once more not be proven.

Results of evaluation/keywords	Unmet needs and hidden morbidity in practice of family doctors; positive effects of the transfer of geriatric screening and assessment in the outpatient sector; supportive outcomes of social advice centre; but also this project was carried out without a control group for reasons of cost, thus, real effectiveness could once more not be proven.

A3: Praxisnetz Nürnberg Nord e.V., HomeCare Nürnberg

Name	Praxisnetz Nürnberg Nord e.V., HomeCare Nürnberg
Provider	Praxisnetz Nürnberg Nord e.V., HomeCare Nürnberg is a regional association in the city of Nuremberg (Bavaria) consisting since 1998 of about 140 physicians in private practice.
Objectives	• To build a comprehensive, integrated care system with the provision of services particularly for older persons in need of care. • Linking the available provisions and services in the health system and assistance for the elderly, by interdisciplinary quality management and the use and development of state-of-the-art information and communication technologies.

	• A coordination point serves to communicate appropriate, quality-controlled information and assistance to stabilise the quality of life in the home for those in need of assistance. • Also cost savings are expected, resulting in particular from the optimisation of provision (geriatric advice, with consequent reduction in the length of hospital stays and avoidance of inpatient admissions).
Target group	All elderly people needing social and health services in a region (25,000)
Number of staff involved	1 Coordinating Team with scientific staff (2 employees) and 1 secretary as a call-center for elderly people; association of ca. 140 physicians in private practice; 1 hospital and diverse health and social care providers in cooperation
Methods	Case Management, Disease Management, Database with Information Platform, Screening, Assessment (pilot study)
Strengths and weaknesses	The advice centre and data bank of service providers and network of participating doctors has already been set up but no information is available as yet about the point reached in establishing the case management as still no evaluation has been published.
Results of evaluation/keywords	Not yet available

325

A4: The Association Structure for Geronto-psychiatric Services in Brandenburg

Name	Gerontopsychiatrische Verbundstruktur Brandenburg (The association structure for geronto-psychiatric services in Brandenburg)
Provider	Brandenburg Alzheimer Society and the Fachhochschule (University for Applied Science) Lausitz in Cottbus
Objectives	• To develop an association structure for geronto-psychiatric services, in a rural region (Oberspreewald-Lausitz) and a city constituting its own administrative district (Cottbus) to improve the provision of information, advice, treatment and care of persons suffering from geronto-psychiatric problems,

	• relieve the burden of their informal caregivers, • improve communication and cooperation between relevant health and social care providers, • improve knowledge regarding diagnosis and treatment of dementia, • fill any gaps in provision with services of appropriate quality.
Target group	Persons suffering from geronto-psychiatric problems – especially dementia – and their informal caregivers
Number of staff involved	1 project manager and 2 social workers (one for each region), health and social care providers in Oberspreewald-Lausitz and Cottbus
Methods	• Collection and documentation of individual requirements for assistance, using assessment instruments • Advice and Case Management • Monthly case conferences • Implementation and evaluation of association conferences (Verbundkonferenzen) for relevant service providers in the region • Production of a handbook of provisions for all partners • Implementation and evaluation of further training courses • Development of common quality standards for advice, attendance and care provided to dementia sufferers • Analysis of gaps in the provision of health and social care • Development of innovative ways of care
Strengths and weaknesses	• Involvement of *all* relevant actors (e.g. medical doctors, service providers, caregivers) • Comprehensive approach • Taking into consideration regional differences (rural versus urban) • Implementation of association conferences as measure to improve cooperation and communication • Special emphasis on persons suffering from dementia as the largest group of geronto-psychiatric patients and their informal caregivers • Evaluation of all measures
Results of evaluation/keywords	Not yet available

A5: Wiesbaden Geriatric Rehabilitation Network

Name	Wiesbaden Geriatric Rehabilitation Network
Provider	City of Wiesbaden (Hesse)
Objectives	<ul><li>To advise or support the elderly,</li><li>to keep them independent and</li><li>to reduce or remove their need for care.</li><li>To this end, cooperation is to be improved with a view to *geriatric rehabilitation*; in particular, the elderly have guaranteed access to this from their own homes.</li></ul>
Target group	Fragile elderly risking the loss of self-sufficiency (selected by standardised screening). The selected target group are people over 70 years of age who suffer from multiple diseases that limit their functioning. In particular, the criteria are: change in lifestyle or health problems in the past 6 months, e.g. need for domestic help or application for provisions from the LTCI; a fall in the past few months; several inpatient stays during the past 6 months; or application for admission to a nursing home. If at least one of these criteria is fulfilled, the "standardised selection" is applied by the 8 advisory centres for independent living of the elderly. This is drawn up in an agreement between the older person and the family doctor.
Number of staff involved	1 project bureau for 3 years with 3 employees (2 scientific, 1 secretary) and the chief manager with 3-5 hours a week; 8 municipal advisory boards (not only for elderly) are associated with 16 employees (social workers) and about 10-20% of total workload is spent for the target group.
Methods	Project parts: 1) Screening and Case Management, then geriatric rehabilitation in special geriatric hospital units (N=81 in 18 months) and support of access to general medical services. 2) Support discharge management and coordination between services; no progress is reported after 3 years due to enduring conflicts (N=0) after 3 years. 3) Support and advice for voluntary and honorary caregivers or assistants for the elderly (N=85).
Strengths and weaknesses	Besides some basic information still no evaluation results have been published.
Results of evaluation/ keywords	Not yet available

327

Providing Integrated Health and Social Care for Older Persons in Greece

Aris Sissouras, Maria Ketsetzopoulou, Nikos Bouzas, Evi Fagadaki, Olga Papaliou, Aliki Fakoura

1   Introduction

In Greece, until recently, the role of the state towards the elderly has been limited to the care of individuals with special needs, the financially weak, and constituted a part of a more general policy against poverty manifested mainly in the form of subsidies. Care for the elderly has been a "family affair". Today, certain positive steps have been taken for the provision of community care services; nevertheless, the development of social services is still limited. It has also to be stressed that the domain of social welfare in the country is characterised by an uneven development with respect to organisation, personnel and spending compared to the two other basic sectors of social protection (social security and health protection).

Indeed, when it comes to examining the system of care for the elderly one has to consider the cultural basis. In the Mediterranean model, the family generally plays the central role in the process of care and in many instances it is considered as the most effective institution for offering an "integrated" balance of health and social care to the older person. Socially and psychologically the old person gains from the fact that s/he feels "secure" and that there is always somebody around to respond to an emergency (health) need.

In the area of formal social and health services, there are two distinct features to observe as determining factors for the (under)development and scarce organisation of public services. One of these reflects the cultural characteristic mentioned above, in that for many years this "informal type of care" acted as a substitute (and in some cases a "deterrent") to committing the state for developing formal services. Only voluntary organisations such as the church, in particular, again within the realms of a special charitable concept and culture, were developing care services for the elderly (a corresponding concept to the *"principle of subsidiarity"*). The second factor refers to the way welfare and social protection services are organised in Greece in that there is a split between what is provided to the elderly through social security funds, which are numerous with different and unequal coverage, and what is provided by the welfare section attached to the Ministry of Health and Welfare, designed exactly to fill the gap in long-term care for older persons by developing new and more comprehensive programmes of care.

It is on the latter programmes that this report is focused, particularly in order to identify "strengths and opportunities" for an integrated type of health and social care for older persons.

2 Legal and Structural Framework and the General Discourse on (Integrated) Care Provision

2.1 Structure of Provision

The structural framework within which care for the elderly is instituted in Greece today is the usual "tripartite" nature of services: the statutory public services, the voluntary and interest organisations and the informal type of care, besides family care.

In the public domain two Ministries have a statutory responsibility for care for the elderly.

- The Ministry of Health and Welfare (MHW) which is the main responsible public body not only for the provision of health care but also for the realisation of constitutive arrangements of social care ensuring a descent standard of living for those who are confronted with particular problems such as the elderly, the persons with special needs, minorities, socially excluded persons, etc.

- The Ministry of Labour and Social Security (through various social insurance funds), which beyond pensions provides certain social and care services within the framework of the contributory state of responsibility.

The MHW provides services through two main mechanisms: the National Health System (NHS) and the National Social Care System (NSCS). They have been developed and implemented separately and not based upon the interface principle, in different time spans and distinct laws rule their objectives, organisational aspects and administrative structure.

More specifically, the NHS was initiated in 1983 under the auspices of L 1397/1983 aiming at the provision of full health coverage to all citizens. Due to important regional imbalances in the accessibility of health services and the centralised decision-making procedure the system was transformed in order to be more efficient at regional level *via* L 2889/2001. According to this law, the whole NHS is divided in 17 Regional Health Systems headed by a Director and an Administrative Body.

On the social care side, the NSCS was established by L 2646/1998 as a merge of pre-existing social welfare organisations, such as the National Welfare Organisation, aiming at the provision of welfare services to all persons in relation to their particular personal, family, financial and social needs verified by means-tested procedures.

A very recent Draft Bill concerning the implementation of social care services at regional level, states that the NSCS is discharged to exist as a centralised mechanism and should be embodied in the 17 Regional Health Systems (RHS) as an autonomous department in terms of administrative structure and financial situation under the direct responsibility of each Regional Health System Director and having financial autonomy.

Summing up, it could be said that any overall legislative framework introducing the provision of health services and social care interventions in an integrated manner has not been elaborated in Greece up to now. There seems to be strong evidence now that the recognition of the necessity of integrated provision of health and social care starts to take an operational form. The exact administrative structure, the patient chain, the collaboration between the two sub-systems (interface aspects) in every RHS constitute important issues to be clarified through the parliamentary procedure where the new law is to be discussed soon.

331

2.2 Recent Trends in the Financing of Social Protection[1] in Greece

2.2.1 Overview Trends in Social Expenditures

The Greek Social Protection System (Social Insurance, Health and Social Welfare) has been characterised as a mixed one belonging to the Southern European Social Protection Model (Esping-Andersen, 1996). This diversity in the formation of the system is explained by the fact that it is Bismarckian in the case of provisions, which are mainly based upon the extensive role of the social insurance funds (see Tables 1, 2 and 4 of Annex I) and Beveridgian in the case of financial resources the bulk of which is supported by the state budget (taxes) and insurance contributions (see Table 3 of Annex I).

As a result, it could be pointed out that over the last decade, financial extension of the Greek Welfare State happened at the absolute expense of employees and pensioners, while a relatively higher priority was expressed in favour of unemployment compensation and housing/social exclusion measures. Simultaneously, a lesser priority had been given to sickness/health care and disability actions. This financial pattern of the Greek Social Protection System raises some questions regarding either its future financial viability or the issue of social justice and also its contemporary and future possibilities in supporting the provision of new integrated services for the elderly.

2.2.2 Financing of Health Care

From the very beginning, it should be stressed that there are no secure and accurate data regarding the financial situation and the rate of social needs coverage by the welfare sector in Greece due to the absence of a unified mechanism for its monitoring in terms of costs, resources and number of users. In this respect, social welfare sector's data steaming from different sources are rarely comparable (see Tables 2 and 4 of Annex I), while it is quite impossible either to detect the magnitude of financial resources devoted to health/social care for the elderly or to integrated care for them.

Total health expenditure accounted for 9.1% of GDP in 2000 according to the OECD database (OECD, 2001). Besides the disagreement about the accurate volume of health expenses as a percentage of GDP, it is remarkable that during the last 30 years public health expenditure has performed a more or less steady growth. In current prices, public health expenditures rose as a share of GDP from 2.4% in 1970 to 4.79% in 1990. During the 1990s there has been a growing stabilisation: 4.93% in 1996 (Ministry of Health and Welfare, 1999: 63) and 5.2% in 2000 (OECD, 2001).

The investigation of the relationship between age and health expenditure reveals that a significant proportion of public health expenses – more than 30% (Ministry of Health and Welfare, 1999: 14) – are devoted to the health treatment of the elderly which is mainly due to the fact that their health cost per capita is on average 4.3 times higher (for those over 75 years of age: 5.9% higher) than for the younger population (Ministry of Health and Welfare, 1999: 14).

During the last 30 years the composition of total expenditure on health has exhibited a consistent shift from private to public financing. In 1970, private expenditure accounted for 57.2% of total health care expenditure, while in 1997 the situation had been reversed as public expenditure accounted for 58.1% of total health expenditure (MHW, 1999: 64). The remaining private expenses consist of two parts: on the one hand, by the fees paid by patients for primary health, dentist's services and medicines on the private health market. On the other hand, they include the fees paid by patients to public hospitals and clinics for some medical examinations and the co-payment for medicines, pharmaceutical products, therapeutic appliances and equipment. The percentage of co-payment ranges from 25% for all insured persons to 10% for pensioners. Uninsured older persons living in a situation of need verified by a means-test are exempted from charges.

As regards households, they spent a diachronically increasing proportion of their income on health. In 1987/88, the monthly average mean of health and personal care services/products purchased absorbed a 7.28% of the total purchasing expenditure, while in 1993/94 the respective percentage reached up to 7.88% (National Statistical Service of Greece/NSSG, 1999: 30). In a sense, the extension of private health expenditure may reveal the rate of quantity and quality inefficiencies of the National Health System. Thus, it is apparent that in Greece, there are a lot of chances for NHS improvement in order to provide full health coverage to the whole population.

2.2.3 Financing of Social Care for the Elderly

As exposed earlier, the public funds devoted to *non-contributive social care* constitute a trivial part of total social expenditure. A closer view on elderly welfare institutions' funding sources in relation to their legal status reveals that:

333

1. Public institutions for residential care are funded on a regular basis from the state budget and from daily fees insurance funds pay for every insured person using their services. A minor source of funding are donations, individual fund-giving, etc. Generally, the users of institutional care services of this type are not charged any co-payment. However, there are some exemptions.
2. Non-profit private institutions are supported by insurance funds through daily fees charged for each insured person using their services and by the state budget through subsidies.
3. Private for-profit institutions are almost exclusively dependent on individual financial resources of their clients.
4. The implemented "open care" programmes for the elderly (Home Care and Open Care Centres) are funded through the state budget and Insurance Funds and do not impose any costs on users.
5. The various cash benefits to the elderly (e.g. rent subsidies, heating allowances, etc.) are financed directly from the state budget or Insurance Funds.

Generally speaking, the kind of legal framework to a great extent determines the financial resources and sources for every welfare institution. Institutions functioning as legal entities under the public law draw funds from the state budget, Insurance Funds and the wider society through donations and fund-giving. Legal entities of private law (private for-profit institutions) have a more or less unique funding source: the day fees payments from their clients. On the other hand, the trivial nature of non-contributory financing of the care sector for old people explains to a great extent the magnitude of uncovered social needs and the difficulty in financing a new array of integrated services for the elderly.

2.2.4 The Socio-economic Situation of the Elderly

It is well-established that the ageing of the population in terms of volume and composition by age, is always accompanied by an upward demand for medical and social care services. According to the Household Expenditure Survey (data for 1993/94), the expenditure on medical and personal care shows a positive correlation with the age of the household head. Households headed by persons up to 24 years old spent a proportion of 4.2% of their total consumption expenditure on health, while the respective percentage for households headed by elderly persons 75 years and over climbs up to 9.5% of their total consumption expenditures.

The growth rate of health and social welfare services demand depends upon subjective and objective factors, such as lifestyle or long-term illness and disability.

In Greece, as in the other EU member-states the post-war demographic composition of the population has changed in favour of the elderly who are now proportionally more and live longer than in the past. According to demographic statistical data, in 1971 there were 957,000 persons 65 years and above (or 10.92% of total population), while the respective numbers for 2001 are at 2,031,000 and 18.52%. During the same time period, the proportion of persons 75 years old and over has increased to 6.7% by 2000 ((NSSG, 2002: 3).

In any case, the rising demand means increased cost to meet new medical and social needs. Consequently, the core question regarding the financial ability of the elderly to afford the excess cost burden is unavoidably raised. The rate and the sign of this ability prescribe the volume and orientation of the medical and social care provisions. In general, it is plausible that the weaker the financial situation of the elderly, the more intensive and extensive the social policy support should be.

The well-being of the elderly in terms of income/wealth and housing conditions is of a minor level compared to the total population. Studies and research projects conclude that "on average, in all EU countries the non-elderly appear to be better-off than the elderly" and "the households of the non-elderly tend to be better equipped than the households of the elderly in terms of household amenities and consumer durables" (Tsakloglou, 1996: 288). Additively, "in Greece, Portugal and the United Kingdom, incomes of the elderly are distributed very unequally, and poverty incidence among the elderly is also high" (Heinrich, 2000: 14).

Given that the main income source for the elderly is their pension, which is generally low, there is a direct linkage between low pensions and older persons' low financial ability. At the same time, statutory income transfers to the needy elderly are neither of a significant amount nor do they constitute a "safety net" in terms of financial resources. Greece is the only EU member-state that has up to now neither established an official poverty line as the basis of social policy measures and as a yardstick for their evaluation nor a guaranteed minimum income scheme (European Commission, 1998: 5), in favour of the most vulnerable socio-economic groups.

In this respect, the elderly in Greece constitute one of the most vulnerable socio-economic groups in terms of low incomes and high poverty rates without an adequate support through a guaranteed minimum income scheme. One of the reasons for this vulnerability is also that they are forced to confront the age-related increasing health and care needs to a great extent by their own financial means.

2.3 Process of Care Provision

2.3.1 System of Provision

Historically, Greece has been characterised by a strong centralised structure of the state mechanism and consequently, the formation and implementation of social policy was highly centralised. During the 1980s an effort was made towards strengthening the decentralised administration by the transfer of competencies from the central ministries to the local authorities and the first notable step in the area of social welfare was the establishment of the Open Care Centres for Older People which are operated by local authorities. However, this attempt did not coincide with a simultaneous transfer of resources and the right to make decisions. The local authorities, which are uniquely positioned to provide effective services for the elderly in response to local demands, play an ever-increasing role, but compared to other European countries, their role is still limited in Greece. The main responsibility for social policy lies with the Ministry of Health and Welfare, which has central and regional services on the level of the prefecture (52 in total). Furthermore, certain other Ministries, such as Labour, Education, Agriculture and Justice, have also some competence in the area of social protection.

On the other hand, it has been widely noted at scientific and political level that the provision of social welfare and services in Greece lacks adequate planning and coordination even within single sectors and with respect to what are conceptualised as unidimensional problems of specific population groups. Rather than being based on a unifying philosophy, the social welfare system as a whole has evolved in a piecemeal fashion, without conjunction between ministries, agencies and services. There is growing recognition in Greece of the need for the formation of partnerships and for the effective coordination of various services, institutions and agencies in order to tackle complex multi-dimensional needs, such as the increasing need for social and health care of the elderly. Recently an important step towards cooperation, coordination and development of the welfare services and different providers has been taken through the law reforming the welfare system as a whole, at a time when this system is not well developed.

In this framework, it is difficult to discover an appropriate definition of integrated health and social care for older people in Greece, or some statutory units aiming particularly at the provision of integrated care. However, recently significant efforts have been made towards the development of social care services, which can be considered as "innovative", given the fact that some of these services incorporate elements of integrated care and seem to be the first step towards further integration in this field.

2.3.2 Needs and Availability of Care

The health status of the population in Greece steadily improved during the past decades. According to WHO estimates, Greece showed significant improvement among the EU countries in six main indicators of relevance (WHO, 1998; Ministry of Health and Welfare, 1999: 18). Currently, among the OECD and EU member states, Greece is considered to rank between those with the highest life expectancy (Ministry of Health and Welfare, 1999: 19).[2] Life expectancy increased from 70.4 years in 1960 to 80.6 in 1997. This means that there are more dependent old people and an increasing need for their care, respectively, by relatives or by professionals. The care provision for the elderly and especially for dependent persons constitutes one of the greatest challenges in the sector of social policy.

In Greece, the provision of care has traditionally been a responsibility of the family and many studies have reported the economic and non-economic burdens of care. However, a series of social and economic developments that affected Greece after the Second World War (i.e. urbanisation, industrialisation, a steady increase of the number of women in the labour force) influenced the structure and operation of the average Greek family as well as the relations at the local community level. As a result, the number of people available to provide care is gradually decreasing (Mestheneou, 1996: 442-443; Sissouras et al., 1998: 33). As in Greece a proper welfare state historically did not develop, the major part of care is provided by the family and informal networks. Thus, there is a great need to develop services to support the informal care sector. With the increasing life expectancy this requires more medical care and the development of socio-medical services that would help the elderly to extend their social activities. According to the existing bibliography, the welfare system in Greece, in comparison with other European models, is still in a stage of evolution, despite important positive steps that have been taken in recent years (Sissouras et al., 1998: 61; Emke-Poulopoulou, 1999). This modernisation process, with respect to old-age policies, is based on three fundamental axes:

- medical and preventive education, as well as the encouragement for social participation, training, entertainment etc. in order to preserve the autonomy and improve the quality of life of the elderly,
- support of the elderly and their families through the development of services which facilitate them to live at home, and
- activation and motivation of the family and the broader local community in order to increase the participation in care provision for the elderly (Centre for Planning and Economic Research, 1989).

This policy trend is mainly expressed by the establishment and continuous development of new administratively decentralised social care units which have as a goal to support the elderly in continuing to live in their natural environment, as well as to implement specific health and social care programmes (in a limited extent or on a pilot level).

In Greece, care for the elderly is provided as part of general social welfare and health care services. Exceptions to the above constitute the old-age homes, the Open Care Centres, the programme "Home help for the elderly" and some other services that function on a pilot basis. Social care is provided by the government, the local authority, the church, private non-profit organisations and the private sector. Health care is provided by doctors, general practitioners, specialised personnel (via the insurance funds), public and private hospitals and clinics.

Intermediate units, with the aim to prevent and shorten hospital admissions, do not exist in an organised way, despite existing legislation that facilitates the operation of such units in the hospitals of the National Health System. Care after discharge from hospital is provided by the "Nursing at home" services, to which all age groups are entitled, as well as in the framework of the Open Care Centres for older persons and the home help services. The publicly-owned nursing homes accept only old people who can take care of themselves, while the nursing homes for the chronically ill and the residential institutions have long waiting lists. The lack of places in these residential institutes and the increase of old people with health and care needs have as a consequence an increasing role of the private sector (Emke-Poulopoulou, 1999: 447; Sissouras et al., 1998: 58).

2.3.3 Health Care

The Greek health care system is a system of compulsory public health in-surance with strong elements of a national health system and an extensive involvement of the private sector. In terms of taxonomy, it is a mixture of the public contract and integrated models; financed by a mixture of social insurance and general taxation, with public and private providers (Minis-try of Health and Welfare, 1999: 40). Older persons – as the rest of the popu-lation – have full access to all levels of health care services which are pro-vided through the National Health System (NHS) and/or through sickness branches of the social insurance funds, while the private sector also plays an important role (Ministry of Health and Welfare, 1999: 40). The National Health Service is responsible for the provision of hospital and primary health care on a universal basis. All citizens are insured in one of the approximately 40 social insurance funds providing coverage against sickness, while the un-insured and the needy are entitled to access to public hospitals, outpatient departments of public hospitals and health centres in rural area.

Primary health care services for the elderly – as for all population groups – are provided through 196 Health Centres in rural areas and the Rural Medical Stations (which operate within the National Health System), poly-clinics of insurance funds, contracted doctors by insurance funds, outpa-tient departments of hospitals and private practitioners. The health insur-ance funds play a significant role in the provision and funding of ambula-tory services. IKA (Institute for Social Insurance), the largest social insur-ance fund (covering 50.7% of the population), is responsible for the funding and provision of health services through its wide and decentralised network of primary health care facilities (over 200 urban polyclinics and clinics). OGA (Organisation of Agricultural Insurance), the second-largest social insurance fund (22.9% of the population), takes advantage of the services of the NHS, i.e. rural health centres (Ministry of Health and Welfare, 1999: 41, 43).[3] However, despite the fact that health services are provided free of charge, people with public insurance, especially under IKA, the main public insur-ance fund, suffer big discomforts and problems of service and quite often persons who can afford to pay prefer health services either at home or pri-vate hospitals and clinics. However, this approach is inaccessible for the majority of pensioners.

Hospital care is provided by NHS public hospitals, public hospitals outside NHS (including those owned by insurance funds – IKA) and pri-vate for-profit hospitals.

The public hospitals (which operate within NHS) include 120 general and specialised hospitals totalling 40,555 beds and 9 psychiatric hospitals totalling 7,440 beds. Outside NHS there are 13 military hospitals, the cardiological centre "Onassio", 5 hospitals of the insurance institute (IKA) and 2 small teaching hospitals. The number of private hospitals (predominantly small clinics) is 234 with a total of 15,397 beds (Ministry of Health and Welfare, 1999: 42, 44). A significant development in the private sector is the establishment, since 1985, of a great number (more than 200) of "diagnostic centres". Rehabilitation services and services for the elderly (geriatric homes) are predominantly offered by the private sector. However, in terms of the total number of beds, Greece has a relatively low bed-to-population ratio among EU countries (5 beds per 1,000 inhabitants in Greece, while the EU average was 8.1).

Emergency Pre-Hospital Care is provided by the National Centre of Emergency Care (EKAB), a NHS agency. All emergency care, including all care necessary after an emergency, is available to everyone, while transfer to the hospital by EKAB is free of charge.

Regarding the Health Manpower, Greece figures as one of the countries with a high number of doctors – 3.9 doctors per 1,000 inhabitants. The opposite is true for the nursing professionals – with 2.6 nurses per 1,000 inhabitants, Greece finds itself at the bottom line among the EU countries (Ministry of Health and Welfare, 1999: 69). It should be mentioned, however, that the service of nurses, which is essential for the heavily ill and those in need of care, is very expensive and only in some cases partly covered by insurance funds.

Despite the important positive developments in the health sector during the last 20 years, in general studies show a low satisfaction of clients with the services, in particular concerning the organisation, the administration, the management and the quality of infrastructures (Mossialos, 1997: 109, 116). There is, however, relatively high user satisfaction regarding scientific and professional services.

Due to the weakness of the public health sector, the private health sector was marked by important investments. Still, these private health services are inaccessible to the low-income pensioner without any additional source of income.

2.3.4 Residential Care

With less than 1% of the total number of older people, the proportion of older people living in residential care institutions is by tradition very small (Ministry of Health and Welfare, 1999: 12). One of the main reasons is the insufficiency and the low quality of care provided by these institutions. In addition, the low level of institutional care in Greece, compared to most other European countries, clearly shows that the largest part of care for the elderly is still provided by their families, relatives and in general, by informal networks. However, as the structure of the Greek family is changing – mainly due to socio-economic changes, the declining size of the family, the increasing participation of women in employment etc. – the role of the family in caring for the elderly will be negatively affected. Also, recent studies show that the needs and demand for residential care increased over the last years.

Residential care for the elderly is provided by the state and private profit and non-profit organisations. The residential services include old-age homes and institutions for chronically ill.

- *The state-owned institutions* mainly accept individuals with low incomes (co-payments according to income, persons without any means are accepted free of charge,). The state-owned institutions, so-called "nursing homes" for the chronically ill, provide for 2,600 places only (Ministry of Health and Welfare, 2002: 9); the majority of these homes are situated in the big cities of the country.
- *The private non-profit sector* operates 57 institutional care units for older persons and about 2,800 individuals aged over 60 are living in these institutions. As in the state-owned, these organisations accept old people with low income. The Church plays an important role – it runs over 60 "houses of serenity" providing help to indigent older people (Ministry of Health and Welfare, 1999: 18).
- The insufficiency of places and the need for better quality of services had as a consequence the establishment of old-age homes and clinics run by the *private (for-profit) sector.* These units often operate as intensive rehabilitation services for persons with health problems. Some insurance funds cover part of the care expenses for private clinics and hospitals for a limited time, while the expenses for private old-age homes are not covered. Regarding the volume of services provided, no data are available; there is an estimation that these units provide hospitality to about 3,200 individuals aged over 65 (Ministry of Health

and Welfare, 2002: 9). The living conditions in some of these old-age homes are difficult, often unacceptable. The operation conditions of private homes are regulated by law, however, it seems that 300 of these homes continue to function without any authorisation in the region of Attica in 1997 (Emke-Poulopoulou, 1999: 449).

One of the policy priorities is to reform and improve the institutional care provided by the state but mainly by the private sector. Recent regulation (1995) made it possible to intervene more effectively, particularly in the private sector. The new law on the National Health System (1997) as well as the law reforming the welfare system, set instruments and measures for the operation and improvement of the institutional care services.

2.3.5 Informal Care for Older Persons

In Greece the majority of older people live alone in their home or with their children. Persons with special needs and health problems continue to accept help from family, friends and neighbours. The family plays a key role in the whole range of care for the elderly in Greece. Today, certain positive steps have been taken for the provision of community care services; nevertheless, care for the elderly is still a family affair. Carers are usually the women of the family. In Greece, there is no direct support from the state or the local government to the family carers. The cost of care is covered by the older person, either from his/her savings or from the pension, or by the family. In recent years some pilot programmes supporting the carers have been implemented. In the framework of the Programme *Ageing Well Europe,* the Gerontological and Geriatric Institute since 1996 implemented a programme for preventive health services and psychosocial support to older people and their families. Similar programmes are implemented in some regions on a pilot basis (Emke-Poulopoulou, 1999: 439, 440).

In order to help families, but also to preserve family ties and to strengthen intergenerational solidarity, special attention is given to the development of Home Care Programmes for the elderly. In addition to these programmes, the government in recent years implemented the following measures (especially for older people) in the framework of a general policy focused on strengthening the low-income groups and promoting social solidarity (Ministry of Labour and Social Security et al., 2001: 25, 26):

- The *Social Solidarity Supplement for Pensions (EKAS)* has been introduced since 1996 for low-rate pensioners whose income falls below a certain level. The grant is paid to approximately 350,000 beneficiaries. Also, EKAS pensioners are entitled to reduced co-payments for medicines.

- The *Allowance to the Uninsured* older people is granted by OGA (the Social Security Fund for the rural population). This means-tested flat rate allowance is offered to 43,000 poor uninsured persons aged over 65 and is equal to the pension granted to those insured by the OGA Fund. In addition, individuals benefiting from this allowance are also entitled to free medical care in the National Health System.
- *Housing assistance supplement* is granted to the uninsured elderly (singles or couples) without pension, with no other income in order to meet their housing expenses.

It is interesting to note that, during the last years, the problem of home care for dependent older persons seems to be "resolved" by an additional strategy, i.e. by the employment from the part of the family of (low-paid) economic immigrants, who are usually unskilled, but capable to provide domestic support. However, this way – by which the middle class generally tries to cope – is considered to curb the further development of integrated health and care services by public policies (Emke-Poulopoulou, 1999: 424).

2.3.6 Community Care as a Form of Integrated Health and Social Care Services

During the last two decades the welfare system in Greece has attempted to increase community and open care services for older people as an alternative model, in order to meet the care needs of the ageing population through policies supporting independence, autonomy and participation. The goal is to maintain the elderly in their traditional environment – home and community – as long as possible, in order to ensure independence, quality of life and social integration of elderly. This goal has been attained mainly through the development and successful implementation (by local authorities) of programmes of Open Care Centres for the Elderly (KAPI) and Home Help for the elderly, which will be extensively described in the next section as a "model working programme".

OPEN CARE CENTRES FOR OLDER PERSONS

The Open Care Centres for Older Persons are state-financed programmes that have been elaborated by the Ministry of Health and Welfare and implemented by the local authorities, aiming at the provision of preventive health services and psychosocial support to older persons in order to help them to continue living in their own environment (Sissouras et al., 1998: 43, 44; Emke-Poulopoulou, 1999: 432; Ministry of Health and Welfare, 1999: 15, 16). Currently they are spread all over the country with a total number of 607 Centres. The Open Care Centres are staffed by a team comprising social workers, medical staff, visiting nurses, occupational and physical therapists and family assistants. The Centres provide a range of services to any older person, such as preventive medical care, physiotherapy, assistance to the person in need or to their family, home help for the lonely elderly, organised entertainment and participation in various social activities. They operate in proper houses and can entertain about 300 persons on average. The establishment of these Centres is considered an innovative and successful intervention.

HELP AT HOME

Some programmes of "home help" for the elderly have been implemented over the last 20 years by public agencies and non-governmental organisations in close collaboration with the Ministry of Health and Welfare, the Church, the local authorities (autonomously or in collaboration with some open care centres) and voluntary organisations (Sissouras et al., 1998; Emke-Poulopoulou, 1999; Ministry of Health and Welfare, 1999: 17, 18).

The systematic development of home help for older persons was realised by the municipalities in collaboration with the Open Care Centres since 1998. The programme is directly supervised by the Ministry of Health and Welfare. Its aim is to provide home care to the elderly – mainly to those in need of care and/or living alone – in order to improve their autonomy and independence, to keep them active, and to reduce institutional/hospital care. Specialised personnel (a social worker, a nurse and a family assistant) regularly visit the old persons in their home. These services are offered essentially in an integrated approach for persons who are not required to stay in hospitals. The programme got enriched by the establishment of "Units of Social Care" in various municipalities – supported by the Ministry of Labour and Social Security – to further enhance the integration of health and social services.

Currently, home services are being implemented in 253 municipalities and have served 9,000 persons for the period 1998-2001. These services cover approximately one third of the individuals with needs (KEDKE, 2002: 48).

NURSING AT HOME

As mentioned before, "intermediate units" to which older persons are admitted after hospital discharge are not functioning systematically. *Nursing at home* plays an important role in this case. In Greece, home nursing was enacted by law in 1992, which determines the terms and conditions of operation. Staffs of these units comprise doctors, nurses, social workers, and other specialised personnel offering integrated health and social care services to the whole population. However, it is important to note that these services, as an organised unit, are exclusively provided by the Greek Red Cross with the exception of only two hospitals that offer this kind of services.

Day care hospitals, especially for older people, offering the necessary medical help to individuals with health problems did not exist in Greece until recently[4] (Emke-Poulopoulou, 1999: 409). In the framework of the National Social Care System (established in 1998) *Day Protection Centres for the Aged* have been developed (National Action Plan for Social Inclusion, 2001). These are small-scale units providing daily opening hours during family working hours. They are interconnected with the Open Care Centres (KAPI) and cooperate with local bodies providing social services, as well as with Health Units. In exceptional cases they have the capability to provide hospitality on a 24-hour basis. They address senior citizens with chronic or temporary physical or mental health problems, who are unable to care for themselves, have insufficient financial means and face social problems. Plans provide for the development of 80 such Centres in all regions. There are great benefits from the operation of these Centres – problems can be anticipated, medical-social problems are dealt with within the community thus preventing costs to the hospital system.

OTHER SERVICES

The National Centre for Immediate Social Assistance addresses individuals facing emergency situations and problems. The Centre's services operate on a 24-hour basis aiming at immediate handling of problems and intervention. They possess an SOS hotline, provide individualised social support and consulting services, and undertake the provision of direct interconnection with the competent services. The 21 structures developed in Athens and Thessaloniki include Admission and Support Centres, as well as short-term care facilities (Ministry of Labour and Social Security, 2001: 26).

345

The National Welfare Organisation, which through recent legislative regulation has been incorporated into the newly-established National Social Care Organisation, has been active in a variety of special programmes for the elderly, aiming at recreation and psychosocial support.

Summer camps and social tourism is a programme providing free of charge summer vacations to elderly persons aged 60 years and over.

2.3.7 Regional and Municipal Variations in Care Provision

The infrastructure and quality of the health system, as well as the provision of community care were improved during the last two decades. However, health and social care services in Greece are still characterised by an unequal distribution as regards regions and municipalities.

The regional distribution of secondary level hospital beds tends to be uneven, with the urban areas of Athens and Thessaloniki being better served. The construction of new hospitals and the renovation of public hospitals in areas distant from the major urban areas, in more recent years represent an effort to address this problem.

In the case of tertiary care, 7 of the 13 regions are covered by at least one large NHS hospital, while the remaining regions are covered by the hospital(s) of the neighbouring regions. In addition, the absence of a referral system and the freedom of patients to refer themselves to virtually any NHS hospital draws patients to the major urban centres, which have a concentration of hospitals with relatively higher standards (Ministry of Health and Welfare, 1999: 52).

Social care services are still limited and are located mainly in the big cities of the country (see Table 5). In the future these services could play an important role constituting an intermediary mechanism between hospital and social care. Nursing at home serves a small share of individuals who actually need it and is often implemented on a pilot basis. Home help services and the Open Care Centres for the Elderly do not cover all municipalities: roughly a third of them is being covered by home help services, while there is an approval by the central government to extend these services to 50% of the municipalities. The Open Care Centres operate approximately in half of the municipalities. However, there are 14 prefectures (the total number of prefectures being 52), as well as islands and remote municipalities without any kind of social care services (KEDKE, 2002). The regional variation of the social care services is presented in the following table.

Table 5: Distribution of Open Care Units for the Elderly and the Population 65+ by Region

Regions	Open Care Units**						Population 65+***(1997)		
	Home help		Open care centres		Day care centres				
	n	%	n	%	n	%	n	%	share*
Northern Greece									
East Macedonia and Thrace	43	6.02	45	7.45	4	15.38	93,549	4.84	19.87
Central Macedonia	127	17.78	216	35.76	7	26.92	300,819	15.57	19.23
West Macedonia	38	5.32	27	4.47	3	11.54	52,284	2.70	20.98
Thessaly	48	6.72	59	9.77	3	11.54	133,018	6.89	22.32
Central Greece									
Epirus	74	10.36	15	2.38	-	-	66,010	3.42	26.83
Ionian Islands	26	3.64	8	1.32	-	-	44,486	2.30	28.45
West Greece	42	5.88	16	2.64	2	7.69	116,041	6.00	22.56
Central Greece	58	8.12	23	3.80	-	-	104,826	5.43	26.14
Peloponnisos	23	3.22	12	1.98	-	-	126,365	6.54	28.32
Attica	110	15.40	133	22.02	-	-	704,591	36.48	20.49
Islands									
North Aegeon	39	5.46	10	1.65	-	-	49,730	2.57	31.87
South Aegeon	21	2.94	9	1.49	2	7.69	37,172	1.92	18.72
Crete	65	9.10	31	5.13	5	19.23	102,515	5.30	24.23
Total Greece	714	100.00	604	100.00	26	100.00	1,931,406	100.00	21.80

Note/Source: *) in relation to the population 14 years old and over; **) Ministry of Health and Welfare (2002), http://shell187.mohaw.gr/Dbsearch/Report.jsp; ***) National Statistical Service of Greece (NSSG) (1997) "Labour Force Survey 1997" (unpublished data).

347

3   Model Ways of Working

3.1   State of Evaluation Research

In Greece, a considerable effort has been made to evaluate and distinguish some "best practices" in the field of care of the elderly. The focus is almost exclusively on two most interesting and advanced programmes, namely:

- the "Open Care Centres for the Elderly" and
- the "Home Help" and Care for the Elderly.

Evaluation studies were predominantly undertaken by the Institute of Social Policy at the National Centre of Social Research (Amira et al., 1986; Teperoglou, 1990).

Furthermore, a more recent evaluation study on the Open Care Centres was carried out by the National School of Public Health (Georgoussi et al., 2001). A general review and a presentation of studies related to care for the elderly in Greece goes back – unfortunately – to 1994: "Health and Social Care for the Third Age" (Kyriopoulos et al., 1994).

3.2 Models of Integrated Care in Greece

3.2.1 The Open Care Centres for the Elderly (KAPI)

In 1979 the Directorate for the Protection of Elderly Persons of the Ministry of Health and Welfare, in cooperation with the Association of Volunteer Workers set up a pilot Open Care Centre for Elderly Persons (called hereafter "KAPI", following the Greek abbreviation). A year later, these centres were institutionalised and by the end of 1981, eight relevant programmes were operating with the contribution of volunteer organisations, the Greek Red Cross (GRC) and the Christian Youth Organisation (CYO). With Law 1416/84, article 68, the state transferred the responsibility of their management and operation to the local authorities. Ever since, their operation has flourished and now their network covers most of the country.

KAPI are public legal entities managed by a board of directors with seven members. They are funded by the municipality to which they belong and have their own budget. A representative of the elderly participates in the board of directors.

The creation of KAPI aims at preventing isolation of the elderly and at contributing to their remaining active members of society. In order to achieve this aim, KAPI should be an interaction channel connecting the elderly to their social environment, rather than a socially closed provider of services. KAPI were considered an innovative and successful intervention since, contrary to traditional services, their action focuses on the application of innovative programmes aiming at socialisation of the elderly, keeping them active, fit and healthy and creating awareness in their social environment (Amira et al., 1986: 15).

KAPI, as open care centres, were set up in order to cover a set of basic needs for as big a proportion of the elderly population as possible. However, various studies have shown that KAPI have attracted specific categories of elderly persons: "younger" elderly people who are relatively healthy and the majority of whom live with their families. This means that a considerable number of elderly persons do not participate in or are excluded from KAPI activities, which led to the conclusion that such programmes must be extended to include the elderly who live alone, have limited mobility and need care (Hatzigianni, 1996: 483).

Despite these obstacles, the role and contribution of KAPI have been widely recognised, especially by the elderly themselves, who declare that KAPI have contributed positively to the improvement of their everyday life. This conclusion is drawn from the results of two past studies undertaken by the National Centre for Social Research (NCSR), one of which related to the study of various socio-economic problems of the areas selected for the creation of KAPI (pre-operational survey – 1986), while the other assessed the opinions of elderly people concerning KAPI programmes (1990 – Evaluation of KAPI contribution).

More specifically, according to the results of the "Evaluation of KAPI contribution", elderly persons declare that KAPI mainly provide them with entertainment and company. The majority (89%) is satisfied with KAPI operation and programmes. It must be noted, though, that a higher percentage of elderly persons over 75 declare themselves satisfied, while elderly persons between 65 and 75 would like to see the programmes to be improved. Furthermore, 42% of the sample declares itself entirely satisfied with the programmes provided, not requiring additional services. Most of the requests for extra services concern health care and recreational activities (Teperoglou, 1990: 155).

Support and acceptance of the elderly for KAPI resulted from studies undertaken during the first years of operation of the centres, but later there were no similar studies concerning the satisfaction of the elderly, at least not on a wider scale. Nevertheless, an evaluation research for KAPI was recently undertaken by the National School of Public Health concerning the range and the frequency of providing services, the number of personnel, the profile of the users (Georgoussi et al., 2001: 164).

However, it is necessary to create a mechanism both for adapting to the constantly changing needs of the elderly and for the evaluation of KAPI contribution to satisfy these needs.

Nowadays, 604 KAPI operate all over Greece, while the completion of existing structures and the development of new KAPI in areas where they do not exist or in which there are increased needs not covered by existing

349

arrangements, are in the implementation stage (Ministry of Health and Welfare, 2002: 13).

This model way of working for the care of the elderly reveals some interesting issues and policies which are contributing to an integrated way of care delivery:

- A well-targeted environment is created where active elderly are exercising their opportunity for integration in social life with the support of an "integrated programme of care", which caters for health and social care needs.
- The scheme enhances the participation of the community and the development of voluntary work as many places in KAPI are covered by volunteers and vice versa, a number of active elders (8.8%) take part in voluntary work in the community, e.g. kindergartens, school keepers etc.
- In the area of "cost containment" for health and care expenditure, a more rational use of resources is exercised and a control of unnecessary demands from elderly (drugs, treatment, visits to health centres etc.)
- There is scope for a more integrated type of programmes on prevention, health promotion, social integration etc.

3.2.2 "Home Help for the Elderly": The Case of (Multiple) Public Involvement

In Greece, *"Home Help for the Elderly"* was institutionalised with Law 2082/ 92 and is implemented by the Ministry of Health and Welfare in cooperation with local authorities, the Church and non-governmental voluntary organisations. From the beginning of the 1980s, however, the Ministry of Health and Welfare had begun to implement and fund, from time to time, home help programmes in some municipalities of the country, independently as well as in cooperation with the Greek Red Cross.

In 1998 the implementation of a five-year pilot programme began, which was based on a "tripartite model" bringing together the Ministry of Health and Welfare, the Ministry of Public Administration and Decentralisation and the municipalities as the third actor responsible for organising and providing the services. To this extent the scheme is an interesting experiment of public policy and public cooperation. The plan is to achieve nation-wide coverage by the end of 2003 (1,000 home care programmes). Home

Help Programmes are closely linked to Open Care Centres for the Elderly of each municipality, while the programme as a whole is coordinated and evaluated by a monitoring committee.

Home help is a right of every elderly citizen, since it ensures his/her being able to remain at home and within the community s/he has chosen to live when s/he faces self-sufficiency problems. The aim of the programme is to promote, maximise and restore, to the greatest possible extent, the independence of elderly persons, providing them with support and help so as to avoid physical disability, exclusion from social participation and confinement.

In the framework of primary care, the services provided by the programme aim at supporting elderly persons and their families so they can cope with the increased needs of their condition, temporary or permanent, and continue to be together with their families' part of the social environment.

The programme organises activities relating to:

- social services (counselling and psychosocial support, information concerning the rights of the elderly and connection to health, welfare and insurance organisations),
- health care services (medical and nursing care, health education and prevention, medication prescription, physiotherapy at home, transfers, e.g. to see the physician), as well as
- family assistance (home and personal care, feeding, chores, befriending, etc).

In order to provide organised and systematic help to the elderly and their families, the programme employs a number of specialised scientists and trained professionals, among which social workers, nurses and family assistants. At the same time, it also makes considerable use of volunteer initiatives, thus promoting the development of social solidarity.

DEVELOPMENT STAGES OF THE PROGRAMME / MAIN ACTION PHASES

A major precondition for the development of the programme is the mapping of the municipality in which it will operate: recording and processing of health and social care needs of elderly persons living in the area, as well as of existent social infrastructures at the local level. The main information sources for potential users of the programme are KAPI, the Church, the neighbourhood, the family, the hospital and other competent institutions.

The next step includes classification of the health and social care needs of elderly citizens (relief, prevention, rehabilitation, psychosocial problem prevention, everyday life support, personal hygiene, etc.) and when deemed necessary, intervention from the specialists employed by the programme. More specifically, the type of required service is identified, followed by the frequency of need, the time period during which this service is required, cooperation with family, volunteers, etc. and referrals to health services and other bodies. When the intervention plan has been completed, a meeting with the family – if any and if willing to contribute – is arranged to inform the relatives about the programme and discuss the particulars of coopera-tion. Data are collected and recorded all through the programme. These data relate to services provided at each visit/meeting and help to assess the type and frequency of intervention in case it needs change.

It must be noted that if the need for hospitalisation of an elderly pa-tient arises, the people in charge of the programmes contact the social serv-ices of hospitals and nursing units for chronic diseases and refer the elderly person to one of those providing the competent authorities with informa-tion about his/her condition. They follow-up his/her progress and take on care again when s/he is released from hospital.

Nowadays, there are 714 operating units/programmes of "Home Help for Elderly Persons". Simultaneously with the Home Help Programme, there are the so-called Social Care Units, financed by the Ministry of Labour and Social Security. These units also provide home help services to elderly per-sons and usually operate in an ancillary fashion to cover existing gaps. There are 211 such units nation-wide.

EVALUATION OF THE PROGRAMME

In 2001, three years after inception of the pilot programme "Home Help for the Elderly" (1998-2003) and while the programme had already expanded, a first evaluation of its contribution was attempted with the participation of 100 municipalities, on the basis of out-turn reports relating to its quality and management control.

The monitoring committee of the programme decided to perform an evaluation of its three-year operation in order to get feedback on planning and on the methods used to assess its effectiveness and to identify its weak-nesses. This evaluation was based on data collected by professional carers. More specifically, information was processed from various documents and questionnaires that were used for assessing the needs and social history of each elderly person participating in "Home Help" in order to provide tailor-made care.

According to the evaluation results, the residents of the areas involved in the programmes responded quite positively to this new service, which they supported either through voluntary work or by offering money and other commodities.

During its first three years of operation, the programme provided services to 9,000 elderly persons. This number is considered satisfactory given the limited extent of the programme. From the total of persons served, 47% were living alone and 34% were in need of care (KEDKE, 2002: 48).

Types of care provided to the elderly participating in the programme included social work services, nursing care and family assistance. The majority of elderly persons participating in the programme (39%) benefited from social work. With regard to nursing care, the services mostly used by the elderly were treatment interventions and health education (26% and 24% respectively). Finally, with regard to family assistance, the highest percentages of use were recorded for company and household work (28% and 27% respectively) (KEDKE, 2002: 38).

With regard to the frequency of use, in the majority of cases social work was required fortnightly (38%) or weekly (34%), while in the remaining, the service was required more often (2-3 times per week or daily). Nursing care and family assistance are requested more frequently or at least once a week (34% and 41% respectively). When deemed necessary, however, all types of services can be provided daily (KEDKE, 2002: 43-46).

An important parameter of the programme is the annual cost estimation for the provision of each programme: on average, 35,000 Euro are necessary to cover the needs of 60 elderly persons. This amount approximately corresponds to the maintenance of two older persons in a residential care unit. In addition, it must be underlined that thanks to the services provided by the programme there has been a potential reduction of the use of outpatient departments in hospitals.

The programme is presently developing with an utmost commitment from the three actors involved and with an exceptional political support. The framework and the process for monitoring and evaluating the programme do already exist. There will be a particular focus on assessing the elements of an *integrated* type of approach, along the main features of the programme which:

353

- made elderly persons living alone feel more secure,
- provided the necessary nursing and support care to persons, which otherwise would have been provided by outpatient departments,
- organised the performance of laboratory tests for patients that otherwise would have been referred to outpatient departments or even to inpatient units,
- contributed to stop the progress of certain diseases thanks to a close follow-up of the patients and frequent administration of the necessary medication,
- eased down the burdens of family dependency, and
- has given the opportunity to test the creation of care teams, which can assure the effective development of the concept of integrated care.

3.2.3 The Red Cross "Home Help Programme": A Case of Non-public Involvement

In 1988, the Greek Red Cross (GRC) started the implementation of a programme called "Home Help" in five districts in the centre of Athens with the cooperation of the Ministry of Health and Welfare.

The proposed services include social services, medical and nursing services and various other events organised by volunteers (keeping company, feasts and celebrations, recreational activities). These services are organised and offered to elderly persons by an interdisciplinary group of specialists consisting of social workers, physicians (general practitioners), psychologists, nurses, physiotherapists, family assistants and social welfare volunteer workers (Liakou, 1998: 203).

Noteworthy is the development of a tele-alarm service. This service is proposed to lonely or non self-sufficient elderly persons participating in the GRC programme. Once this service is activated, the elderly person has the possibility to communicate at all times in case of emergency with a centre and explain what his/her problem is.

PROCESS OF ACCESS TO THE PROGRAMME

With regard to referral and inclusion of elderly persons to the programme, it must be noted that a first step is to record applications for help and to include elderly persons living in the districts covered. An alternative route is to be referred to the programme by other "Home Help" programmes implemented by the local authorities. The programme also provides information about other existing services and structures in order to help the elderly to cover needs not addressed by the programme.

Newcomers are first individually interviewed, at home, by a social worker. The aim of this interview is to identify the older person's needs. Then, the elderly are informed about the services/facilities provided by the programme and about the way in which the various bodies involved should cooperate in order to enhance the services received.

EVALUATION OF THE PROGRAMME

From October 2001 to February 2002 an evaluation study was undertaken concerning the "Home Help Programme" services on the basis of a sample of 100 older persons living in the districts of Exarchia, Kipseli and Patissia. The sample consisted of persons having used almost all services provided by the programme for a long period of time.

According to the evaluation data, the majority of elderly persons participating in the programme are either living alone (49%) or with their companion (13%) and are lacking family support for company or in case of illness. With regard to their health status, 40% are self-sufficient and 49% partly self-sufficient. The majority of elderly persons participating in the programme (88%) are women, whose financial position is precarious. With regard to the age of older persons participating in the programme, the majority are over 70 years old (60%). These persons face serious economic problems and either cover their basic needs with difficulty (44%) or cannot satisfy these needs by themselves so that they are dependent on help from their children or from other relatives (30%) (Greek Red Cross, 2002: 1-32).

The profile of elderly participants in the programme indicates that they have to cope with more than one serious problem, such as illness, poverty, loneliness, bad relations with their families, etc. Without support provided by the programme, these problems would lead to their social exclusion. The continuation and extension of these programmes is under way along with assessing new and emerging needs, so as to plan early for new services.

3.2.4 The Programme of the Hellenic Association of Gerontology and Geriatrics: The Case of a Special Group of Patients

The Hellenic Association of Gerontology and Geriatrics (HAGG) was founded in 1977, in order to promote the creation of structures and to provide consultancy services on issues relating to old age.

In this framework, the HAGG is striving to create a network for Alzheimer's disease (AD) in order to permanently inform health professionals on the latest developments concerning AD, thus helping persons with dementia and their families. It has also played a leading role in the creation of the Alzheimer's Caregivers' Association. This association was founded in 1997 to provide information on existing structures and new therapeutic approaches. At the same time, in 2001 the HAGG founded the psycho-geriatric association "Nestor", the aim of which is to provide services relating to dementia and other psychiatric problems linked to old age.

In Greece there are no institutions specialised in dementia. Patients are referred to the outpatient departments of certain hospitals (organic psychiatric syndromes or memory clinics), to hospitals with psychiatric, neurological clinics or specialised psycho-geriatric clinics, to private psychiatric clinics and to nursing homes for the chronically ill. It must be noted that both general hospitals and specialised psychiatric hospitals are health service providers and not welfare institutions. This means that they lack hospital beds for chronically ill patients suffering from AD, since their role is to diagnose the problem, suggest possible ways of treatment and then consign the persons to their families for care. Hospital beds for chronically-ill patients are available, in limited numbers, at nursing homes for the chronically ill and at some private psychiatric clinics. Greece also lacks open day care structures for this type of patients, with the exception of day centres for psychiatric incidents, which accept persons suffering from mild dementia (Mougias, 2001: 168-170).

It is obvious that structures for patients with dementia are insufficient and for this reason the three associations mentioned above are planning to jointly operate from 2003 onwards two Alzheimer centres (each consisting of a Day Centre, a Boarding House and a Family Assistance Team). One of these centres will open its doors in Athens and another one will operate, on pilot basis, on the island of Chios, co-funded by the EU and the Ministry of Health and Welfare. The Day Centre will be open morning and afternoon and employ specialised experts (psychologists, psychiatrists, social workers, psychotherapists, labour therapists). It will provide day care and short-stay services. Day care services will include labour therapy, physiotherapy, direct medical care and entertainment. The Boarding House will be staffed by 21 persons of the same specialities as the Day Centre and have a capacity of 15 beds. Furthermore, it is expected that the Association of Psycho-geriatrics "Nestor" will develop, in 2003, a psycho-geriatrics clinic and a training programme addressing general practitioners.

Meanwhile, contributing to the efforts to draw up a common European policy, the Hellenic Association of Gerontology and Geriatrics (HAGG) has participated in recent years in a number of European programmes co-financed by the European Commission such as the:

- Health Education Programme on Cardiovascular Diseases
- Information and Awareness Programme on Issues relating to the Improvement of Elderly Persons' Health
- Programme on Nutrition and Alzheimer's disease
- "Alzheimer's Disease Network" Programme
- Programme relating to resolving legal issues of Alzheimer patients.

This programme offers the chance to look for the development of programmes of care for special groups of the elderly. The nature of integrated care requires a different view particularly because it involves a range of different factors.

3.2.5 Care for the Elderly by the Greek Church: The Case of a Non-governmental Organisation[5]

Care for the elderly by the Greek Church has had ever since a prominent place in the Greek welfare system.[6] Its activities are focused on the following measures:

- In Greece, which is administratively covered by the authority of the Greek Orthodox Church, apart from the Archdiocese of Athens, there are nowadays 74 care institutions for older persons, hosting about 2,700 persons. These are directly managed by the Holy Metropolitans.
- Voluntary working groups focus their activities on finding lonely older persons, in order to provide them with the best support in every respect on the level of the parish.
- In the majority of the parishes daily meals are being offered to Greek and migrant older persons. In special cases these people can be supported by organised home deliveries.
- Extra financial support is being offered to persons with low pensions.
- Many of the Bishops of the Greek Orthodox Church are elected as presidents of not only church-owned care institutions, but also of those owned by other organisations of the Third Sector.

The role of the Athens Archdiocese in social care for the elderly has to be especially highlighted:

- In each of the 144 parish churches of Athens there are donations to all needy older people.

- There are 78 "Christian Centres" where 3,580 older persons are provided with food and care.
- There are 30 parish churches with specialised psychologists who help lonely old people to find psychological support.
- There are 19 care institutions with about 490 older persons.

It is very important to mention that all the above services, medical treatment and social care, are completely free of charge. The Church's social care for older persons is based on the following principles:

- All institutions must be built in separate regions close to the natural environment of older people.
- The Church's care institutions must operate as small units, so that there is an opportunity to build on strong bonds and healthy relationships between all people that use these facilities.
- Volunteers' work should be developed in coordination with the principles of the "Social Economy".
- There should be no discrimination (religion, nationality, colour, sex, etc.).
- The social care and health needs of elderly people should be taken care of.

The care scheme provided by the Church presents an interesting case: firstly, because it shows that the religious tradition continues to include welfare and social protection in its activities and, secondly, for the high number of persons served and care centres supplied. In fact, recently a debate has started to further examine the "model" of care provided by the Church, in particular the type, quality and nature of this "integrated" concept. The PROCARE project could include this concept – provided by a voluntary organisation – and attempt to "transfuse" its principles and practice.

4   Conclusions and Policy Considerations

The previous exposition leads us to a number of conclusions, which can provide the basis and framework for the development of policies and programme actions.

Greece is following the European pattern of a growing ageing population. Currently, national policies – reinforced also by European Union policies – are mainly focused on "solving" the pressing problem of pensions and social security. Greece, too, has responded to this issue of pensions and has "consumed" plenty of time and efforts until this year a drastic reform of the pension system has been decided in Parliament. However, it is equally high time to develop respective policies in the area of a comprehensive system of health and social care for the elderly. In this respect, the European Union policies have started to become more elaborated and we may count much on the process being developed by the Social Protection Committee. The first investigations and policy recommendations are depicted in two very important documents, namely *"The future of health care and care for the elderly: guaranteeing accessibility, quality and financial viability (COM2001 723 final)"* and the follow-up of this communication, entitled *"Supporting national strategies for the future health care and care for the elderly"*. Of high importance are also the documents provided by all Member States as a response to a (well-designed) questionnaire on *"Health and Social Care for the Elderly"*, on the basis of which the second document mentioned above was drafted.[7]

The traditional *model of "informal care" mainly at the family level,* has started to recede due to new "cultural and lifestyle" developments of the Greek family backed up by income improvements of the typical household. This has led to a policy of shifting to residential care for elderly, developed by both the public and the growing private sector. Therefore the demand for a "regulated" mechanism for the evaluation of these services by the state is a new claim from the "taxpayer" who now "recognises" more the value and the obligation of the state for welfare services.

The organisational and institutional arrangements and the split between the "contributory" and "non-contributory" funds, i.e. general budget and social insurance funds providing health and social care for the elderly, must be solved. While the social insurance funds should develop a more comprehensive system of benefits (in cash), the public authorities should promote a likewise comprehensive system of public care institutions and services, in which health and social care are organised by integrated processes and programmes. *The financing of care for the elderly* thus has to be based on strategies that facilitate integration. The allocation of resources should be based on a "mixed model" that will ensure the appropriate financial sustainability. Thus, provision by *statutory authorities, social insurance, voluntary organisations, family*, and *private* organisations (contracting-in) have to be regulated. Currently, efforts are being made to develop such steering mechanisms and contractual arrangements, in particular with respect to statutory funding of voluntary organisations and private enterprises.

A critical consideration concerns *the evaluation and monitoring* of special programmes, particularly the "Open Care Programme" and the "Home Care and Help Programme" in which the government is investing to improve social integration and health of older people. Besides, a new experiment of coordination is being tested between public and local authority services, where the programmes themselves act as "catalysts" in developing social care policies at municipal level. Thus, an information system is to be introduced in the "Home Help" programme in order to assess the *quality of care* offered.

In this report it became evident that in Greece there currently exists a spectrum of services scattered around the country, operating under different administrative structures and at different levels of functioning and effectiveness. During the last two years a major project has been undertaken in the Ministry of Health and Welfare, *to develop a "Master Plan" of these services*. This plan will be the basis of a reform that should give way to a new organisational structure with a respective redefinition of responsibilities, particularly with respect to the integration of health and social care services at the regional level.

360

Notes

1   The functions of social protection are: *Sickness/Health Care* (includes, *inter alia*, paid sick leave, medical care and the supply of pharmaceutical products); *Disability* (includes, *inter alia*, disability pensions and the provision of goods and services, other than medical care, to the disabled); *Old-age* (includes, *inter alia*, old-age pensions and the provision of goods and services, other than medical care, to the elderly); *Survivors* (income support in connection with the death of a family member, e,g. survivors' pensions); *Family/children* (includes support, other than medical care, in connection with pregnancy, childbirth, maternity and the care of children and other dependent family members); *Unemployment* (includes, *inter alia*, unemployment benefits and vocational training financed by public agencies); *Housing* (includes interventions by public authorities to help households meet the cost of housing); *Social exclusion* (not elsewhere classified [n.e.c.]) (includes income-support benefits, rehabilitation of alcoholics and drug addicts, and various other benefits [other than medical care]).

2   Ministry of Health and Welfare, 1999, based on United Nations, OECD Health Data 1998, and National Statistical Services in Greece.

3   The rest of the funds provide health care services to their beneficiaries mainly through contracts with private physicians for the ambulatory sector, and public and private hospitals for secondary and tertiary health care services.

4   There exist two units of health day care, from which the older citizens are excluded. The private sector tried to cover this lack in services. The first centre was established in 1998 and operates under excellent conditions.

5   This extract has been prepared by G. Diellas who works as an advisor in the Welfare section of the Ministry of Health and Welfare.

6   The creation, formation and administration of the institutes and general legal entities, which provide social care services on behalf of the Church, are regulated in the Law 590/1977 (Charter of the Greek Orthodox Church); financial resources and expenditures are publicly controlled.

7   These documents and particularly the "Questionnaire Request" are important references to the PROCARE project.

References

Amira, A./Georgiadi, E./Teperoglou, A. (1986) *The Institution of Open Care of the Elderly in Greece.* Athens: National Centre for Social Research / Ministry of Health and Welfare.

Centre for Planning and Economic Research (KEPE) (1989) *Welfare State for the Programming Period 1988-1992,* Athens.

Emke-Poulopoulou, I. (1999) *Greek Old Citizens, Past, Present and Future.* Athens: Ellin.

Esping-Andersen, G. (1996) *The Three Worlds of Welfare Capitalism.* Cambridge: Polity Press-Blackwell Publishers.

European Commission (1998) *Commission Report on the implementation of the recommendation 92/441/eec/of 24 June 1992 on common criteria concerning sufficient resources and social assistance in social protection systems, Com (98) 774 final.* From the World Wide Web: http://europa.eu.int/comm/employment_social/soc-prot/social/com98-774/com774_en.pdf

European Commission (2002) *The Social Situation in the European Union 2002,* Luxembourg: Eurostat Directorate-General for Employment and Social Affairs.

Georgoussi, E./Economou, Ch./Danielidou, N./Kyriopoulos, J. (2001) 'Evaluation of the Provided Services by Open Care Centres for the Elderly (KAPI) towards Health Prevention and Promotion', pp. 164-182 in: Dimoliatis, G./Kyriopoulos, J./Lagas, D./Filalithis, T. (eds.), *Public Health in Greece.* Athens: Themelio / Society and Health.

Greek Red Cross (2001) Directorate for Social Welfare, *Report: Home Care Programme – 2001.* Unpublished Manuscript.

Greek Red Cross (2002) Directorate for Social Welfare, *Evaluation of the Home Care Programme for the Elderly by the Users.* Unpublished Manuscript.

Hatzigianni, A. (1996) 'The Incorporation of the Elderly in the Society and the Role of the Protective Institutions', pp. 479-487 in: Kotzamanis, B./Maratou-Alipranti, L./Teperoglou, A./Tzortzopoulou, M. (eds.), *Ageing and Society –Minutes of the Panellenic Congress of National Centre for Social Research (EKKE).* Athens: EKKE.

Heinrich, G. A. (2000) *Affluence and Poverty in Old Age: New Evidence from the European Community Household Panel. CEPS/INSTEAD,* Luxembourg, pp. 1-28.

(KEDKE) Central Union of Municipalities and Communities of Greece (2002) *The Programme "Home Care for the Elderly".* Athens: KEDKE.

Kotzamanis, B./Maratou-Alipranti, L./Teperoglou, A./Tzortzopoulou, M. (eds.) (1996) *Ageing and Society –Minutes of the Panellenic Congress of National Centre for Social Research (EKKE).* Athens: EKKE.

Kyriopoulos, J./Georgoussi, E./Skoutelis, G. (eds.) (1994) *Health, Social Protection for Third Age.* Athens: Centre for Health and Social Sciences.

Liakou, M. (1998) 'Home Care – Greek Red Cross Programme. Dimensions and Perspectives', *Social Work 52:* 203-209.

Marlier, E./Cohen-Solal, M. (2000) 'Social Benefits and their Redistributive Effect in EU: Latest Data Available', Eurostat, *Statistics in Focus,* THEME 3- 9/2000, Luxembourg: 1-7.

Mestheneou, E. (1996) 'Who Cares', pp. 442-443 in: Kotzamanis, B./Maratou-Alipranti, L./ Teperoglou, A./Tzortzopoulou, M. (eds.) *Ageing and Society – Minutes of the Panhellenic Congress of the National Centre for Social Research (EKKE)*. Athens: EKKE.

Ministry of Health and Welfare (1999) *Health Care in Greece*. Athens: Ministry of Health and Welfare.

Ministry of Health and Welfare (1990) *Social Budget 1990*. Athens.

Ministry of Health and Welfare (2000) *Social Budget 2000*. Athens.

Ministry of Health and Welfare (1999) *The Elderly in Greece. Policies and Actions.* Athens: Ministry of Health and Welfare.

Ministry of Health and Welfare (2002) The Hellenic Response to the EPC/SPC Questionnaire on Health and Long-term Care for the Elderly. From the world wide web: http://www.europa.eu.int/comm/employment_socioP/soc-prot/healthcare/eP-healthreply-en.pdf

Ministry of Labour and Social Security (Coordinator), Ministry of Health and Welfare, Ministry of Interior, Public Administration and Decentralization, Ministry of Education and Religious Affairs and Ministry of National Economy and Finance (2001) *National Action Plan for Social Inclusion 2001-2003*, Athens.

Mossialos, E. (1997) 'Citizens' Views on Health Care Systems in the 15 Member States of the European Union', *Health Economics*: 109-116.

Mougias, A. (1998, 2nd ed.) *Alzheimer Disease, Timely Diagnosis, Help for the Family. A*thens: Hellenic Association of Gerontology and Geriatrics.

Mougias, A. (2001) *Alzheimer Disease. For use of Health Professionals and Carers.* Programme "Psychargos": Hellenic Association of Gerontology and Geriatrics, Tripoli.

National Statistical Service of Greece (1999) *Household Expenditure Survey 1993/1994.* Athens.

National Statistical Service of Greece (2002) *Greece in Numbers 2002.* Athens. From the World Wide Web: http://www.statistics.gr/gr_tables/hellas_in_numbers.pdf

OECD (2001) *Health Data.* Paris.

OECD (1996) *Ageing in OECD Countries: A Critical Policy Challenge.* Paris: Social Policy Studies, No. 20.

Papaliou, O./Fagadaki, E. (2002) 'The Profile of Health and Welfare in Greece', pp. 89-110 in: Mouriki, A./Naoumi, M./Papapetrou, J. (eds.), *The Social Portrait of Greece – 2001.* Athens: Institute of Social Policy, National Centre for Social Research (EKKE).

Sissouras, A./ Ketsetzopoulou, M./Bouzas, N. (1998) *The Elderly in Greece: Analysis and Proposals for a National Programme.* Athens: Institute of Social Policy, National Centre for Social Research.

Triantafilou, T./ Mestheneou, E. (1993) *Who Cares?* Athens: Sextant.

Tsakloglou, P. (1996) 'Elderly and Non-elderly in the European Union: A Comparison of Living Standards', *Review of Income and Wealth*, 42 (3): 271-291.

Visko, I. (2000) *Welfare Systems, Aging and Work: An OECD Perspective.* Banca Nazionale del Lavoro Quarterly Review.

Teperoglou, A. (1990) *Evaluation of the Contribution of the Open Care Centres for the Elderly.* Athens: National Centre for Social Research / Ministry of Health and Welfare.

Teperoglou, A. (1993) 'The Institution of Open Care for the Elderly: Stagnation or Evolution?', pp. 293-300 in: Kyriopoulos, J./Georgoussi, E./Skoutelis, G. (eds.), *Health, Social Protection for Third Age.* Athens: Centre for Health and Social Sciences.

Tsaoussis, D./Xatzigianni, A. (1990) *Social and Land-planning Conditions for the Operation of the Open Care Centres for the Elderly (KAPI).* Panteion University of Social and Political Sciences/Ministry of Health and Welfare.

World Health Organisation (1998) *Highlights on Health in Greece (Draft).* Copenhagen: WHO.

362

Annex I: Financial Data

Table 1: Social Protection Expenditures as Percentage of GDP:
          Greece and EU-15 (1990 and 1999)

	1990	1999	+/- %1999-'90
Greece	22.9	25.5	11.35
EU-15	25.5	27.6	8.23

Source: European Commission, 2002: 123.

Table 2: Social Protection Expenditure by Sector: 1990 and 2000
          (Current Prices)

Sectors	1990		2000	
	in million euro	%	in million euro	%
Social insurance*	6,232.1	84.48	21,007.5	87.14
Health**	945.5	12.81	2,391.7	9.92
Welfare***	199.4	2.71	709.2	2.94
Total	7,377.0	100.00	24,108.4	100.00

Sources: Ministry of Health and Welfare, 1990:13 and 2000: 21.
Notes: *) Social Insurance Funds provisions include expenditure on: pensions, health care, welfare benefits
           and administrative support.
           **) This headline includes the funds, which are transferred from MHW to public hospitals.
           ***) Financial funds transferred from MHW to welfare institutions. Also, it must be noted that
           the Greek MHW offers a variety of social services and cash benefits to needed families, vulnerable
           groups and in cases of physical disasters.

Table 3:   Receipts of Social Protection by Type of Contributors (as Percentage of
            Total Receipts: Greece and EU-15, 1990 and 1999)

	General Government Contributions		Employers		Social Contributions		Other	
	1990	1999	1990	1999	1990	1999	1990	1999
Greece	33.0	28.6	39.4	37.7	19.6	23.4	8.0	10.3
EU-15	28.8	35.7	42.5	37.9	24.6	22.7	4.1	3.7

Source: European Commission, 2002: 123.

Table 4   Social Benefits by Groups of Functions: Greece and EU-15
            (1990 and 1999)

	Old age survivors		Sickness, health care and disability		Unemployment		Family and children		Housing and social exclusion	
	1990	1999	1990	1999	1990	1999	1990	1999	1990	1999
Greece	51.7	50.7	33.2	31.0	4.1	5.7	7.5	7.6	3.4	5.0
EU-15	45.9	46.0	36.1	34.9	7.3	6.8	7.7	8.5	3.0	3.8

Source: European Commission 2002: 123.

Annex II: Project Abstracts

A1 Open Care Centres for the Elderly (KAPI)

Provider (organisations involved)	Local Authorities (Municipal Social Services)
Objectives	• To provide services focused on prevention, treatment and rehabilitation of the biological, psychological and social problems of the elderly, so that they remain independent, active and equal members of society. • To inform the public opinion and all competent bodies about the problems and needs of the elderly and earn their support. • To promote and support the family principle and the possibility for the elderly to continue to live in their social environment. • To promote socio-medical research on issues related to the elderly.
Target group and number of clients	Registered members should be at least 60 years old, men and women living in the KAPI reference area; irrespective of their financial status (they pay a "symbolic" annual membership fee). The number of active members of a KAPI depends on the size of its area of responsibility. There are usually more women than men.
Number of staff involved	Each KAPI has a scientific team consisting of the following specialised personnel: social workers, nurses, health visitors, family assistants, physiotherapists and labour therapists. In some cases it is possible to have a leaner team with less specialised personnel.
Methods	The actions taken to promote inclusion and stay of the elderly in the community are the following: • Social participation actions, through which the team tries to alleviate the feeling of loneliness of the elderly by providing them with opportunities to discuss, communicate, develop various hobbies and feel useful and necessary for their families and for society. • Preventive medicine, divided into primary (vaccinations, advice relating to healthy eating habits, etc) and secondary (performance of medical tests aiming at early diagnosis in order to avoid frequent lengthy treatments). • Active participation of the elderly through the creation of activity teams corresponding to their interests (theatre, choir, traditional dances, and gym).

365

	• Staging of cultural and recreational activities (excursions, camping, attending various events, etc).
	• Turning their skills and experience to advantage.
	• Promoting awareness of the community and solidarity between generations.
	• Creation of links and cooperation with other bodies (Popular Education Committees, schools, cultural associations) in order to jointly organise activities and bridge the generation gap.
Strengths	Local authorities, which have first hand knowledge of the needs and particularities of the elderly living in their area, are responsible for the development and implementation of this institution.
	• The elderly have expressed positive opinions and have welcomed the creation of KAPI.
	• The KAPI network covers most of Greece.
	• There is significant participation of the elderly in recreational and cultural activities.
	• KAPI are linked to the "IKA" (Public Insurance Fund) in order to cover their members' needs, no matter which insurance fund they originally belong to.
Weaknesses	Lack of a mechanism of study, recording and permanent follow-up of the elderly population, in order to identify their needs and accordingly complete or modify the services provided.
	• Insufficient staffing as regards scientific personnel.
	• Problems related to the buildings used (difficult access, inappropriate buildings).
	• Lack of appropriate information in order to attract new members.
	• Limited financial resources impacting on the quality of available programmes, number of employees and opening hours.
Results of evaluation/keywords	Nation-wide expansion of the network
	• Securing of funds to improve KAPI operation.
	• Completion of services and activities and enhancement of KAPI programmes.

A2 "Home Help for Elderly Persons"

Provider (organisations involved)	This programme is supervised by the Ministry of Health and Welfare and jointly co-financed by the Ministries of Health and Welfare and Public Administration and Decentralisation. After 2003, the programmes will be entirely financed by the municipal authorities. Local authorities, through their KAPI (Open Care Centres for the Elderly), have undertaken its implementation.
Objectives	• To enable the elderly to remain in their homes and to improve their quality of life. • To provide care to elderly persons to help them maintain their independence and their physical and psychological condition to the greatest possible extent. • Minimalisation of recourse to care homes. • Support to persons or families taking care of elderly relatives. • Sensitisation of the neighbourhood and of society in general to promote support of the elderly and development of voluntary services at municipal level.
Target group and number of clients	From 1998 to 2001 9,000 elderly have been included in the programme. Priority of participation was given to persons that: • were not entirely self-sufficient, • required special care, • lived alone, • had insufficient resources.
Number of staff involved	The programme employed more than 300 personnel (social workers, nurses and family assistants). Furthermore, it received assistance from 1,200 trained volunteers.
Methods	The "Home Help" programme has been implemented by municipalities, which already operate a KAPI, since Open Care Centres for the Elderly are the major source of information and referral to the programme. The programme also includes a study of the health and social care needs of the elderly and the collection of data relating to services provided and frequency of use. Furthermore, it communicates/cooperates with other institutions (such as hospital, municipal clinics, care homes, etc) to cover cases in which the changing needs of the elderly require their referral to other competent structures.

Strengths	• Positive response of the elderly. • Significant degree of satisfaction of their needs. • Alleviation of family members caring for the elderly. • Mobilisation of volunteers. • Exploitation and organisation of various sources of aid (citizen donations in the form of food, clothing, pharmaceuticals and nursing material.
Weaknesses	Lack of a network covering all municipalities in Greece and especially insular and mountainous areas (60% of such programmes being run in Attica and Central Macedonia). • Insufficient satisfaction of the needs of isolated communities due to lack of specialised staff. • Lack of coordination of programmes and services in favour of the elderly at municipal or prefectural level. • Overloading of the personnel, since the existing needs are quite considerable and each programme covers a significant number of elderly persons (60 on average). • Lack of specialised personnel in certain categories (physiotherapists, labour therapists, psychologists, psychiatrists, etc), which are indispensable for effective implementation of the programme.
Results of evalua- tion/keywords	Ensuring the continuation and expansion of these programmes to cover the entire country. • Adopting a favourable policy to support the elderly (legislation, funding, extension of benefits). • Coordination between the programme and local authorities, welfare structures, health units, the church, etc. to avoid overlaps and cover existing gaps. • Enriching the programmes with personnel from other specialities.

368

A3 The Greek Red Cross "Home Help for the Elderly"

Provider (organisations involved)	The Directorate of Social Care of the Greek Red Cross with the cooperation and financial support of the Ministry of Health and Welfare.
Objectives	• To provide specialised services to elderly people who are isolated and suffering from temporary or permanent social, health or economic problems, and/or from loneliness. The aim is to help them maintain their independence and stay within their own environment • To provide support services to families who are caring for elderly family members
Target group and number of clients	These services are addressed to elderly persons and their families. 618 persons made use of the programme's services in 2001.
Number of staff involved	Services are offered by a specialist team of social workers, doctors, health visitors, carers, physiotherapists, psychologists and volunteers. The number of staff involved is 16 specialised persons and 18 volunteers.
Methods	The aim of the evaluation was to measure the degree of satisfaction of people making use of these services, to upgrade services and to plan new services timely adapted to emerging needs. The evaluation was performed on the basis of a representative sample of 100 persons taken from 3 out of the 5 programme districts, which had used the services provided by the programme for a long period of time. The sample includes people participating in the programme from its inception to present day (1988-2001).
Strengths	80% of people availing themselves of the services provided by the programme declared that the programme entirely covered their needs (if the programme did not exist, they would not be able to cope in an alternative way). • The service used most is social work (90% of the total cases). • 95% declare that their lives have significantly improved thanks to their participation in the programme (46% feel safer, while 37% have seen their lives improve in relation to satisfaction of everyday needs). • 89% declare that their cooperation with the personnel is satisfactory.
Weaknesses	The programme was solely applied in a small area in the centre of Athens. • The services provided must be enhanced (help during moving, more recreational activities, employment of more family assistants).

369

Results of evalua-tion/keywords	Extension of the programme to other areas. • Exploitation and organisation of sources of support. • Re-assessment of the services provided. • Assessment concerning the operation of special units (for example care of persons with dementia, etc.).

A4 Network for Alzheimer's disease

Provider (organisa-tions involved)	• Hellenic Association of Gerontology and Geriatrics • Alzheimer's Caregivers' Association • Psychogeriatrics Association "Nestor"
Objectives	• Development of actions and services relating to dementia and other contiguous disorders afflicting the elderly. • Informing health professionals and carers of persons with dementia about effective tackling of problems linked to this disease.
Target group and number of clients	These services are addressed to all elderly persons suffering from dementia and other contiguous disorders (it has been calculated that they represent 4-5% of the total population of 65+) and to the persons caring for them.
Number of staff involved	These services are provided by a specialised team of psychiatrists, psychologists, neurologists, social workers, etc.
Methods	Organisation of open meetings to provide information and support to elderly persons suffering from dementia and their carers. • Tailored consultant services relative to dealing with legal and insurance issues as well as to coping with health issues. • Development of cooperation with public and private non-profit scientific organisations in order to provide solutions to problems faced by the elderly. • Publications providing information on issues concerning the elderly and their carers (nutrition, depression, Alzheimer's Disease). • Setting up of a help telephone line on dementia. This help line will provide information and advise relating to the proper diagnosis and care of patients with dementia.
Strengths	Covering the existing gaps in specialised care in order to cover the needs of elderly persons with dementia and their carers. • Creation of open and residential care structures for persons suffering from dementia (Day Centre, Home Help) in order to provide specialised care to patients and support to their families.
Weaknesses	These programmes must be financially reinforced so as to ensure their continuation.

370

Providing Integrated Health and Social Care for Older Persons in Italy

Giorgia Nesti, Stefano Campostrini, Stefano Garbin,
Paola Piva, Patrizia Di Santo, Filomena Tunzi

1 Introduction

In Italy the problem of integrated health and social care exists since the national health system was eventually given birth in 1978 thus overcoming the old corporatist system with assistance assigned to the mutualistic agencies of the various professional categories. The foundation of a health system on a universal basis (L. 833/1978), however, was not able to trigger an equally strong impact on the development of social services. As we will show in this contribution, Italy does not dispose of an integrated health and social system, but of a health service system with more or less stable organisational ties with a structurally distinguished social service system.

In order to understand the difficulties of integrated health and social service provision it is necessary to keep in mind that, when the public health system was born in 1978, Italy still lacked a complete system of social protection on the national level. In particular, social services had not been regulated universally and homogeneously until 22 years later when, in October 2000, the legal framework and the financial basis for a national development of social services was endowed – 100 years after the first Italian law on social assistance, commissioned by the liberal government of Minister Crispi (1900).

In the following we would like to, first, outline the process towards integration from the health reform until today, in order to show the problems that are still unsolved on the theoretical, financial and managerial level. Section 2 will then describe the legal and structural framework of health and social service provision, while section 3 will illustrate some model ways of working that, in future development, are to guide general improvements in integrated health and social service provision.

1.1 Historic Development

In theory, the integration of health and social care services constitutes one of the main objectives of the public health system in Italy. With its introduction in 1978, Local Health Authorities (USL) were established as decentralised management bodies: close to the people, and controlled by the municipalities. In those years, democratic participation in managing the public health system was considered an indispensable prerequisite for integration as it was the municipalities that were responsible for the organisation and provision of social services.

Thus, during the 1980s, many municipalities followed the first steps towards integration. However, the available resources were modest and, above all, it was not easy to combine the operating paradigm of the health system with the social paradigms. Many professionals still consider the cultural diversity between the social and health sector as the main reason for the failure of health and social services integration. Moreover, within the health system it was rather the hospitals that regained more and more importance, rather than community health care that should have assumed a leading role. The former attracted a great part of public investments, structures and technological innovations, and medical specialisation increased within the hospitals while primary health care had to deal with limited resources. Investments in preventive medicine and interventions based on the collaboration between professionals and informal caregivers were neglected.

Therefore, the integration of health and social care would have risked to remain only a theoretical option if it was not for two important events in Italian health policies: the psychiatric reform and the national planning of objectives.

The reform of psychiatric treatments (L.180/1978) had important consequences both from a cultural and from a practical point of view, as it helped

372

to show both the feasibility and the effectiveness of integrated working. In this connection we would like to remind of the important cultural drive that accompanied the reform of psychiatry. Although this transformation – taking place in the same year as the health reform – was a very Italian feature, it was reflected all over Europe and launched a health care paradigm strongly centred on outpatient treatments. It was based on the following improvements:

- all asylums have progressively been closed down,
- patients with mental health problems are mainly supported by home care services and day centres with a wide range of operating models (ambulatory, job and rehabilitation centres, sheltered housing, etc.),
- patients are entitled to subsidies for social inclusion,
- patients are accepted in hospital wards only during an acute crisis, with a maximum permanence of 15 days, and an authorisation by the mayor if the patient is resistant to this kind of intervention (TSO = obligatory health treatment),
- the mental health department has the task to coordinate all health and social services.

373

The radical content of this reform caused immense controversies. Associations of patients' relatives up till today blame the deficiency of provisions, and claim for services that are able to support not only the patients but also their families. Time and again several political forces propose legal reforms. Nevertheless, professionals working in the sector have always sustained that it was not necessary to change the laws, but rather to put them in practice by providing adequate means and resources. In 1988, ten years after the reform, while the controversies in relation to the reform had yet again been inflamed, the Ministry of Health embraced this guideline and decided to focus all national planning towards an expansion of community health care.

The "National Public Health Plan" was considered as an indispensable instrument for the central government to steer the whole system. In order to overcome the disparity of resources among the regions, the national government was determined to improve its planning capacities by emanating legal guidelines containing projects and objectives in six fields in which the integration of health and social care was considered as particularly essential, i.e. in those areas in which social factors were to be found both at the origin and in the solution of pathologies: prevention, protection of mental health, protection of maternal and children's health, protection of the elderly, drug addiction, and AIDS.

The regional governments, having the task to organise hospitals and the Local Health Authorities (USL), were to create special departments for each of these six fields of intervention. In reality, however, this task was thoroughly implemented only with respect to the Department of Mental Health and the Department of Prevention (structural departments). Although proper services were created to tackle the remaining areas of intervention, these did not dispose of a real organisational autonomy (functional departments). In many local health authorities even a special organisational unit dealing with care for the elderly is missing.[1] Outside the hospitals, care for the elderly has been entrusted, on the one hand, to the general practitioners and, on the other hand, to community care services organised by the municipalities. Due to the scarcity of resources, community care has usually been restricted to home help at minimal levels. At the same time, demand grew significantly due to the growing number of older persons in need of care.

To summarise, the Italian pathway towards health and social integration is complex and fragmented for structural, cultural and economic reasons. Legal deficiencies but, in particular, implementation problems of definitely interesting and innovative policies or regulations (e.g. Law no. 833/1978; or the project "Objective: Ageing Persons") are the main causes for a still extremely fragmented system of health and social care.

2 Legal and Structural Framework and the General Discourse on Integrated Care Provision

Italy's establishment of health and social integration was marked by a lengthy delay in drawing up and implementing the necessary legislation. The national health service was slow to arrive, and when it did, it focused on integrated services for disabled people, whilst completely overlooking ageing and chronic diseases. Indeed, national regulation was not introduced into the social sector until 2000 (Law 328/2000). Nor was any coherent legal and organisational framework set up to deal with extensive changes in demographic trends, family structures, and the organisation of the national welfare state. This brought about a proliferation of varying approaches to long-term care, both in terms of territory and organisation. At least until the 1990s, Italy had no clear concept of the problems inherent to elderly people with care needs, nor was it clear which services were required to maintain their health.

The lack of in-depth analysis of demographic trends and elderly people's care needs, combined with a dearth of administrative specialists to plan, manage and evaluate health and social services, has meant that each region has introduced its own system. The vast array of regional situations, as well as the different functions performed by institutional bodies, associations, and families, are a constant influence on the organisation of integrated services for elderly people within a territory.

National health reform in 1992 began to rationalise the regulation of both financial and organisational resources. Target groups, needs structures, integrated care service types, and specific organisational methods for integrated and coordinated work procedures were defined. A health care decree, no. 502/1992, the "Objective: Ageing Persons" project, and Law no. 328/2000 pertaining to the creation of an integrated care and social services system are now the national normative framework for the definition and promotion of an integrated health and care system. Although this legislation established projects and structural arrangements – a step towards the promotion of integrated health and social care – it still leaves some crucial questions unanswered, such as the diverse range of activities in the territory and the problems of coordinating the different bodies within the care system.

375

2.1 Legal Framework of Integrated Care

The Constitution of the Italian Republic (1948) declares that health has to be protected as a fundamental individual right and interest of society and that Italian citizens have the right to free care and free health care (Article 32). The individual and equal right to welfare, and the principle of universality, are reiterated by Law no. 833/1978, which established the National Health Service (NHS). This Law states that all Italian citizens, regardless of their individual or social status, are entitled to receive equal treatment by the State, Regions, and Local Authorities.

Law no. 833/1978 is the first coherent Italian health care act, but it does not deal with the question of integrated health and social care. In fact, the first relevant normative framework pertaining thereto was Decree no. 502/1992 and its amendments (Law no. 419/1998 and Legislative Decree no. 229/1999), Law no. 328/2000 on Social Care, and the "Guidance and Coordination related to Health and Social Integration Act" (2001). Firstly, Decree no. 502/1992 states that *integrated health and social services* are "*any activities geared towards the fulfilment of individual welfare needs through integrated care, and the assurance of continuous, long-term care and rehabilitative services"* (Art. 3).

This national legislative framework defines some fundamental guidelines for the establishment of an integrated care system, namely the institutional levels involved in health and social planning (State, Regions, Local Councils and Local Health Units), the tools available to plan activities (Targeted Projects, Health and Social National Plans, Local Health and Social Plans), the main contents of integrated health and social services (e.g. temporary admissions to Health Centres and Integrated Home Care Services).

Uniform and Essential Levels of Care (ELCs) and targeted projects have to be declared by the triennial National Health Plan. ELCs are "areas or sectors protected by the national welfare system with specific services (see DPCM 29/11/2001): health care, quality of life, integrated care, emergency assistance. Targeted projects are specific documents issued by Parliament which cover specific issues. For instance, the Project "Objective: Ageing Persons" – one of the specific projects mentioned in the Directive no. 502/1992, approved by the Italian Parliament in 1992 – seeks to solve the problem of health and social care for elderly people by setting goals, establishing local organisation and forms of assistance (see section 2.3).

Regions are expected to plan health and social care with the Regional Health and Social Plan (RHSP) and to implement it through the Local Health Units (LHUs). Each Unit is subdivided into territorial districts encompassing at least 60,000 inhabitants. They have to provide prevention, information, counselling and care to disabled people, terminal patients, and elderly people.

The RHSP establishes general goals and programmes for specific thematic areas in order to achieve long-term aims. A second level of organisation, Local Executive Plans (LEPs), sets goals and strategies for each Local Health Unit. Each LHU District adopts its LEP through Territorial Executive Plans (TEPs), which contain specific goals, and implementation guidelines. Alongside the LEPs are Zone Plans for social care, drawn up by local councils, which either manage social care directly or delegate it to Local Health Units.

The main types of integrated activities are health services with social importance; social services with health importance; and health and social services with highly integrated health importance. The first tend to promote welfare, and to recognise, prevent, remove or monitor the invalidating and degenerative consequences of individual pathologies. These services are the Local Health Units' responsibility and are provided by outpatient departments, or within home care and home nursing programmes. The second encompasses social activities designed to support disabled or socially excluded patients: housing services to cope with and to maintain persons with care needs at home, temporary admission to nursing homes for elderly people with limited autonomy. Local councils are in charge of social services with health importance, which are financed by local councils and client fees. Finally, the third set of provisions represents all the activities with particular medical importance. These are the Local Health Units' responsibility and are financed by the National Health Fund; they are provided by outpatient departments, home care and home nursing programmes.

2.2   Financing

Decree no. 502/1992 states that integrated health and social care is to be financed by the Regions, which arrange the budget of Local Health Units on the basis of an individual quota related to the type of local resident citizens. The Regions finance their health and social services with tax revenues and state subsidies (the so-called "National Health Fund"). The Italian National Health Service is financed with specific contributions paid by employers and self-employed workers to the National Institute of Social Security, which then shares it among the 22 Regions. Every year, the National Financial Law calculates the National Health Fund and fully finances it through the national budget. Individual regional budgets are then calculated using coefficients of resident population, health mobility, consistence and conditions of wealth, and the technological infrastructure. Finally, the Regions set their own regional taxation and client fees on the basis of local needs assessment. The "Guidance and Coordination of Health and Social Integration" act (2001) established that the National Health Service is responsible for home care in the event of intensive care; for long-term home care, the service has to be financed equally by the National Health Service (50%) and Local Councils (50%). Regarding the Integrated Home Care Service, medical, rehabilitative and nursing care are the responsibility of the National Health Service, while administrative services are the responsibility of both the National Health Service (50%) and Local Councils (50%). Home help services are to be financed entirely by Local Councils.

   Elderly people could pay for part of their health and social care with financial subsidies distributed by the State, Regions and Local Councils, e.g. pensions, vouchers and care payments.

2.3   Process of Care Provision

2.3.1 The National Situation

In the beginning of the 1990s, the project "Objective: Ageing Persons" tried to set the objectives, the organisational framework and the competencies of integrated health and social care for elderly people in Italy. Overall, these services focus on improving elderly people's well-being by prevention, and by promoting and maintaining their autonomy. The care system is supposed to be organised into a network which encompasses a range of services with clear, common goals, processes, instruments and evaluation methods tailored to elderly and disabled people's needs.

Regions represent the institutional level devoted to define more general and strategic goals for the local integrated network; they plan local care provision and are responsible for the financial and economic management of the integrated system. Local Health Units and their Districts, in particular, are responsible for providing health services and for planning individual care. Local Councils are, in turn, responsible for coordinating the entire network and for providing care. In order to enter the integrated care system, elderly people have to contact a social worker at the Local Social Service or their General Practitioner (GP). The social worker and the GP forward the request to the needs assessment district. This district employs a multiprofessional team, a Geriatric Assessment Unit,[2] which comprises an array of professionals (geriatrician, physiotherapist, professional nurse, physician and social worker) in order to:

1.   assess an elderly person's autonomy with integrated and multidimensional tests;
2.   set goals;
3.   draw up an individual care plan specifying the goals and services required for its success;
4.   oversee the implementation of the care provision process and the individual care plan, as well as to monitor and assess the goals achieved.

The services provided by the territorial network are:
- *Home care* (community care): with social importance (home help, meals and personal care); with health importance (medical, rehabilitative and/or nursing care); integrated.
- *Integrated home care service*: is a combination of integrated and coordinated health and social activities which seek to keep an elderly person

at home as long as possible. Health services are medical care (geriatric, psychiatric, physiotherapy), nursing, rehabilitation, medicines and prosthesis supply. Social services are: personal care, meals, house work, laundry, administrative services.

- *Day centre*: semi-residential structure, within the District, which hosts disabled elderly people for a short-term period (they are open during the day, 5 days a week, 7 hours a day, and admit 20 elderly persons). They provide health care services (prevention, therapy, and rehabilitation), and social care services (personal care and promotion of personal autonomy, entertainment, job therapy, and social activities).

- *Nursing home:* residential structure, organised into small groups ("nuclei"), which provides health care, social care, and functional rehabilitation for people with disabilities. Patient care can be extensive or intensive. The first area comprises temporary accommodation for long-term care and rehabilitation (while hospitalisation is limited only to the acute stage). The second area comprises intensive rehabilitation, with high medical importance, plus a hospice for terminal patients that provides palliative care (reduction of pain; social protection for patients and their family; family support). Doctors, nurses, social workers and psychologists are available at the nursing home.

The integrated social and health care services require GPs or social workers to send elderly people in need of care to their local District. The district's Geriatric Assessment Unit assesses the patient's needs, establishes an individual care plan and evaluates the goals achieved. Local services have different degrees of care intensity, but the general objective is to help the elderly person to live at home.

2.3.2 Regional Variations

Italy's integrated health and social care system for elderly people is a general framework set up by national legislation which the Regions have to implement with a certain degree of autonomy in order to cater fully for local needs. Each region differs vastly in terms of the demand for integrated health and social care due to the wide variety of ages and to different local care traditions.

Demographic records rate Italy as having one of the highest percentages of elderly people in Europe. In 2000, there were more than 10 million people over 65 (18% of the entire population), of which 22% were over 80

379

years. According to the *Biennial Report to the Parliament about the Condition of Elderly People* (1998-1999), there are almost 2 million disabled elderly people: 9% between 65-74, 20.7% between 75-79, and 47.5% over 80 years old. Elderly people do not only have to face disease, but also social hardships. The Report highlights that 40% of disabled people have financial difficulties, 25.6% live alone, often far from families (23%), and without central heating (21.3%). In territorial terms, there is a deep divide between North Italy, where elderly people live in better conditions, and Italy's islands – Sicily and Sardinia – which have the highest percentages of chronic diseases and disability.

Recently, however, care provision methods have become more uniform throughout Italy. During the 1990s each region had a vastly different system; over the last few years, however, almost all Italy's regions have implemented similar care supply frameworks. In 1996-1997 there were eight Geriatric Evaluation Units within the Districts; now almost all regions have them, with the highest number in Lombardy (109), in Veneto (84) and in Lazio (61). Each team contains a number of professionals including GPs, nurses, social workers, geriatricians, and therapists.

Furthermore, Integrated Home Care Services have been set up in each Region: 177 out of Italy's 197 Local Health Units provide Integrated Home Care for 240,105 people (79.8% of which are elderly).

There are 4,383 Nursing Homes (1,605 in the North-West, 1,149 in the North-East, 750 in the Centre, 421 in the South, and 428 on the islands) with a total of 212,624 available places.

Geriatric Evaluation Units and integrated care are, therefore, available throughout Italy, even though the number of services in the Central North greatly outweighs those in the South. Care provision methods have become increasingly uniform because north and central Italy have shared their policies with the rest of the country. Indeed, the creation of a care network system in the north, regulated by a public service – which assesses, plans and coordinates activities – has achieved positive results in user terms by improving quality of life and in organisational terms by optimising local financial and structural resources.

2.4 Stakeholders

As mentioned before, health and social care services are regulated by public authorities at the national, regional and local level. A special role is given to the Geriatric Assessment Units (GAUs), working within Health Districts. Services are provided by the municipalities themselves or by other actors, mainly in the form of municipal contracting-out to Third Sector organisations (cooperatives). In some areas there are also private for-profit providers directly paid by users. The main actors of the integrated care system are, therefore:

- Users and their caregivers, or informal carers;
- Geriatric Assessment Units, and their staff: geriatricians, nurses, GPs, social workers, and sometimes also other professionals;
- Professionals from the public and the Third Sector;
- A small number of private for-profit providers.

Individual planning and the provision of services are taking place on two distinct levels, with different actors involved, thus triggering that need for coordination in order to guarantee seamless and efficient care provision to older persons. In theory, the GAUs are in charge of planning, coordinating, monitoring and evaluating the individual care plan by means of a case manager (usually the social worker).

In practice, the lack of coordinating activities provided by the GAUs represents a general weakness of the system, both within the GAUs and at the interface between them and other providers, thus triggering a kind of "twofold cleavage" and respective inter-professional conflicts:

- Within the GAU, conflicts between social and health professionals may be explained by differences in status, career patterns, training, and by a different level of legitimisation within the integrated health and social system. In theory, the presence of different specific competencies should guarantee effective and high quality services. In practice, it touches upon the crucial question of how to foster the integration of different professionals. In the Italian context, this is even more difficult for the lack of a clear legal background that would clearly define members, roles and procedures of the Unit.
- Between public actors, the GAU and private/third-sector operators, providing services. In this case, the main critical points are related to the different organisational structure adopted by the public sector as supervisor and third-sector organisations as providers of services.

In any case, successful integration could only be achieved if all members agree upon a common objective and mutually agreed methods. The experiences made at the regional level underline, however, the difficulty to communicate among different professionals who are divided by status, ideological professional views (in particular between health and social sectors), and their capability to work together as a team.

In Italy, job profiles for the social sector were accepted only recently: in Veneto, for instance, social workers were recognised not earlier than in 2001 (Regional Law n. 20). Only with this law social workers' competencies, education, training, and criteria for selection were defined, requesting the following health and social capabilities: s/he should be able to provide care directly to users, to support health staff, using common information tools, to promote quality development, to communicate with users and their caregivers, and to work in a team. However, GPs, geriatricians and nurses remain to have great privileges with respect to education, training and payments. This different level of influence and legitimisation often creates antagonisms between health staff and social workers that are reflected in daily practice.

One of the crucial questions in the practice of integrated health and social care services is how to define the result that is to be achieved by the intervention(s). Thus it seems most important that multi-professional teams use multi-dimensional assessment tools in order to foster the dialogue among professionals and to create a basis for joint working during the whole process of care provision: first, when needs are assessed and goals to be achieved are defined; subsequently, during the implementation of commonly agreed measures, and finally, when results pursued have to be monitored and evaluated.

Another relevant aspect to make coordination work concerns the capability to steer complex processes, to manage, aggregate and motivate persons, and to achieve results. In the Italian case, one fundamental problem in providing "Integrated Home Care Services" is how to integrate the municipal social services and the District of the Local Health Unit, which should provide health and nursing care. Generally, defined institutional guidelines and, above all, clear legal responsibilities are lacking. Regional experiences show that, in particular, the lack of an integrating professional, i.e. a case manager assuming the role as a coordinator, is a main obstacle to real integration. The multi-professional team and multidimensional assessment tools alone are not enough to guide complex processes, to manage, aggregate and motivate persons, and to achieve results. As the team is not coordinated by a case manager, an integrated management of the Integrated Home Care Service – based on shared objectives and a shared individual care plan – is hardly ever realised due to internal professional cleavages and disperse responsibilities.

A most important player in the Italian care system are the families, in particular female siblings and partners. According to the national system of social care, the public service performs a relevant function during the initial stage (in-take, definition of the individual care plan). Nevertheless, the process of real hands-on care provision has developed within the families and the local communities. In Italy, as in most other countries, informal care networks, in particular the family, are the core resource in care for the elderly, as also the Law n. 328/2000, the Social Plan 2001-2003 and the local legislation have underlined. In this connection, two features are of utmost importance: first, the family networks guarantee a real and continuous process of care provision; second, the family dimension of care is based on the right to choose the preferred care arrangement. Thus, the family is the crucial actor. Due to its flexible structure, it is easy to involve in the process of care provision, and it is at the core of society, where individual interests are protected. Even if the public sector is present in Italy, most of the "Integrated Home Care Services" have nevertheless been "transferred" to families, paradoxically without preventing economic and psychological long-term consequences on carers. Family carers would need their role to be socially recognised, and they need information, education and counselling on practical features connected to social care.

383

In a situation of high physical and emotional engagement, due to a continuous and consistent effort, caregivers need psychological support, listening and dialogue about their problems, decision-making, the management of changes and coping strategies, in order to prevent situations of burnout. Moreover, carers need to "take a breath", to take care of themselves and to be temporarily supported. To give respite to family carers is the aim of more recent and innovative national and regional policies. If a huge amount of care load depends on families, it is important to define – beside the care provision to the older person – policies supporting informal care networks such as economic provisions for families (vouchers and payments for care), day centres as special support to home care services, and respite by means of temporary admission to nursing homes. This represents a challenge to the local care system as it adds up to its organisational complexity. On the one side, the temporary care by professionals is to be organised as smoothly as possible, both for the older person who might feel abandoned, and for the carer who might feel inadequate and/or a sense of guilt. On the other side, it seems crucial to involve the family into the process of care provision, through the participation in defining the personal care plan, and to link formal care provision with the informal care system.

The Third Sector represents another important actor in an integrated care system, due to the diffusion of welfare policies in Italy that are pointing at the establishment of quasi-markets and outsourcing of service provision. In particular, "Integrated Home Care" is increasingly contracted out to third-sector organisations. As the Italian institutional context is marked by an elevated public debt and an inflexible public administration, contracting-out seems to be a suitable solution to reduce costs and to make bureaucratic processes more flexible. Moreover, the Third Sector in Italy has a long-standing and culturally rooted legitimisation. In Veneto and Emilia Romagna, for instance, the public sector collaborates with organisations working in these regions since many years, though based on different traditions: catholic co-operatives and voluntary associations, in the first case, communist organisations, in the second. However, the Third Sector has not been able to encourage the process of integration as, although it has gained quite a strong position in the social sector, it is hardly visible in the health system. Furthermore, in Italy, as a regulatory framework and criteria for the selection of providers have been missing, local monopolies were fostered, rather than competition and a high qualitative standard of provision. This restricted relationship between the public and the private non-profit sector also avoided that users became directly involved in selecting services to satisfy their needs. The implementation of the Law 328/2000, therefore, is fundamental in order to promote market competition among providers and to improve the quality of services.

A further critical group of stakeholders concerns the increasing number of immigrants who are privately "employed" as carers. The general demographic, social and economic transformations (increase of one-person families, increasing female labour market participation and increasing mobility) had as a consequence that family care has considerably changed its characteristics. National surveys put in evidence that 15% of the Italian families with an older person in need of care, make use of private (informal) carers for more than 20 hours per week, with an average expenditure of 320 Euros per month (in a range from 240 € in South Italy to 400 € in the North).

It is important to stress that this kind of private care provision seems to be very fragmented and scarcely regulated, mainly based on direct relationships between families and single workers without professional guarantees. Generally speaking, workers involved in private care are often irregular workers, especially immigrants, with low levels of professional qualification. Private care, therefore, represents a way to externalise family care and to achieve a flexible response to complex needs – with a high risk for both the privately paid worker (illegal payments, no defined rights etc.) and the quality of care.

3 Model Ways of Working

Following the reform of the National Health System at the end of the 1980s, the above-mentioned obstacles for integrated care delivery have actively been confronted, focusing on unsatisfied demand of persons with chronic diseases, persons with disabilities and older persons in need of flexible and effective health and social care services. In connection with a parallel modernisation of the public administration, the 1990s thus gave birth to a number of model projects developing innovative care services, especially at the regional level. In particular, new integrated care services were established, combining modern organisational approaches (project management, managerial culture, empowerment, quality system) with client-oriented attitudes. Once again, regions such as Veneto, Emilia Romagna and Tuscany turned out as most innovative, due to their specific local civic culture, political, administrative and entrepreneurial capabilities.

385

In the following, five examples of "good practice" are presented, i.e. integrated health and social services that represent new modes of planning integration and promoting quality. The first two models (3.1.1 and 3.1.2) constitute examples of how quality could be improved by the integration of different organisational structures and the utilisation of new technologies to create a system for rapid information exchange within local provider networks.

The second type of models (3.2) illustrates ways of process integration by means of multidimensional needs assessment (3.2.1) and multi-professional teams (3.2.2) pushing health and social workers towards joint working.

The last two models testify how a qualitative integration could be promoted by a goal-oriented organisation. In the first case, integration is encouraged through the implementation of quality management within the service (3.3), in the second case (3.4) seamless care is promoted for a special target group with mixed health and social care needs – persons with Alzheimer's disease who should move within the network without disruptions and tailored to their specific needs.

3.1 Integration by "One-window" Approaches and Shared Information Systems (Valdarno, Empolese Valdelsa)

3.1.1 The Project "Single Information Point for Home Care" (see Annex A1)

The integration of different functions and services, and between different professionals is crucial when the health status of older persons gets worse and his/her stay at home requires constant health and social assistance. The plurality of services and their affiliation to different bodies and organisations makes it difficult for the older person and his/her family to apply timely for the services that s/he needs often from one moment to the other.

To simplify the access to home care services is therefore the specific objective of an experimental project carried out in the Valdarno and Empolese Valdelsa area. Single information points, where all the requests for home care – including the protected discharge from hospital – are collected, were made available within the area covered by the Local Health Agency.[3] It is important to underline that the existing service network had already been widely integrated. However, the objective is to add two new instruments that will support the collaboration among staff and create synergies between services. Apart from the single information point for home care a standardised information system for all interventions within the territory was introduced. Thus the efficiency of home care (following hospital discharge), the quality of life of the elderly, the general welfare and the survival rate of the client/patient were to be increased. The average stay in hospital was to be decreased for those types of pathologies that could also be treated by means of home care services, i.e. hospitalisation was to be restricted to the acute phase.

The project is promoted and coordinated by the Department of Primary Care of the Local Health Agency 11 (Empoli) and should be an example for a "friendly health service that adopts a strongly client oriented approach". Furthermore, 15 municipalities and the General Practitioners were involved.

In practice, the territory of the Local Health Agency was divided in three homogeneous areas each of which created one "Single Information Point" where all requests for access to home care services, including hospital discharge, are gathered. By directly involving the General Practitioner, a project of integrated home care is defined for each individual client. More complex cases are handed over to the Territorial Assessment Unit (multiprofessional team). All information and each single step of the process are recorded and monitored by special software helping to coordinate the different resources working in the area (see 3.1.2).

The project's objectives have been realised, not least by the solid managerial integration of health and social services, given that 10 municipalities out of 15 delegated the responsibility for social services to the Local Health Agency (with the remaining 5 municipalities an efficient agreement between the Local Health Agency and the Municipal Social Services was concluded).

The project is still in progress and also promotes the development of new services. For instance, three new front offices were opened to guarantee better information and to simplify the bureaucratic procedures to access home care services. The creation of "Single Information Points" also accelerated the procedures to access home care services after hospital discharge, simplifying the relationship between the hospital and community care services.

Still, during the experimental phase some problems occurred due to the vast area in which the project had to be implemented, in particular with respect to the general coordination of the experiment, and the large number of staff dispersed in the territory. Furthermore, a weakness of the project is the lacking involvement of voluntary organisations that are quite active in Tuscany, in particular in the area of tele-help.

3.1.2 The Project "Information System for All Activities Carried out in the Territory" (see Annex A2)

One of the organisational elements to realise social and health care services' integration is concerning the access to shared information that is collected during the different phases of the care process about the patient/client by all the different services and respective staff. To this behalf, the Local Health Agency 11 Valdelsa and Valdarno has complemented the project "Single Information Point" for home care with an adequate information system. The initiative has linked all social services, the health districts, the hospital, general practitioners and specialists, and home care services.

Furthermore, a database has been set up that provides the most important information for those older persons who would like to apply for home care services, economic support and other welfare provisions.

The project was born by the need to monitor medical and pharmaceutical expenses in the territory, starting from the general practitioners' prescriptions. Once started, the Department of Primary Care realised that this was an opportunity to link all primary health care services, including social services. Now, all data of citizens who are treated by a general practitioner, supported by social and health services or hosted in hospitals, old-age and nursing homes can be searched and tracked down in a single database that is continuously being updated. The database is accessible for all staff of the territory, thus supporting joint working and reducing the time for information exchange between different agencies and organisations.

Approximately 500 workers in health and social care services are involved in the experiment, which started in 2002 and has already achieved some remarkable results:

- all administrative and bureaucratic procedures have been simplified;
- data are inserted only once for each citizen, data entry can be accessed by all staff;
- the database can be accessed by any staff member, if authorised by the citizen him-/herself (MPs and some other key staff may access at any time);
- the provision of both health and social services has been accelerated;
- different staff and services working on the same territory are collaborating;
- the hospital has been linked to the community care services;
- the software is user-friendly and can be easily exported.

It should be mentioned, however, that it is still not easy to overcome some staff members' cultural resistance towards joint working and/or the use of personal computers. The already mentioned cultural cleavages between health and social care workers have been experienced also in this project, not least due to the large number of persons involved and also the geographical distance between staff members.

3.2   Integration by Inter-professional Teams

3.2.1 The Multidimensional Assessment District Unit
(Veneto; see Annex A3)

The region of Veneto represents a forerunner concerning the introduction of inter-professional teams. The "Multidimensional Assessment District

Unit" (MADU) is the functional unit of the District that assesses the needs of older persons and thus is responsible for the in-take of eligible clients, for choosing and implementing the best solution for his/her needs, using local resources. On request, the MADU gathers the Chief of the Health District who is responsible for the Unit, the GP in charge of the person, the social worker of the municipality or, in case of delegation, of the Local Health Unit, a geriatrician, a physiotherapist, a professional nurse, and administrative personnel. The MADU has to:

1. assess the older person's situation in a multidimensional way, through the preliminary collection of information about the user made by the social worker or by the GP, filling in the regional multidimensional assessment form, called S.V.A.M.A.;
2. define the individual care plan within 30 days from the presentation of the request;
3. implement the project, that has to be started within 20 days;
4. audit the implementation of the project;
5. keep documents related to the assessed persons;
6. define the case manager, who will follow the user and his/her individual project, and represents the link between the user and the Unit.

In order to assess users' needs in a multidimensional way, the MADU uses the S.V.A.M.A. form to collect personal data, the type of request, pathologies, results from the cognitive and functional assessment (Short Portable Mental Status Questionnaire; Barthel Index), results from the social and environmental assessment. These data might be supplemented, if appropriate, by other information from members of the Unit, and represent the basis for the individual care plan. This individual care plan defines the community care services required (home help, home nursing, etc.). Once the care plan and the case manager have been defined, the District Unit starts to implement it and evaluate results achieved. The experimentation of these instruments and respective processes has produced relevant results:

- Within the service organisation: the cooperation among different professionals involved in the needs assessment; the elaboration of a care plan tailored to users' needs; the ability in managing critical moments during the process of service provision.
- Within the network of services: community care resources have been optimised and controlling processes have been improved.
- Concerning users: goals achieved are now also evaluated; communication became more transparent and effective.

Weaknesses of the model are strictly connected to its organisational complexity creating the risk of bureaucratic rigidity and an exceeded formalisation of processes. Furthermore, the coordination among staff is difficult and inter-professional competition can still be observed.

It has to be stressed that the territorial network involves different governmental levels: the regional government, Local Health Units and municipalities. Local experiences give evidence of how difficult it is to coordinate different institutional levels, in particular as effective instruments (financial incentives) are missing. For instance, the MADU are to guarantee the integration between different professional figures. In reality, however, these units are not always present at the local level nor do they always involve all different professionals. The assessment is a most critical activity during the whole process (in-take, monitoring, evaluation of results) and would thus need more than a "virtual" unit of various professionals who are employed with different entities. Furthermore, specific instruments for joint working, communication and data analysis would be needed as well as funding for innovative solutions. Above all, the members of the Unit must have the capability to analyse the outcomes of the process of care provision critically and to correct the individual care plan, if necessary. The Region Veneto, for instance, implemented the MADU in 1994, but it was not before 1999 that the multidimensional assessment form S.V.A.M.A. was introduced, due to the lack of a "culture of evaluation" in the field of health and social care.

Concerning the user's role, it has to be pointed out that this kind of integration does not foster the users' participation. First, the MDAU is activated by the GP, though on user's request. Secondly, the lack of any evaluation of the units' activities and of results achieved, e.g. by means of questionnaires or interviews with clients, have thus far avoided the evaluation of users' satisfaction and their perception of seamless care.

3.2.2 The Working Unit for Continuous Care (Local Health Unit 4: Alto Vicentino, see Annex A4)

A particular example of good practice is given by the "Department of Continuous Care" of the Local Health Agency 4 (municipalities from Alto Vicentino) that, since 2000, has started the first Italian "Working Unit for Continuous Care" (WUCC).

The WUCC is, in fact, a Geriatric Assessment Unit, composed by health and social workers but it is organised within the hospitals of Thiene and

Schio, rather than being organised by the Health District. The WUCC has the duty to guarantee the older person's hospital discharge, by organising and providing continuous and integrated health and social care, departing from the hospital.

The WUCC is managed by the Director of the Geriatric Department and comprises also a professional nurse (responsible for data collection and nursing assessment), a physiotherapist, and the social worker from the hospital. Such a social worker, uncommon within Italian hospitals, represents the interface between the hospital and the territory. Her fundamental role is to keep in touch with caregivers and with the Municipal social worker in order to plan and prepare the older person's discharge from hospital.

Figure 1 below represents the WUCC flow of working. The process starts with the identification of older persons at risk by hospital staff. Persons who need rehabilitation, integrated health and social care, terminal care or short-term care while waiting for a regular place in a Nursing Home are referred to the WUCC staff. The WUCC takes over to assess users in a multi-dimensional way (using the regional assessment instrument S.V.A.M.A.), to contact the competent Health District and to inform the patient's GP.

Figure 1:   **Flow-chart of the WUCC**

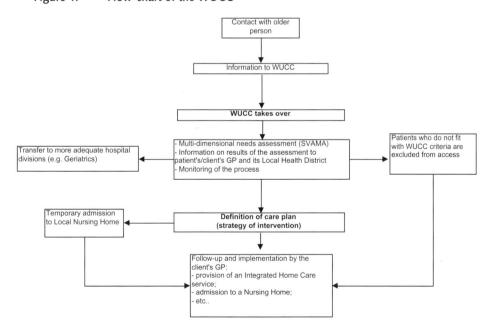

In case of complex pathologies, s/he is transferred to the appropriate hospital division. Otherwise the WUCC plans a solution that usually includes a temporary admission in the nursing home annexed to the hospital. After two months, responsibility for follow-up and further implementation steps is transferred to the user's GP and to the Health District. The older person could then be taken in charge by the integrated home service or by local nursing homes.

The WUCC represents an innovative approach to integrated care with regard to several points of view:

- Organisationally, the in-take by means of an inter-professional team is different from the GAU as the WUCC can dispose of a social worker who is properly taking over the case management function.
- The WUCC has introduced a very innovative idea of "taking in charge" by taking care of "users and guiding them within the care pathway. The very WUCC defines an adequate care plan, by integrating the hospital's resources and those of community care.
- Methodologically the project is interesting as, first, the care plan is the result of an interdisciplinary effort, and secondly, because it represents a real project as it takes into account all the resources actually available in the area, rather than drawing on an ideal but unrealistic solution.

Directors from all hospital departments like to collaborate with the WUCC because it also helps to improve the communication and integration between the departments. Moreover, the WUCC has achieved relevant results. For instance, avoidable hospital admissions have been reduced from 123 to 83 during 2002. The WUCC, in fact, automatically starts its job as soon as the older person is discharged from the hospital, because physicians themselves request its intervention. On the contrary, the GEU is set off by users and caregivers. The older person is, therefore, followed as soon as s/he has been dismissed from the hospital, avoiding his/her inadequate re-admission. The older person, in fact, after the hospital discharge, might stay for some time in the nursing home attached to the hospital while waiting for the organisation of an appropriate solution in the community or the admission to a regular nursing home.

The WUCC represents a good model way of work that tries to combine strengths from professional integration (e.g. interdisciplinary structure and multidimensional evaluation) with a user-centred approach, aimed at guaranteeing seamless care.

During the first two years of experimentation, the WUCC has achieved excellent results. Nevertheless, in the long term problems might rise with respect to the loss of flexibility, increasing conflicts among staff within the hospital but also between the WUCC and community care services. Another weakness is the lack of evaluation of users' satisfaction, in contrast with its declared user-oriented approach. Finally, it is important to notice that the WUCC is an innovative and recent project, launched by the local service itself. Such a bottom-up approach fostered its success until now. The question is whether this model will gain structural support, independently from its current managers and staff turn-over.

3.3 Integration by Quality Management: The Project "Quality of Integrated Home Care" (Annex A5)

"Emilia Romagna" is one of the most advanced Italian Regions concerning the provision of welfare services, in particular with respect to the integration of social and health services for older persons. One of the various local experiments was carried out in the District of Correggio under the title "Quality of Integrated Home Care". The District is part of the Local Health Authority (AUSL) of Reggio Emilia, including six municipalities (Correggio, Fabbrico, Campagnola Emilia, Rio Saliceto, Rolo, San Martino in Rio) for a total of 45,204 inhabitants. Older persons over 75 represent 21.4% of the population. In 2000, the share of registered persons with disabilities was 6.21% of the population. The experimental project started in 1996 and ended in 2000 with the introduction of some new innovative strategies, in particular the implementation of a quality guideline (in compliance with ISO 9000) and a "global" and "holistic approach" of Primary Health Care. The project provided for an integration at institutional, managerial and vocational levels.

At the institutional level the collaboration was formalised by programme agreements and contracts signed by all organisations involved:

- the local health agency and their respective departments and collaborators (local hospital, general practitioner, specialist's outpatient treatments, home nursing services),
- municipalities (social care, social services),
- voluntary organisations providing social services, and
- the University of Modena and Reggio that planned and carried out a training programme for all staff, in order to support the adoption of a quality management approach.

At the professional level the project was to achieve a shared approach among all workers involved. According to the planning documents of the WHO (Alma Ata, 1978; Alma Ata revisited, 1994), the service chose to adopt the "holistic approach" to satisfy patients' needs. According to that approach physical, psychological and social needs both of the patient and of his/her family have to be considered. Particular attention is given to the referring relative (*caregiver*) who may encounter physical, psychological and economic problems due to the constant and often heavy assistance offered to his/her relative. "Global approach" means using the integrated social and health district services in order to assist the patient and to support the family contemporarily.

The specific objectives of the project were:
- to create a network of territorial health and social services,
- to favour constant care (also by means of "protected hospital discharge"), and
- to activate a functional service of "Integrated Home Care" (ADI) according to quality criteria (fairness, timeliness, suitability of level, effectiveness, efficiency).

The project, addressed to the over 65, was carried out in different phases and started with the involvement in vocational training of social and health care staff to develop shared objectives, methodologies and results.

In a second stage institutional protocols were drawn up between different services and bodies and an effective model of the service was defined. These procedures were then activated by an experimental multiprofessional team before being evaluated from a quantitative and economic point of view.

The activities were carried out by health care staff and social workers providing for the multiprofessional needs assessment (social and health care needs), the elaboration of an individual project shared by the family and the staff, the activation of the service(s) in relation to the expressed needs of the clients and their family, and the monitoring/evaluation of the individual project.

In order to provide adequate information to all participants of the individual project, a common "diary" was used to fill in all health and social care activities that were carried out by the different staff members (the general practitioner included). The "diary" was entrusted to the client or the family member to be kept during the whole period of service provision.

During the experimentation phase a quality handbook for "Integrated Home Care" (ADI) was realised containing the mission of the service, the vision and the quality indicators shared by all the involved health and social care workers.

The project's strength lies in the fact that it achieved to integrate all organisational levels (institutional, managerial and professional). Furthermore, the strong institutional convergence on the objectives of the project and the delegation of the social functions of the municipality to the AUSL of Reggio Emilia favoured the integration of responsibilities. The small dimension of the experimental environment favoured its management and allowed for a decent coordination of the different phases of the project.

Moreover the experiment inspired the Health Council of the Region Emilia Romagna in the development of the Directive "Criteria for the reorganisation of home care" (DGR 124/1999). It also helped to put in practice the accreditation system for home care services that had been endowed by recent regional legislation (DL 229/1999 and LR 34/1998).

Among the weaknesses it has to be mentioned that investment in constant training of staff is indispensable to create and develop a shared culture in home care to motivate staff. Indeed, the widespread opinion among professionals still is that care at home is only a way of "reducing expenses", rather than a rational and user-oriented choice. In this connection, also the participation of the families in planning and managing services is still to be developed in a constant process of cultural change with respective conflicts and time-spans.

395

3.4   Integrated Services for Special Target Groups: The Alzheimer Day Centre "Stella del Colle" (Annex A6)

One of the most interesting examples of integration between social and health services concerning elderly Alzheimer patients in Italy is represented by the project "Objective: Older Persons" in the Region of Tuscany. The Regional Health Plan 1999-2001 promoted the creation of a network of integrated services (day centres, primary and secondary health care, and social services provided by municipalities, social enterprises and voluntary organisations) to offer an articulated alternative to nursing homes as an answer to the increasing number of persons suffering from dementia and chronic-degenerative pathologies.

The Day Centre "Stella del Colle" is an excellent example for this innovative approach. It is organised by the municipality of Florence that had launched an experiment of community care for this target group in 1989, in collaboration with the Institute for Geriatrics and Gerontology, the Clinic for Nervous Diseases of the University of Florence, the INRCA (Hospital "I Fraticini") and an association of families (AMA).

Given the complete lack of regional laws and policies in favour of Alzheimer patients, the project was meant to give an answer to an urban emergency as there were about 6,000 supposed cases of persons with dementia in the area of Florence, most of which living at home. The project was thus to avoid the hospitalisation in nursing homes of the Alzheimer patients and to support their families (caregivers).

The project has ever since been carried out by the Consortium "Zenit" while the municipality of Florence and the INRCA collaborate in the assessment, the support to family members (caregivers), and the training of staff. The experiment anticipated the project "Objective: Older Persons" that was approved in January 1992 by the Ministry of Health and defined guidelines for the constitution of a model of integrated care services for persons in need of care.

The Day Centre was included in a network of dementia services provided by the municipality, which was later complemented by the "Integrated Home Care Service" being extended to the whole urban area, and the Alzheimer Units installed in some nursing homes of Florence.

All services are provided by multiprofessional teams (educators, social workers, nurses, physiotherapists, physicians) following the ensuing process: observation, analysis, planning and implementation of the interventions, feedback and global evaluation. Staff members are constantly trained.

The day centre is open seven days a week, all year round. It is organised in a flexible way, adapting to the individual needs of each patient, reaching from part-time arrangements to full-time adhesion (7 days a week). Clients may benefit from a transportation service.

The Centre might be characterised as a "family-like" community. A customised rehabilitation programme is developed for each patient. It includes individual and group activities for the maintenance of relational and communicative skills to face the bewilderment and the confusion that are the cause of the agitation and depression of the patient. Concerning assistance, all services usually offered in a nursing home are granted.

The project was inspired by the Canadian model of constant care that provides for a strong integration between the general practitioner, the territorial health and social services that are responsible for the admission, the hospital and the specialist's health services (see Annex).

During the last 10 years of its activity the Centre has been attended by about 300 guests with an average frequency of 7-8 months. It proved to be a valid alternative to hospitalisation in a nursing home and an important resource at the district level, collaborating closely with other community care services.

The chosen methodology assures an efficient support and relief service for the family that is involved in the rehabilitation project of the elderly and receives training and psychological support to face the situation.

Notwithstanding the good results obtained by the centre the Consortium "Zenit" has not yet overcome the managerial and economical problems, in particular in their collaboration with the municipality of Florence. Thus, the foreseen additional services could not be launched. After a first experimental phase of the professional-caregivers-at-home system, for instance, the municipality of Florence returned to the old home care system (on contract). Furthermore, short-term care facilities in nursing homes were never activated.

397

4 Conclusions

In this contribution we tried to shed light on the growing importance of health and social integration for older persons and respective developments in Italy between 1980s and 1990s. Improvements have developed in a differentiated way and with significant regional variations. The following are the main impediments to the diffusion of a generally integrated approach to the provision of social and health services for older persons in Italy:

- There is no single legal framework concerning integrated health and social care at the national level, but health and social matters are regulated by separated legislation. This distinction is also reflected on the regional and local level, thus increasing the complexity of any coordination efforts between the two sectors.
- This structural complexity can be observed both at the vertical and at the horizontal level – at the vertical level this concerns federal and regional policy-making (legislation), at the horizontal level the distinct organisation between health and social services is crucial. National leg-

islation only defines guidelines for the development of integrated health and social care, it describes some basic services that should be present in every region, and defines an organisational framework, but it also delegates the detailed planning of services and activities and the definition of the care network to regional institutions. As we have seen above, this has fostered a strong differentiation in local supply, the creation of territorial divides, which has been harmful to the principle of equal treatment of all citizens. Moreover, this fragmentation hampers the process of mutual learning among regions, and between regions and national institutions, in particular with respect to the promotion of effective organisational and managerial models. Finally, there are variations between regions in terms of economic resources, local culture, and attitudes of public administration towards innovation.

- There are no economic strategies and mechanisms to improve integration between health care, which represents by far the "richer" sector, and social care.

- The deep cultural and professional divide between health and social care systems can be observed both between professionals engaged in care provision but also between health care management and social care management. Within each Local Health Agency, in fact, there are two different managers: one responsible for the health department, and one for the social department – with respective conflicts concerning competencies and decision-making.

The reform law n. 328/2000 was to give an answer to all these cultural, financial, and organisational unbalances and thus formulated the strategic objective already in its title: "Framework law for an integrated system of interventions and social services". The principles introduced by the reform are very ambitious:

- *Universalism*: social services are to be extended to all citizens, with priority given to those who are worst-off; social services are available to everybody without distinction of income, though the municipalities can ask user contributions based on universal criteria.
- The quota of *essential services* that all the Regions have to guarantee is defined by the federal state; as already applies for the health sector the constitutional principle of the right to assistance is to be introduced also in the social field (LEA = essential or standard level of social assistance).

- National planning is to be introduced together with a national social fund that is to *re-balance* the huge gaps that accumulated over time among the various Italian regions.
- The municipality is the first institution responsible for the quality of social services but the management has to be realised by means of association with all other municipalities that cover the area of a Health District; this territory is now called the *"social zone"*.

For the sake of health and social services integration it is important to understand the institutional innovation of the social zone, because it is this entity that deals with the Local Health Agency (ASL) in planning and providing highly integrated services. The social zone (or area) is a recent institution that, in some regions of the North-Centre of Italy, was introduced some years before the reform, while in the South respective experiments started in 2003 only. Generally speaking the associated planning of the municipalities has a history of four years as a maximum. The social zone requires complex agreements between public entities and the private non-profit sector as the legislator wanted to respect three principles that are not easy to combine:

- *Representative democracy*: The reform confirms the municipality as the genuine subject of the functions concerning social interventions carried out in the territory (L. 328/2000). The municipal government is steered by elected organisms that guarantee the control of the citizens on the municipal budget. In order to respect this principle, the assignment of each municipality's social funds to the budget of the social zone must be approved by every single municipality.
- *Managerial rationality*: Small municipalities must associate with others in order to be able to guarantee a level of services that is able to cover the whole range of inhabitants' vital needs. The reform indicates some options for the management of the social zone, e.g. to form a union of municipalities or a consortium, to install an assembly of the mayors, to delegate the management to the leading municipality, or to constitute a special company. Each of these solutions has advantages and disadvantages but they all involve a twofold decision-making process: from the single municipality to the association of municipalities (political subject) and from the association to the management body (administrative subject).
- *Horizontal subsidiarity*: The reform recognises that social well-being originates in the first place from the collaboration among citizens; the

399

social ties that are developed by and within the community are the energy to nurture also social services. Therefore organised citizens – the associations, social co-operatives, and voluntary organisations – are explicitly mentioned as partners, with whom the municipality should share all stages of planning, management and evaluation.

It is important to recall the cultural turning point represented by this law: Italy is modifying the political approach towards social care, social policies have widened their horizon, discovering precious synergies that stem from the integration with the health sector, but also with other public policies. This change was sustained by the Law on childhood and youth (L. 285/1997) that induced the municipalities to develop programmatic agreements with all those territorial institutions that influence the welfare of children and youth. This law in fact helped the institutions and the private non-profit sector in the development of combined plans and interventions, formalised in agreements and budgets to be managed together. The Law 285/1997 is generally considered as a laboratory in which the competencies, the management style and working cultures necessary for the implementation of the social reform were born.

Although the cooperation with the health system is still very important it became more and more evident to align the social services with additional areas such as school, vocational training, guidance, adult education, job centres, active labour policies, cultural centres, libraries, research institutions, sport centres, parks, leisure time institutions, and environmental policies. Some social plans of the zone ("piani di zona") reflect this new scenario and promote the integration between services to the people (protection, care) and those services that develop social capital (positive bonds, entertainment, pleasure). This strategic evolution, however, does not reduce the need to reinforce the axis of integrated health and social services.

Summing up, there are three crucial points for the development of integrated health and social care in Italy:

1.   *Funds:* In Italy the quantitative importance of the health resources is a hundred to one against resources for social care. In the future, a slow increase of the funds for the social sector and a contraction of the expenses for the health sector can be predicted. In this framework, the increase of highly integrated health and social services depends mostly on the conversion of hospital-based structures and human resources – with respective risks in terms of conflicts and managerial problems.

2.   *Management:* The territories covered by the Local Health Agencies are generally about four to five times larger than those of the social zones.

400

Moreover, they consistently diverge in their organisational and managerial structures. While the Local Health Agencies are a unitary subject, with a general manager elected by the regional government that is directly transferring the budget, the social zone consists of multiple subjects and is funded by the various municipalities that belong to it.

3.   *Working culture:* The health sector has experienced a progressive specialisation characterising the professionals' approaches, while the professional cultures in the social sector are more fluid and open to new common paradigms in terms of a global approach to people's welfare.

Although these factors are rather critical to the integration of health and social care services, they have not prevented the blooming of many projects and experiences focused on integration. In particular, some stakeholders have taken initiative based on different rationales, for instance:

* *administrators* who consider the integration of health and social services as a strategic factor qualifying the system and overcoming financial gaps (principle of effectiveness/efficiency);

* *professionals* who are convinced that they cannot produce satisfying results if they do not increase the collaboration among the various professions (principle of technical effectiveness); and, last but not least

* *citizens* who become aware of their complex needs and claim for more coherence of the supply system (principle of strategic effectiveness).

401

Notes

1   The difference between a "structural" and a "functional" department concerns the autonomy of the department's head in relation to the distribution of resources – a "functional department" does not dispose of a proper budget. Thus problems arise, for instance, as the head of the department is not in charge of the human resources that are managed by the general manager of the Local Health Authority (USL). Moreover, investments are strongly limited as the head of the department is lacking contractual power within the Local Health Authority. In general, managers of community care departments assert that decision-making is mainly influenced by medical doctors, in particular by those employed in hospitals.

2   Depending on the region, this team is known under different titles: in Veneto, for instance, it is called "Multidimensional Assessment District Unit".

3   The experimentation is based on the following legal guidelines: Deliberation of the Regional Council of Tuscany of 9/4/2002, n. 60 (Health Plan 2002-2004); L.R n. 72/1997 ("Organisation and promotion of a system of citizenship rights and of equal opportunity: reorganisation of integrated social and health services"); Deliberation of the Regional Council of Tuscany as of 24/7/2002, n. 122 (Integrated Regional Social Plan 2002-2004).

References

AA.VV. (2000) 'Il carer e l'operatore nella gestione dell'anziano non autosufficiente', *La Rivista di Servizio Sociale*: 217-242.

Belloni, M.C. (1997) 'Le politiche dei tempi della città', in: Belloni, M.C./Bimbi, F. (a cura di) *Microfisica della cittadinanza. Città, genere, politiche dei tempi*. Milano: F. Angeli.

Benedetti, L./Donati, D./Fazioli, R./Maffeo, R. (1997) *Valutazione e riforma dei servizi sociali*. Milano: Franco Angeli.

Bertin, G. (ed.) (1995) *Valutazione e sapere sociologico*. Milano: Franco Angeli.

Bimbi F./Prestinger F. (a cura di) (1985) *Profili sovrapposti*. Milano: Franco Angeli.

Bracco, L./Baroni, A./Gori, G./Piccini, C./Notarelli, A. (1993) *Day – Hospital per dementi*, Atti della Giornata Anno Europeo dell'Anziano.

Calcioli, S. (2001) *L'assistenza agli anziani*. Milano: Franco Angeli.

Casagrande, S. (2001) 'L'ADI: il punto e le prospettive', *Prospettive Sociali e Sanitarie* 1: 2-6.

Cave, M./Kogan, M./Smith, R. (eds.) (1990) *Output and Performance Measurement in Government – The State of the Art*. London: Jessica Kingsley Publishers.

Cerasa, F./Lucchetti, M. (1998) 'Donne anziane sempre più sole: il caso delle Marche', *Prisma* 7: 23-48.

Cerasa, F./Lucchetti, M. (1998) 'Il tempo e gli interessi degli anziani', *Qualità-Equità* 11: 119-124

Chiesa, S. (2000) 'Integrazione dei servizi socio – sanitari', *Prospettive Sociali e Sanitarie* 12: 10-12

Chiesi, A. (1993) 'Diseguaglianze sociali nell'uso del tempo', in: Paci M. (a cura di), *Le dimensioni della diseguaglianza*. Bologna: Il Mulino.

Cimbelli, P. (2001) *La malattia di Alzheimer e il caregiver professionale nella rete integrata dei servizi*. Zenit Editore.

Cnel (1998) *L'assistenza ai non autosufficienti: azione pubblica e meccanismi di mercato*, Indagine richiesta dalla Camera dei Deputati, Rapporto n.1, Roma: Cnel.

Costanzi C./Ferrari F. (a cura di) (1997) *Progettare la qualità negli Istituti per anziani*. Milano: Ediz. Franco Angeli.

Cremoncini, V./Vernò, F. (a cura di) (1983) 'La via del Distretto come occasione di integrazione fra il sociale e il sanitario. Il ruolo degli operatori sociali', *Servizi Sociali* 3: 36-53.

Cucinotta, D. (1992) *Curare l'anziano*. Milano: Ediz. Sorbona.

De Vincenti, C. (ed.) (2000) *Gli anziani in Europa – IX Rapporto CER-SPI*. Bari: Laterza.

Di Iorio, A./Ferrucci, L./Del Lungo (1996) 'Tipologia degli utenti dei servizi in ADI: indagine multicentrica nazionale', *Giornale Gerontologico* 44: 44-72.

D'Orazio, E. (1994) *Studiare da grande*. Roma: Edup.

D'Orazio, E. (1996) 'Il terzo settore nel sud', *Qualità Equità* 4: 26-43.

D'Orazio, E. (1998) *L'economia della solidarietà. Terzo settore e sindacato*. Roma: Ediesse.

Egidi, V. (1997) 'Anziani: prospettive demografiche e problemi sociali', in: da Empoli, D./Muraro, G. (a cura di), *Verso un nuovo stato sociale, tendenze e criteri*. Milano: Franco Angeli.

Giordano M. (2000) *L'integrazione possibile*. Ediz. Lavoro

Giunco, F. (ed.) (1994) *Anziani e Centri Diurni*. Milano: Franco Angeli.

Gori, G./Cimbelli, P./Pientini, S. (1999) 'Il Centro Diurno: un'esperienza fiorentina nel trattamento della demenza', *Toscana Medica*: 8-20.

Gori, C. (a cura di) (2001) *Le politiche per gli anzini non autosufficienti*. Milano: Franco Angeli

Gruppo di Lavoro della Fondazione Smith Kline (2000) 'Un contributo al dibattito sulle politiche per gli anziani', *Tendenze Nuove* 2: 45-72.

Gruetzner, H. (1991) *Alzheimer: una malattia da vivere*. Milano: Ed. Tecniche Nuove.

Lamura, G. (1999) 'Le politiche per la salute degli anziani in Italia', pp. 193-213 in: Colantonio, R./Lucchetti, M./Venturelli, A. (a cura di) *Ambiente ed invecchiamento*. Milano: Guerini.

Lazzarini, G. (a cura di) (1994) *Anziani e generazioni*. Milano: F. Angeli.

Levorato, A./Rozzini, R./Trabucchi, M. (1994) *I costi della vecchiaia*. Bologna: Il Mulino.

Lesemann, F./Martin, C. (1994) *Assistenza a domicilio. Famiglia e anziani*. Milano: F. Angeli.

Longo, R. (1997) 'I servizi per gli anziani: una rete di aziende in un gioco competitivo a somma negativa. Ipotesi per un sistema di relazioni', *Mecosan* 23: 18-35.

Lucchetti, M./Rossi, L./Cerasa, F. (1997) *Primi risultati economico-gestionali dell'Assistenza Domiciliare Integrata*. Ancona: INRCA/Dipartimento Ricerche Gerontologiche.

Lucchetti, M. (1998) 'Assistenza domiciliare, sanitaria, sociale, integrata. Modello organizzativo e funzionale', pp. 31-43 in: Gaetti, R. (a cura di), *I nuovi orizzonti della Geriatria*. Ancona: ed. Anniballi.

Lucchetti, M. (1999) 'Qualche rovello, due nuove idee e un approccio operativo a proposito di Assistenza Domiciliare Integrata', *La Rivista di Servizio Sociale* 4: 43-52

Lucchetti, M. (2001) 'L'assistenza Domiciliare Integrata basata sull'utente. Il modello operativo GIADA per la gestione degli utenti, degli operatori e per il controllo della spesa', *Giornale di Gerontologia* 4: 155-160.

Magistrali, G./Cagnolati, G./Fava, S. (a cura di) (1998) *Gli anziani, la città e i servizi*. Milano: Franco Angeli.

Maguire, L. (1999) *Il lavoro sociale di rete*. Trento: Ediz. Erickson.

Marcolini, M./Donnini, L./Lucchetti, M. (2001) 'Studio delle caratteristiche socio-economiche di fragilità associate a condizioni di salute precarie per gli anziani che vivono soli', *Salute e Territorio* 127.

Ministero della Sanità (1995) *Tutela della salute degli anziani: materiali e indirizzi per l'attuazione del progetto obiettivo*. Roma: Ministero della Sanità.

Pace, D./Pisani, S. (1998) *Le condizioni economiche degli anziani*. Roma/Bari: La Terza.

Piazza, M. (1993) 'Il tempo per sè. Un anello forte nella costruzione del soggetto', in: Carbonaro, A./Facchini, C. (a cura di), *Biografie e costruzione dell'identità*. Milano: F. Angeli.

Presidenza del Consiglio dei Ministri, Dipartimento per gli Affari Sociali (1998) *Anziani. Relazione biennale al parlamento sulla condizione dell'anziano, 1996-1997*. Roma.

Presidenza del Consiglio dei Ministri, Dipartimento per gli Affari Sociali (2000) *Anziani. Relazione biennale al parlamento sulla condizione dell'anziano, 1998-1999*. Roma.

Rossi, N. (1997) *Meno ai padri, più ai figli*. Bologna: Il Mulino.

Spi-Cgil (1997) *Progetto obiettivo anziani. Dall'assistenza negata alle nuove politiche regionali d'intervento*. Roma: Ediesse.

Saraceno, C. (1989) 'La struttura temporale della vita', in: Belloni, M.C./Rampazi, M. (a cura di), *Tempo, spazio, attore sociale*. Milano: F. Angeli.

Scortegagna, R. (1993) 'Lo stato dei servizi per anziani', *Animazione Sociale* 13 (10): 9-19.

Scortegagna, R. (1996) *Progetto Anziani*. Roma: La Nuova Italia Scientifica.

Scortegagna, R. (1999) 'Lavorare per progetti nell'ambito dei servizi di assistenza agli anziani', *La Rivista di Servizio Sociale* 1: 26-36.

Scortegagna, R. (2000) 'Anziani e politiche per l'invecchiamento in Italia', *La Rivista di Servizio Sociale* 3: 65-74.

Taccani, P./Tramma, S./Barbieri Dotti, A. (1999) *Gli anziani nelle strutture residenziali.* Roma: Ediz. Carocci.

Toniolo Piva, P. (1998) *Vita normale. Guida ai servizi per le persone non autosufficienti*. Roma: Spi-Cgil/Fnp-Cisl/Uilp-Uil.

Trabucchi, M. (1998) *Le demenze*. Milano: Ed. UTET.

Zanetti, E. (1997) *Il nursing delle demenze*. Milano: Ed. Lauri.

Annex: Project Descriptions

A1 Integration by "One-window" Approaches and Shared Information Systems: The Project "Single Point of Home Care"

Provider	Local Health Agency 11, 15 Municipalities (5 of the Valdarno Zone and 10 of the Empolese Valdelsa Zone), Social Co-operatives.
Objectives	• increasing the efficiency and the effectiveness of the home care • increasing the satisfaction of the client/patient • increasing the general welfare • increasing the survival rate • restrict the hospital to the acute phase • decreasing the average length of stay in hospitals for pathologies that may benefit from home care
Description	The experimentation foresees the creation of a Single Point in the Local Health Authority/Company 11 where all the requests for home care come together (including the protected hospital discharge) where the home care plan is set up directly involving the General Practitioner. The "Unit of Territorial Evaluation" (UVT) takes in charge the most complex demands and draws up the plan. A computer programme follows and records the several phases.
Target Group	• All patients discharged from hospitals, RSA (Nursing Home), Day Centres (any "institutional" centre) with particular regard to the elderly in need of care or elderly at risk • All citizens in need of home care
Number of Clients	Approximately 200
Staff Involved	Social workers, professional nurses, social and health assistants, District Physicians, General Practitioners, physiotherapists, specialised physicians
Instruments	For the project evaluation the following indicators are taken into consideration: • Number of contacts • Number of patients discharged from hospital that need home care • Time of latency, counted in days, between the contact and the actual in-take

	• Average hospitalisation of pathologies that can benefit of home care • Number of hospitalisations, even temporary, in RSA (Assisted Sanitary Residence)/Number of reports
Methods	The method in use is that of teamwork within the UVT (Territorial Assessment Unit), the UVG (Unit of Geriatric Assessment) and the UVA (Unit of Alzheimer Assessment), i.e. a multidimensional and multiprofessional needs assessment.
Strengths	Centralisation of requests, with the opportunity of rationalising interventions, assigning resources to the most disadvantaged persons.
Weaknesses	It is difficult to coordinate the interventions maintaining and explicitly taking into account the user's perspective.
Results of Evaluation	Although the project is still in progress, the first important results are already evident: rationalisation of the relationships among hospital, territory, MMG (General Practitioners), municipalities and citizens; decreasing length of stay in hospitals for pathologies that benefit from ADI (Integrated Home Care); continuous support to the family.
Keywords	Centralisation of requests, multidimensional and multiprofessional assessment

A2 Integration by "One-window" Approaches and Shared Information Systems: The Project "Information System for All Activities Carried out in the Territory"

Provider	Local Health Authority/Company 11 of Empoli, Municipal Governments, voluntary service associations ("Assistenze", "Misericordie", the Red Cross, "AUSER Filo d'Argento", Italian League for Combating Cancer)
Objectives	• creating a relational information system covering all services distributed to the citizens in the area • creating a network of care services collaborating with the hospitals on the territory, in particular by involving also those social services of municipalities that have not delegated them to the Local Health Agency • re-assigning to every citizen, and therefore to his/her MMG (General Practitioner), all activities/services carried out in the community • re-assigning to every GP the responsibility of all community care services provided to his/her patients either if they have been directly prescribed or if they have been prescribed by others

- favouring communication and the flow of information among all actors by means of adequate software
- realising a kind of DRG (Diagnosis Related Group) system in community care
- gathering information if a citizen is also receiving services by other providers and, if yes, which kind of services are provided
- providing the opportunity for hospital staff to following the further process after a patient's discharge
- connecting General Practitioners to community care services and the hospital in order to exchange information and to accelerate procedures
- creating Diagnostic Therapeutic Courses (PDT) to monitor the health status in the territory, involving municipalities and General Practitioners
- creating a database to also control the double supply of medicines (Law n. 135/2002)

The information system is to provide the following data:

- home nursing carried out by: professional nurses, physiotherapists, district physicians, specialised doctors (e.g. anaesthetists, oncologists, cardiologists, palliativists…), MMG (General Practitioner)
- social care carried out by: social workers, OTA/OSA/OSS
- assistance inside the District Divisions for non-specialised and non-medical services such as those of the professional nurses, physiotherapists…
- management of the single waiting list for temporary/ definitive admission in nursing homes
- activities of the MMG (General Practitioner)
- screening directly carried out by the MMG (General Practitioner)
- services carried out by the District and/or Territorial Divisions

Description	The project is to install special hard- and software to manage all social and health activities carried out in the territory by the Local Health Agency, the Municipalities and the GPs). Once the citizen's data are registered by the respective office of the Local Health Agency it will be possible to re-assign all services provided to the citizens in relation to their GP. This information should also help to better monitor budgets and costs in General Medicine and community care.
Target Group	All residents in the territory of the Local Health Agency 11, in particular older persons and persons at risk.
Number of Clients	Approximately 500
Staff Involved	• Social service and community care professionals • Administrative staff in the Health Care Agency and the municipalities

	• Home care staff (nurses) • Rehabilitation units • General Practitioners • Hospital Units (physiotherapy, geriatric, oncology, reanimation, orthopaedics, cardiology) • Units for oncology screening of II° level (pathological anatomy, digestive endoscopy, radiology, obstetrics and gynaecology) • Working Unit administrative support • Technical Units (maintenance, electromedical equipment, great works • Hospital and territorial pharmaceutical departments • Voluntary services ("AUSER", "Pubbliche Assistenze", "Misericordia", the Red Cross, the "Italian League for Combating Cancer")
Instruments	In the evaluation the following indicators are taken in consideration: *Process indicators:* • No. of GPs connected to the information system (% of computerised GPs) • No. of health and social staff using the information system, i.e. entering and updating data (% of data entry by all staff and by single professional groups) • % of cases receiving community care entered in the information system by respective staff *Result indicators:* • % of decrease of the average length of stay in hospitals for persons with pathologies that might be treated by community care • mortality rate standardised on the population for pathologies as object of screening • business savings (meaning minor absorption of resources and appropriateness of the treatment plans) on the bases of the P.D.T. (Diagnostic Therapeutic Process) shared by GPs and specialists
Methods	"Cluster Method": all single services "cluster" around the client
Strengths	• software may be applied in every situation and territory • other agencies may benefit from solutions found in the project • stronger integration of all stakeholders and improvement of the interface hospital-community care • better organisation and motivation of staff, and involvement of GPs
Weaknesses	• necessity of a special software and an intranet solution • resistance of staff both to the working method and to the use of information technology

Results of Evaluation	• simplification of all the administrative and bureaucratic processes
	• single entry of the citizens' data in the system available to anyone
	• creation of a database, available to anyone, if authorised by the citizen him-/herself or by the responsible of the service, e.g. the GP
	• acceleration of the supply of both health and social services
	• real integration among the mutually linked services
Keywords	Information System, simplification of administrative processes

A3 Integration by Inter-professional Teams: The Multi-dimensional Assessment District Unit ("Unità Valutativa Multidimensionale Distrettuale")

Provider	Each Health District within each Local Health Agency in the Veneto Region
Objectives	To assess older person's needs, defining and implementing the best solution available, if possible in the community; specific tasks are: • multidimensional needs assessment using the S.V.A.M.A. form; • elaboration of an individual care plan within a month • implementation of the individual project within 20 days after the care plan validation • monitoring and final evaluation of goals achieved • data collection
Target Group	Older persons in need of care (residents of the Veneto Region)
Type of Staff Involved	• Manager of the Health District • General Practitioner • Social Worker from the Municipality involved or, in case of delegation, from the Health District • Geriatrician • Nurse • Administration
Methods and Instruments	Needs assessments using S.V.A.M.A., a form for the multi-dimensional assessment which collects personal data, pathologies, requests, outcomes of cognitive, functional (Short Portable Mental Status Questionnaire; Barthel Index) and social assessment.

Strengths	Interdisciplinary team; Transparent way of working; Goal orientation; Effective projects; Quality evaluation; Budgeting; Improvement of the care network; Risk management
Weaknesses	Structural complexity; Difficult coordination; Inter-professional conflicts; Bureaucratic rigidity; Lack of follow-up in relation to the results of evaluation
Results of Evaluation	*not available*
Keywords	Inter-professional team, Inter-disciplinary assessment, Project Management

A4 Integration by Inter-professional Teams: The Working Unit of Continuous Care/WUCC ("Unità Operativa di Continuità Assistenziale")

Providers	Hospitals of Thiene and Schio; Health District ASL 4; Municipalities from Alto Vicentino; Local Nursing Homes
Objectives	To guide older persons from hospital toward the appropriate care service
Target Group	Older persons discharged from hospital
Staff Involved	Hospital: Head Physicians, Geriatrician, Nurses, Social Worker, General Practitioners, community care service staff
Methods and Instruments	• Definition of eligibility criteria and needs using the assessment form "S.V.A.M.A.", developed for multi-dimensional assessment, which collects personal data, pathologies, requests, outcomes of cognitive, functional (Short Portable Mental Status Questionnaire; Barthel Index) and social assessment • Definition procedure for WUCC taking in charge
Strengths	• In-take by hospital staff, Multi-stakeholders approach; detailed care planning • Integrated work: within the WUCC, the hospitals, the territory • Innovative methodology: experimentation of seamless care • Outcomes: reduction of avoidable hospital admissions (from 123 to 83 in 2002) • Effectiveness: reduction of avoidable hospital admissions; awareness about resources available on the territory • Shared information system

409

Weaknesses	<ul><li>Lack of evaluation: on customer's satisfaction; on the service</li><li>Target strictly focused on older persons</li><li>Health-oriented approach</li><li>Conflicts between WUCC and other hospital divisions</li><li>Conflicts among professionals (cultures, methods, goals)</li><li>Shared responsibility</li><li>Formalism</li></ul>
Results of Evaluation	Reduction of avoidable hospital admissions (from 123 to 83 in 2002): 30% of discharged persons went to Nursing Homes for temporary admissions (2 months), the others moved back home.
Keywords	Inter-professional team, interdisciplinary assessment, project management, programmed (accompanied) hospital discharge; seamless care; community care

A5 Integration by Quality Management: The Project "Quality of Integrated Home Care"

Provider	Municipalities of the District, the Local Health Agency (ASL) of Reggio Emilia, the Chair of Public Health at the University of Modena and Reggio Emilia, and some voluntary service organisations.
Objectives	To create a net of territorial health and social services, to favour continuous care (protected discharge from hospital), and to activate an integrated care service according to quality criteria (fairness, timeliness, suitability of level, effectiveness, efficiency).
Description	The project, addressed to the over 65, was carried out in four stages: *1st stage:* interdisciplinary training of social and health staff engaged in integrated home care (ADI) to create shared working instruments and methods. *2nd stage:* developing the Quality System for integrated home care by creating a net of health and social services (signed protocols and agreements; outline of an operating model). Activation of an Operating Territorial Centre in order to assure the quality of admittance to the territorial care regimes (home care, residential, semi-residential). Development of a computerised information system for the collection and the elaboration of data. *3rd stage:* activation of an experimental team for integrated home care.

	4th stage: evaluation of the quantitative and economic aspects of the scheme
Target Group	9,600 persons over 65 (plus 100 patients suffering from cancer)
Number of Clients	927 cases (1997-2001)
Staff Involved	Health and social staff (32 general practitioners, paediatricians, 10 professional nurses, 17 care assistants, social workers, specialised physicians (oncologist, neurologist, cardiologist, surgeon, internist, physiotherapist).
Instruments	During the experimentation a handbook on the quality of integrated home care (ADI) was realised containing shared quality indicators: • rate of home services for the elderly and terminal oncology patients • frequency of protected discharge processes (i.e. organised discharge in coordination with the GP and home care services) • Waiting time for admission • Efficiency (average activity of the home care staff by number of integrated home care clients) • Suitability (index of care intensity: days of actual care/ waiting time before admission) – number of persons admitted to hospitals/number of integrated care services' clients • Acceptability (satisfaction index, based on a questionnaire) • Reliability: number of warnings/total patients in integrated care
Methods	Teamwork, information system, quality development
Strengths	• Small dimension of the experimental environment • The project supplied cues to the Health Council of the Region of Emilia Romagna in drawing up the Directive *"Criteria for the reorganisation of the home treatments"* (DGR 124/1999) • The project has provided indicators for Integrated Home Care that, in the light of recent norms on accreditation of services (DL 229/1999 and LR 34/1998), were used to define accreditation criteria in the Region of Emilia Romagna.
Weaknesses	It is necessary to continuously sustain the motivation of staff. Integration, the idea of responsibility of the families, their participation, are the results of a cultural change that requires long periods of time and continuous conflict management.
Keywords	Integrated home care service (ADI); hospital-community care interface; quality criteria

411

A6 Integrated Services for Special Target Groups: The Alzheimer Day Centre "Stella del Colle"

Provider	The Municipality of Florence launched an experimentation of territorial care for dementia patients, provided by the Consortium "Zenit"
Objectives	• to provide rehabilitation targeted to prevent progression of the disease • to avoid unnecessary admittance in nursing homes • to support the family during the phases of medium and high gravity (4°, 5°, 6° of the Reisberg Scale) • to study the difficulties of staff to grant suitable care to dementia patients • to study the problems of families caring for a person suffering from dementia • to study new care models
Description	The service is continuously opened from 7.30 a.m. to 8.00 p.m., 7 days a week all year round. Users can be brought by family members or use a transportation service organised by the Consortium. In the Day Centre individual and group activities are organised according to the personal (life and working) experiences of the patients. The number of operators is related to the number of guests, according to the conventions and regional standards. On the care level all the services of a nursing home are granted. The project was inspired by the Canadian model of continuous care.
Target Group	To dementia patients and especially to Alzheimer patients.
Number of Clients	During the last 10 years, the Centre has been attended by about 300 guests with an average frequency of 7-8 months.
Staff Involved	The Day Centre employs professional social educators, social workers and health professionals (nurses, physiotherapists, physicians). At the moment, the following professionals work in the Centre: 1 neuropsychiatrist (Medical Director of the Consortium), 1 geriatrician/IRCCS researcher, some professional educators, 1 rehabilitation therapist, 1 professional nurse, 1 musicotherapist, 6 social workers, drivers
Instruments	All activities and results of the Day Centre are evaluated during a constant monitoring process with the aid of specific instruments, i.e. an admission form sent by the social services, the Centre's admission form, information schedule, monthly meetings with family members, weekly meetings with staff and monthly meetings between staff and the Centre's geriatrician.

412

Methods	• R.O.T. Gentle Care by Moira Jones • Validation by Naomi Feil • Integrated Psycho-relational Method elaborated by the team of the Centre
Strengths	• The Day Centre is a valid alternative to the nursing home • The patient is supported in his/her psychological, relational and cognitive skills • The family takes part in the rehabilitation project • The family is supported to face the situation with less stress and anxiety
Weaknesses	The complementary service of *"professional caregivers at home"* was not established; after some years the Municipality stopped to use it, preferring the mainstream services of contracted organisations. The complementary service of *"short-term care in nursing homes"* was not established, notwithstanding respective proposals to the Municipality with the full support of the families. The service was meant to grant relief and support to family caregivers during absence and/or sickness of the caregiver.
Results of Evaluation	• support of the patient in the family, even for very long periods of time, despite the acute degree of the disease • decrease of family stress (30% reduction of the Burden Instrument score) • decrease of psychothropic drugs together with mitigation of the disturbing behaviours, improvement of the motoric performance, re-balance of the waking-sleeping rhythm, promotion of socialisation skills, adaptation and simple learning in seriously ill patients
Keywords	Alzheimer Day Centre, CAD, Continuous care

413

Providing Integrated Health and Social Care for Older Persons in the Netherlands

Carine Ex, Klaas Gorter, Uschi Janssen

1   Introduction

This report is to tackle the question whether the Dutch policy concerning elderly citizens directs the care system towards an integrated provision, and whether the care system is capable of delivering an integrated supply of health and social care. Following Kodner/Kyriakou (2000), integrated care may be defined as: "A discrete set of techniques and organisational models designed to create connectivity, alignment and collaboration within and between the cure and care sectors at the funding, administrative and/or provider level." For the clients these techniques and models should result in getting the care they need, that means adequate amounts of the right types, and delivered in the appropriate order and at the right moment in time. This may be regarded as a definition of integrated care *from the client's perspective*.

1.1   Trends in the Demand of Care

In an exposition about care for the elderly in the Netherlands, the *Algemene Rekenkamer* (2002) states that the overall demand for the amount and types of care is influenced by various factors that we shall pass in review:
*   demographic developments (with respect to population growth and ageing);

- social-cultural developments relating to:
  - the desire to remain living at home as long as possible,
  - changes in the relation between intramural and extramural care,
  - the articulation of a hitherto hidden care demand (in connection with cultural changes),
  - a postponed demand for care (considering the waiting lists).

The Netherlands has about 16 million inhabitants. According to predicted demographic developments, the number of elderly people will strongly grow. The increase of life expectancy will lead to a percentage of the population over 55 years of age, amounting from presently 23% to 35% in 2030. Especially the number of very old people (over 85) will grow. This demographic trend implies an increase of chronically intermittent disorders, for which a flexible supply of care is required, consisting of an acute component and a long-term component, and of health care and social components (housing, care and additional provisions). In an integrated system those various components should seamlessly connect to each other. This is especially the case with chronic disorders that demand a clustering of various knowledge and abilities in the medical, paramedical, nursing, caring, and social fields. Influenced by the relative growth of the number of chronically ill, public attention for care, next to cure, has increased (*Raad voor de Volksgezondheid en Zorg*, 2001). However, the current approach of the health care system lags behind demographic developments and is still too much targeted at acute rather than chronically intermittent disorders (Delnoij et al., 2001).

Today, elderly people are increasingly active and vigorous to a greater age; they are better educated and, as a consequence, have become more independent and responsible. On top of that, many elderly have achieved a state of (relative) prosperity. As a result, they demand a greater say in matters concerning their health and welfare and expect a wider range of services (Van Ewijk, 1999).

Since the 1980s, independence has become an essential element of the life style of many in the new generation of elderly. The general trend has become to keep older persons as long as possible in their own homes as this is what they want themselves, rather than having to move to a nursing home. Many "new" elderly also want assistance contributing to a meaningful participation in social life. As a result, "old" care facilities which were introduced during the 1970s are, wherever possible, replaced by professional home care services cooperating with family and other informal carers.

416

Moreover, the expectations of patients towards the health care system increase, and may best be summarised as: "more, better, faster". There is also a larger need for differentiation. The care system should be organised in such a manner that (a) the increasing need for differentiation can be met, and (b) those groups of society, who have not yet been able to acquire skills for acting as critical, well-informed patients, continue to get access to the care system.

The new creed is, that the elderly themselves have to be able to decide where and how to live, and which services they will utilise if their need for care increases (Lammers/Driest, 2002). Within this scope, the term *"custom-made care"* is often used. This concept is closely connected to integrated care. "Custom-made" expresses that the supplied care should match the needs of the person. And because the needs of the elderly often bear upon multiple areas (like problems with health, functional limitations, housing and transport), an integration supply of services from these sectors is necessary.

The Social and Cultural Planning Board (*Sociaal en Cultureel Planbureau*, SCP) that publishes a comprehensive report on the living situation of the elderly every two years, confirms this view on the position of the elderly. The latest report concludes that most elderly in the Netherlands are doing well, and that their position has improved rather than deteriorated in the 1990s. Nevertheless, there still are groups of older persons for whom a definite policy for care and protection is urgently required. This applies, for instance, to elderly with severe physical or mental impairments, who depend on others, and to elderly who dispose of limited resources: people with a low level of education or income, or people with a small social network (De Klerk, 2001).

To what extent does the supply of care cover the demand? Recently, *demand-oriented care* has become a central theme for policy-makers, i.e. the supply of care should adapt to the demand for care, rather than making demand dependent on supply. However, the present care demand of the elderly is still insufficiently known. Regarding the demand for facilities, three categories of persons can be distinguished: those who get the care to which they are entitled, those on waiting lists, and those who have not yet expressed their need. The latter indicate a hidden care demand. The group on the waiting list can be divided into two sub-categories, namely those "simply" on the waiting list, and those who are on the waiting list but meanwhile receive transitional ('bridging") care, e.g. in the form of home care. As a result, however, waiting lists tend to grow in the home care system, too (*Algemene*

Rekenkamer, 2002). It is expected that the home care by 2004 will be considerably short in staff: 18,000, i.e. more than 10% of the present workforce (Nivel, 2002).

The information about care supply (utilised capacity) is also insufficient. Neither "influx", "through-flux", nor "outflux" of clients are fully known. The lack of clarity as to how many people may utilise the existing care supply hampers the policy that aims at attuning demand and supply of care provisions (*Algemene Rekenkamer*, 2002). That the match between the two is far from perfect becomes only too obvious from the existence of waiting lists.

1.2 Trends in the Supply of Care

The organisation of the care system in the Netherlands used to be arranged according to target groups: people with a mental disability, people with a physical disability, people over 65, and people who are chronically ill. Based on this arrangement, diverging care systems developed for separate groups of clients or patients. Recently, a different approach arose, which increasingly determines the general discourse: one should not so much take the target group as a point of departure, but rather the functional limitations the individual experiences from his/her illness or disability. Thus, the orientation shifts from the traditional target group to the consequences of an impairment. Furthermore, this implies not to operate anymore from the viewpoint of supply for a particular target group (separate provisions for specific impairments or age groups), but to start from the client's needs which may be satisfied by any relevant institution or service.

During the last decades, various solutions have been worked out in order to arrange the care system in such a manner that the older person may receive appropriate care. Since the 1960s, residential homes and nursing homes for the frail elderly were established and extended. In the period 1963 to 1980 the number of nursing homes increased from 106 to 325. The distinction between somatic nursing homes (primarily for elderly with severe physical disabilities), psycho-geriatric nursing homes (primarily for elderly with dementia) and residential homes (primarily for elderly with less severe disabilities) is diminishing. This results from changes in admission: residential homes increasingly function more or less as nursing homes, by receiving people with severe disabilities. Moreover, mergers have taken place between nursing homes, and between nursing and residential homes. These large-scale institutions offer housing and comprehensive care as one full package. In 2001, the expenditures for nursing homes were 3.6 billion €, and for residential homes 3,1 € (van Mosseveld/Smit, 2002: 28).

Over time, increasing resistance has risen against these large-scale facilities, pointing to the loss of independence and freedom of choice for their residents. This resistance was the main driving force behind the development of all sorts of innovations in the direction of down-scaled and more independent types of dwelling for the frail elderly, which are described in section 3.

In 1999, about 7% of the Dutch citizens over 65 lived in institutions for the elderly, 2% in a nursing home and 5% in a residential home. In the last decade, the overall intramural capacity was reduced. This applies to residential homes: in the period 1990 to 2000 the total number of its residents decreased by 18% (from 131,000 to 107,000). The reduction in capacity was mainly reached by scaling down the size of the residential homes. The newly-built homes accommodate considerably less people (the mean is 68) than the old homes which were built before 1970 (the mean is 112). On the other hand, the capacity of the nursing homes was enlarged: In the same period the number of residents increased by 14% (from 50,000 to 57,000). This expansion merely concerns the places for people with dementia; the number of places for elderly with only physical disabilities hardly changed. All in all, the shifts resulted in a net reduction in intramural capacity of almost 10%. This decrease was made possible by a number of developments, such as the "extramuralisation", meaning that many nursing homes and residential homes now also deliver care outside their walls, such as alarm services and meals-on-wheels (De Klerk, 2001: 5, 108, 184, 203; Raad voor de Volksgezondheid en Zorg, 2001: 95-96; Ooms/Ras, 2002: 21-23).

The majority of the elderly with less extensive care needs have been provided home care in the community. In line with the resistance against living in institutions, the government aims to relieve the growing pressure on residential care services by encouraging older people to continue living in their own home and by promoting arrangements for informal care and assistance-at-home. Professional community-based care at home encompasses all types of care, nursing, supervision and monitoring of people who require assistance at home (Goris et al., 2002). As a consequence, much has happened in the home care sector over the last ten years: demand increased and became more complex, supply and its organisation became more flex-

419

ible and more customer-oriented (e.g. services were extended to intensive home care with 7 days/24 hours accessibility), and competition between home care providers increased, by giving room to commercial home care providers. The home care sector is by far the most important supplier of professional social care for the elderly living on their own. In 1999, about 14% of them received home care (De Klerk, 2001: 196). In 2001, the expenditures in home care for all age groups (about 80% of the clients being of old age) amounted to 2.8 billion €. From 1998 to 2001 the expenditures increased by almost 40%. The total expenditures for the most important care sectors (nursing homes, residential homes and home care) were 9.5 billion €, reaching almost the total budget for cure in hospitals (10.9 billion €) (Van Mosseveld/Smit, 2002: 28).

Some ten years ago, institutions started providing care services in the homes of elderly living in their neighbourhood. This development was made possible by changes in policy and legislation, yielding an increased responsibility to provincial and local governments, and to involved organisations (such as financiers and care providers, housing corporations, patients' associations and elderly people's unions).

2 Legal and Structural Framework

In the Dutch system of care for the elderly three parties are involved: the authorities who formulate the policy, private non-profit or profit organisations who provide the care, and interest organisations who influence the policy.

While the national government is responsible for health care and income, the local authorities are responsible for housing, well-being, and mobility. The provinces have a task in the regional planning of facilities such as care and nursing homes. Together, public policies share the vision that the elderly no longer must be treated as a separate (categorial) group, even if they require more care, but as a regular part of society.

2.1 Policy at the National Level

In the Netherlands, the care policy for the elderly is pursued by several ministries, particularly by the Ministry of Health, Welfare and Sports (*Volksgezondheid, Welzijn en Sport, VWS*), the Ministry of Social Affairs (*Sociale*

Zaken en Werkgelegenheid, SZW) and the Ministry of Housing, Planning and Environment (*Volkshuisvesting, Ruimtelijke Ordening en Milieubeheer, VROM*). The responsibility of the national government includes legislation and issuing of regulations, making financial means available, and supervising the efficient performance of the care system (*Algemene Rekenkamer*, 2002).

The central target of the policy on the elderly is to prevent their social exclusion, where one may think of their health, care, financial situation, housing, and living surroundings. Moreover, the policy frameworks, which the various ministries have formulated, are more or less identical. This policy framework presents a vision of steering, in which the roles of the various actors in the care sector are specified: on the national level the government determines the framework within which the finance agencies, providers and interest organisations must take their responsibilities. These tasks and responsibilities have to connect with each other, so that a good accessibility of the care system may be realised (Rijkschroeff et al., 2002).

2.2 Policy at the Regional and Local Level

The regional responsibility is expressed by the fact that provinces and municipalities together are in charge of the regional planning of care facilities. Within the framework and support set by the state government, and together with organisations of clients, care providers and regional administrative care offices, the provinces and municipalities define which kind of care should be delivered. They periodically produce a policy document (called *regiovisie*) in which they present their views and objectives concerning care, housing, welfare, and transport for the elderly and disabled people in the region.

During the last two decades, the municipalities have been increasingly involved in matters concerning care for the elderly and disabled people. It was expected that decentralisation could better address local differences, and improve the attuning of supply to demand (De Klerk, 2001). The responsibility of the municipalities extends to several areas.

First of all, the local authorities execute the "Facilities for the Disabled Act" (*Wet Voorzieningen Gehandicapten, WVG*). Previously, this legislation and its provisions were reserved to disabled people under the age of 65. Since a few years, it also applies to the elderly in need of wheelchairs, housing adaptations and adapted transport facilities. By now, the majority of the users of these facilities are above the age of 65.

Since 1988, under the Welfare Act (*Welzijnswet*), the local governments are responsible for the welfare policy concerning the elderly. Three core functions are distinguished in this welfare work:

- social re-activation, i.e. stimulating the elderly to fulfil social tasks and promote their own interests in "self-help organisations";
- social prevention, which involves prevention of social exclusion, support in directing one's own life;
- person-oriented guidance and assistance, which means individual support in retaining or restoring the balance between the person and his/her surroundings.

Since 1997 the municipalities are also responsible for the execution and financing of a part of the so-called "flanking policy", which aims at additional provisions for the elderly. Among other things, the provision of services by residential homes to people living independently is involved, such as the supply of meals and alarm services.

2.3   The Process of Care Provision

2.3.1 Referral to the Care System

Many people address to their general practitioner for acquiring cure and care. The general practitioner is not only the gatekeeper for access to medical care in the hospital, but also an important guide for access to the care system. Increasingly, the general practitioner has to cooperate with several disciplines in the care area.

In acquiring social care and other facilities, the applicant has to deal with several bodies. First, the client has to expose his/her situation and needs at a Regional Assessment Board (RIO)[1], which decides to what kind of care, facilities or support the person is entitled. After a positive advice, the allocation of services takes place at the administrative care office. It is decided whether the required care can be delivered or whether the client must be placed on a waiting list. This procedure applies to most provisions, such as admission to a residential or a nursing home, day-treatment in an institution, several kinds of home care, adapted transport facilities, housing adaptations, "meals on wheels" facilities and alarm services.

2.3.2 Care Providers

From the 1970s to the 1990s, care policies aimed at substitution[2] in the care system (De Klerk, 2001). The objective was to shift usage from relatively intensive and costly care to minor and cheaper provisions. Depending on the situation of the client, this could mean a move from intramural to transmural and extramural provisions, from intensive to extensive care, from long-term to short-term care, from curative to preventive care, and from professional to informal care.

"Extramuralisation" was one of the effects: many nursing homes and residential homes now also deliver care outside their walls. Thus, nursing homes deploy a part of their budgets for elderly who are staying in residential homes. These residents are provided with care from nursing home doctors and other therapists, with the aim of postponing or preventing their transfer to a nursing home. Consequently, the through-flux from residential homes to nursing homes is decreasing. In turn, residential homes deliver extramural care to elderly living in the area, and to elderly in sheltered housing blocks or "leaning houses" (*aanleunwoningen*, independent housing, next to and "leaning" against a residential home). To date, about a quarter of those who receive services from nursing or residential homes live outside the walls of these institutions.

2.3.3 Informal Care

It is still common practice that the informal care sector – defined as assistance in housekeeping and/or personal care by members of the family, neighbours or acquaintances – covers the gaps of the formal care system. When suitable professional care is not available, it is assumed that family, neighbours and friends will step in.

In the Netherlands, the number of households with elderly persons (55+) receiving informal care, amounts to some 11-13%. This share has remained stable over the past ten years (De Klerk, 2001: 192).

2.3.4 Sheltered Accommodation

Sheltered or "protective" types of housing supply a combination of "normal" living and the provision of care services. In the Netherlands, various types of sheltered housing for the elderly are increasingly implemented, for instance as a row of houses near residential units ("leaning dwellings") and sheltered housing complexes (*woonzorgcomplexen*). The number of units per institution is lower at a sheltered housing complex than at residential homes. This indicates a decreasing scale in newly-constructed forms of sheltered housing. 70% of these dwellings are situated near a residential home, 9% near a service centre, and 10% near another form of service. The main reasons for older persons to move to a sheltered type of housing are the unsuitability of the former independent home and the fear of disabling health problems with no help network around (Van Dugteren, 2001).

Residential homes focus on elderly people who are unable to live independently, even with the assistance of home care and informal care. The reasons for moving to a residential home are much more prompted by (possible future) care needs and the heavy burden of having to arrange one's own household. Also, the care supply influences the decision, if home care services and/or the family can no longer cope. Nursing homes focus on those who need the most intensive care and nursing with an increasing share of older people suffering from Alzheimer's disease.

2.3.5 Home Care

Professional home care encompasses all care, nursing, supervision and monitoring of people who require assistance at home. Home care used to be carried out by separate organisations for family care, maternity care and district nursing services. Recently most of them merged into large home care organisations, which combine these three areas of work. People can also turn to home care organisations to borrow or buy (medical) aids. Terminally ill people are offered intensive home care. This may involve day and night care.

In the home care sector more than 175,000 persons are employed (about 60,000 full-time equivalents), delivering various services to about two million clients per year. They serve different target groups, like new-born babies and their mothers, pre-schoolers, disabled persons, mental patients, chronically ill, terminal patients and elderly people. The latter outnumber: in 2001, 80% of the clients were over 65 years of age. The home care organisations are spread over the country. In 1999, there were 104 non-profit organisations and 217 (generally small) for-profit organisations. They delivered on average 2,300 hours of home care per 1,000 people living at home (Nivel, 2002). In addition, people can employ cleaning personnel for their household work. In 1999, 14% of the households with elderly persons (55+)

received home care from non-profit organisations, and 11% received care (usually domestic chores) from a private person or profit organisation (De Klerk, 2001: 197). Elderly of foreign origin (an increasing group in the Netherlands) make relatively little us of the professional home care.

Long waiting lists and the fact that the amount of care is considered insufficient are an important source of discontent within the regular home care system. In 2000, 54,300 people entitled to nursing and care services found themselves on a waiting list. Approximately half of those do meanwhile receive some kind of transitional care.

2.4 Stakeholders

In the preceding sections, the national and local authorities, the several care providers, the insurance bodies, and the assessment agencies were already introduced as the main stakeholders in the Dutch care system. In this section we would therefore like to focus on another most important stakeholder, engaged in interest representation. The General Dutch Union for the Elderly (*ANBO*) is the largest interest organisation. Furthermore – as an expression of the pillarisation – there are unions with Catholic and Protestant persuasion (*KBO* and *PCBO*).

The *ANBO* and the other unions are organisations pursuing independence and freedom of choice for the elderly in housing, care, mobility, and activities, and also availability of affordable facilities in those areas. Together with other organisations, the union dedicates itself at all levels (national, provincial and local) to the improvement of the social, material, and cultural position of persons above the age of 50 in society. With almost 180,000 members and some 575 local branches spread all over the country, they deal with the social integration of and participation by senior citizens of both Dutch as well as other descent.

Concerning care for the elderly, the union emphasises the importance of independent living and functioning. That requires proximity of facilities, safety, and availability of (home) care. It is held that the informal carer should not be a necessity for living at home, but an additional source of care. Furthermore, additional facilities for informal carers are claimed.

The union states that elderly people have different desires and needs, and therefore desire freedom of choice. That implies sufficient options for senior citizens in housing, care institutions, and service packages, and an

425

independent needs assessment. They also insist on a sufficient offer of cultural and social-cultural activities, within and without the *ANBO*-organisation.

Scarcity of facilities impedes freedom of choice and independence. Therefore, availability has become an important theme to the elderly. Especially in this area, the union meets with other parties, such as insurers, service providers, and housing corporations. Such contacts concern issues such as the addition of provisions to the basic package of care insurance, removing waiting lists, and gaining clarity as to the measure of actually required and supplied assistance. Furthermore, the union insists on adequately equipped and sufficient housing and care facilities, and suitable housing for the elderly in general. In addition, accessible and frequently operating public transport is stressed as important for the mobility of the elderly.

2.5 Financing Care for the Elderly

In the Netherlands, care for the elderly is mainly funded by the following sources:

- Short-term medical care is insured via the (public) health insurance fund (*Ziekenfonds*) and private health insurances.
- Home care, nursing homes and residential homes for the elderly are covered by the Exceptional Medical Expenses Act (*Algemene Wet Bijzondere Ziektekosten, AWBZ*). The funds stem from special taxes, which all inhabitants in the Netherlands have to pay. Clients are required to contribute an amount of money in proportion to their income. Home care users are charged between 2,20 to 124,60 Euro per week. For the financing of the products, next to the regular sources of income, non-regular sources such as sponsoring, subsidies, donations and gifts, funds, and commercial activities, are exploited. The costs of the residential and home care for the elderly are covered for 84% by the AWBZ, for 15% by contributions of the clients, and for 1% by other sources (Ooms/Ras, 2002: 10).
- The Provisions for the Disabled Act (*Wet Voorzieningen Gehandicapten, WVG*), implemented by local authorities, are financed by the national government from tax revenues.

2.6   Problems in Integrating Health and Care Services

As the previous sections show, a certain degree of integration has been accomplished in the Netherlands. However, integration of the various forms of care services for the elderly may take place at various levels and to various degrees. Delnoij (2001) distinguishes:

- clinical integration which takes place at the micro-level of the primary process, where we have to think of "chains of care" and transmural care;
- professional integration of professionals mutually, and of professionals and institutions;
- organisational integration in the form of mergers, or the creation of networks between institutions;
- functional integration of cure, care, and prevention.

In principle, good pre-conditions have been created for cooperation and substitution within the nursing and caring sectors. In nursing homes and residential homes, a great degree of internal integration is realised at the levels of professional and organisational integration as all disciplines involved in the care process are present at the same place in which the elderly person is living. However, for those older persons who live independently, this kind of integration is much more difficult to achieve. In practice, the clustering of capacities is insufficient in the cooperation between hospitals, specialists, and general practitioners on the one hand, and the nursing and caring staff on the other hand. Nevertheless, cooperation is increasing. Examples are the "liaison nurse" from the home care that is posted in the hospital to coordinate the transition of the patient to the home, and the office hours of district nurses in outpatient clinics. But patients who are discharged from hospitals and still find themselves in need of home care or institutional care are often confronted with waiting lists. So, the through-flux in the hospital is not only dependent on internal processes, but in particular also on the (limited) capacity of all other (extramural) facilities.

It is increasingly possible to organise specialist care and knowledge outside hospital walls, in the form of care at home and transmural care. Transmural care demands more intensive cooperation between the hospital and its specialists, and community care. However, cooperation is hampered by the increasing specialisation in medical care.

Care for the elderly increasingly extends over various assistance providers, institutions, and insurance compartments. In order to promote the interests of individual clients, the assistance provider not only has to know what to provide, but also what others have to offer, and under which terms of insurance and financing that care is accessible to the client. Functional integration constitutes a major problem in its concrete implementation at an institutional level as the overall design of the care system is still too much aimed at acute care, rather than at chronically intermittent diseases. In addition, the system of care, cure and prevention does not sufficiently adapt to the rapidly changing needs of the population (Delnoij, 2001).

Other impeding factors derive from flawed lines in the financing system. The Dutch system shows a dichotomy between the so-called primary and secondary health care, which was established in the 1960s and 1970s. In the Memorandum on Primary Care (*Nota Eerstelijnszorg*), general practitioners and district nurses, together with social workers and home carers, were acclaimed the four core disciplines in the front line. Hospitals and nursing homes are secondary care facilities. With that choice a strong bond of the professionals to these distinguished care sectors has developed. General practitioners are active in the primary sector but not in hospitals or nursing homes. At the same time, specialists in the hospital are not considered and / or considering themselves as a referral point in the care system. This "echelonisation principle" has been institutionalised in the referral system of the health insurance fund. The partitions that have developed in the financing and organisation of the care system, now constitute the major demarcation lines impeding the development of integrated care. Care has mainly been financed from the Exceptional Medical Expenses Act (*AWBZ*), while cure is funded by the private and compulsory health insurances. As a result of this separation in the financing structure, organisational integration mainly occurs between nursing homes and residential homes. However, the increasing number of the elderly and the chronically ill also demands a cooperation between cure and care (especially as concerns nursing and caring), and between health care and social provisions. In this context, the *Raad voor de Volksgezondheid en Zorg* (2001) stated: When trying to arrange for a smooth transition between care and cure, i.e. between *AWBZ* (Exceptional Medical Expenses Act) and *ZFW* (Compulsory Health Insurance Act), one runs into a wall of tight regulations, which determine whether a facility will be reimbursed by the health insurance fund or via the *AWBZ*; this impedes a further development of the community care systems.

3   Innovative Models

3.1   Introduction

Due to the described developments and difficulties, the Dutch care system is in motion. It is generally acknowledged that care *supply* should no longer be the point of departure, but the desire of the care requester. In the new perspective, the user should be central: care services have to come to the client. The elderly user, too, should no longer have to rely on just one care institution or organisation, but should be able to make use of a combination of services, like independent housing, welfare and health care services. As far as possible, care for the elderly has to be moved from institutions to districts, enabling independent living. And if admission to an institution becomes inevitable because of severe mental or physical disabilities of the person, a small-scale facility is preferable.

In many areas, innovations have been initiated. At the regional level, the Regional Assessment Boards (*RIOs*) and individual budgets are examples. Locally, municipal initiatives have led to sheltered housing zones, projects in lifetime housing, service centres, and consultants for elderly people. Innovations in the care system occur against the background of social developments in which individualisation, emancipation and increasing (material) welfare lead to higher demands posed on the provision of services. The elderly, too, present themselves ever more often as critical consumers. Reforms in the care system are targeted at offering integrated care, contributing to the client's satisfaction and his/her quality of life. Expressions of these reforms can, amongst other things, be found in the tendency towards the individualisation of the care system (the individual as the point of departure), in combining independent housing with care, in working intersectorally, in the development of care networks, but also in older people's pursuit of participation in society – the so-called "socialisation" of the care system (Coolen et al., 2001), which is also referred to as transmural care or community care (Lammers/Driest, 2002).

3.2   *Regional Assessment Board (RIO)*

In the new care scenario, *receiving* care begins with formulating the correct demand. Since 1997/98 there are regional organisations for the conversion of care needs into care requests, the RIOs (Regional Assessment Boards). They attend to care requests, which they may grant by needs assessment for relief in the area of *care*: nursing and (personal) care, care for the disabled, mental health care, wheelchair, living and transportation facilities. The introduction of an *independent needs assessment*, in which the care need is determined individually, is a manifestation of the trend towards individualisation. Here, independent means: "without being influenced by the parties involved in the needs assessment, financing and care allocation" (Schrijvers et al., 2001: 5).

When the RIO deems the care need to be necessary, the care request is passed on to the *administrative care office* in the region. Which kind of care is required, is determined on the basis of seven functions: housekeeping assistance, personal care, nursing, supporting guidance, activating/advising guidance, treatment, and accommodation (Schrijvers et al., 2001). Subsequently, the administrative care office is responsible for purchasing the required care. But this office, too, has to agree with the allocation of care, because only after a positive decision on the needs assessment, services and aids can be financed from public funds. The administrative office, on behalf of the client, purchases care from a care provider.

Thus, if an elderly and/or disabled person articulates a care need in the area of nursing, home care, or material support (e.g. transport or housing facilities), then (s)he has to turn to a Regional Assessment Board (RIO). In mutual consultation with the client, a special trained "assessment consultant" determines the kind of care that is needed. To assess the care need, consultants make use of a standard , and nationally-used, protocol (the so-called "model protocol") in which criteria for the access to specialised care are formulated. In general, RIOs are responsible for objectively assessing care, attuned to the *request* and *need* of the client. The Netherlands dispose of some 85 *RIOs*, whose functioning falls under municipal responsibility. Recently, there is a trend for smaller RIOs to merge, which will decrease their number.

The introduction of *RIOs* is part of modernising the care system. They have been called into existence to enable the client to choose from various kinds of care through "one window". RIOs are a first step on the way to care integration by rendering different sources of care accessible to a client. They constitute the starting point in the chain of needs assessment, care allocation, and delivery of care. Even in case of heavy care needs it is examined whether, and if so, how they may be addressed by a combination of specific arrangements and facilities (e.g. home care plus housing adaptation). Severely frail elderly or elderly with dementia consult their general practitioner first, accompanied by a family member or intimate.

The RIOs have to meet a number of quality aspects. First, *not* the available care supply has to be the basis of the needs assessment, but the client's request and need – *supply follows demand* being the primary consideration. Clients have to be able to call on the RIO for various forms of care supply – "*integrality*" is the motto. Personal traits of the client and the assessment consultant may not influence the assessment decision – *objectivity* must be guaranteed. The needs assessment, as discussed before, must be free of the influence of municipalities, care agencies, care providers, those passing referrals, and patient interest groups – *independence* must be warranted. The needs assessment decision must be made within a maximum of six weeks (to guard the processing speed), and the number of assessment decisions per assessment consultant must be optimal – *efficiency* is the ambition (Schrijvers et al., 2001).

Presently, the role, mode of operation, and added value of *RIOs* are under discussion. The quality of the needs assessment still needs a lot of improvement, especially with regard to integrality and demand orientation. Furthermore, The question is, for instance, whether RIOs lead to more bureaucracy, and, because of their municipal status, whether they differ too much with respect to the integrated care they offer.

In a first national evaluation study (Jedeloo et al., 2001), which was completed in 1999, it was found that clients were generally satisfied with the advice they received, and with the manner in which their needs were provided for. This is similar to what Knapen (2002) recently has remarked on the matter, viz. that "the system works". Still, the system deserves improvement with respect to instruction and information, during the needs assessment, and with respect to the allocation and implementation of the care plan.

About a quarter of the clients from the above-mentioned study indeed appear only moderately satisfied with the information they received. They desired more information about the time in which care might be expected, and about the number of hours to be allocated to them. Also, they wished to know more about alternatives, in case their care request would be denied. Knapen (2002: 6) notices, that "the response to a submitted care need is structurally suspended, as a result of which no timely solace is offered for short term care needs". Subsequently, a call must be made upon family, volunteers or private care. That also applies to long-term or chronic care needs.

As a result, a part of the care needs or care requests is "structurally papered away", writes Knapen (2002). By the deployment of informal carers – family, friends, volunteers – the real care needs remain hidden, and the real care request does not arise. The outcome of the assessment reveals more about the amount of care the relatives can provide than about the care needs of the patient. Van Vliet et al. (2003: 18) also argue that both the insight in the care needs of the clients and in the burden of informal carers disappear if the contribution of the informal cares is taken for granted.

In determining the *real* care need, the assessment consultant should initially leave partner, family and neighbours out of consideration, and determine in mutual consultation to what extent they wish and are able to contribute to the care (Van Nispen et al., 2002). In assessing the care need, however, the RIO considers care at home to be additional to care provided by family, friends, or volunteers. In case a person is a member of a household, relatives are expected to take part in the care to an acceptable degree. On the national level, the number of people that make a request for care at home, is unknown. Well-known is the fact that the number of people whose care request is rewarded, exceeds the present-day capacity of home care.

The evaluation study (Jedeloo et al., 2001) showed that efficiency can be improved too. In the perception of most clients, the time span between submission and assessment was too long. Moreover, the allocation and realisation of care involve struggling with long waiting lists and waiting times, and bottlenecks around the deployment of temporary solutions for transitional ("bridging") purposes. It are the regional administrative care offices which in the future will become ever more responsible for the waiting list management.

The *RIOs*, that pass the care allowance to the regional administrative office, have to contend with scarcity on the supply side. Until recently home care was bound to a legal ceiling: on average 3 hours per day of home care was applicable, or 21 hours per week (Knapen, 2002). Furthermore, given a care intensity above a certain number of hours, the administrative office will refer a person to a care centre or nursing home, because the costs of care at home far outweigh those of institutional care.

Therefore, the attuning between real needs, assessed care, allocated care, and realised care falls short at various levels. However, an objective, integrated, and functional needs assessment is of great importance, for effective demand-orientation and budgetary manageability, as concludes the IBO (*Interdepartementaal Beleidsonderzoek*, 2002). Such an assessment does occur in formulating the care needs. But often that is as far as it goes. Integration is found to be lacking with regard to their conversion into the client's entitlement to care (Coolen et al., 2002).

To reach demand-driven care and to provide clients with control, other forms of financing are also aimed for, such as "individual budgets".

3.3 *Individual Budgets*

Changes are taking place in the financing of care as well. Individual budgets *(PGB)* for care users have been introduced: a sum of money instead of receiving care in kind. A PGB has been introduced for those people who are in need of long-term care because of chronicle illness, ageing, psychological problems, or a physical handicap.

It is assumed that the introduction of individual budgets *(PGB)* is better geared to innovations in the care system. The regional administrative care office gives the person concerned a sum of money or a bond – a voucher – as a means to pay for public services (upon the consent of the *RIO*). In this case, it is not the care office that purchases services, but the client himself. Individuals may, according to their own views, determine from which provider they will purchase care. The Regional Assessment Board (*RIO*) determines for which kind of care needs money is to be awarded. Various interest organisations of care requesters have intervened in favour of an extension of these individual budgets, which give clients more individual autonomy and flexibility.

With a PGB someone opts to negotiate himself with providers about the care arrangement and the related price (*Ministerie van Volksgezondheid, Welzijn en Sport*, 2001a), or chooses a mediator or agency to do it instead. Moreover, a PGB is individually assigned, and therefore is a personal, client-related, budget. Since the introduction of the individual budget, the number of budget-holders has increased from 4,000 in 1996 to over 16,000 in 2000 (De Klerk, 2001: 195).

Until now there do exist different kinds of PGBs, which are related to specialised forms of care: a PGB (V&V) for care and nursing, a PGB (VG) for intensive home care, and a PGB (GGZ) for mental health care, for instance. In order to meet the care needed, a client may combine different PGBs. In 2003 these different kinds of PGBs will be substituted by one general PGB. For nursing and care, a PGB is limited to a maximum of 136 Euro per day

433

for three hours of care per day. In case the client needs more care than the maximum of three hours (intensive home care), he or she receives another 136 Euro a day, in addition to the PGB provided. Again, the RIO has to legitimate this. A part of the individual budget (called "the drawing right") is reserved at the PGB office of the National Insurance Institute (SVB). This Institute is responsible for carrying out the payments to the care providers on behalf of the client. Another part of the budget (called "the fixed sum") is directly booked to the account of the client (1,089 Euro a year) and can be spend on care and mediation facilities in accordance with her or his view.

In case of an "individual-trailing budget" (*PVB*) the client receives care in kind, and is free to compile a care arrangement at a care provider he or she wants, or may enter into a care arrangement compiled by the care provider (and which is contracted by the insurer). In this case, the payment "trails" the client. The regional administrative care office pays the providers for the care they have delivered to the client. In both cases (PGB or PVB), the needs assessment is identical, and should be aimed at the required care, and not at the supply (*Ministerie van Volksgezondheid, Welzijn en Sport*, 2001a).

With the introduction of this form of financing, the decision power moves more into the hands of the individual. In principle, the recipient may determine how and where specific services are purchased. Furthermore, someone may opt for a more fanciful type of care than the needs assessment prescribes. In this case, however, the client will have to pay for extra costs. For the care providers, this implies thinking and working more market- and client-oriented (Knapen, 2002). Nursing and residential homes may for instance begin providing care outside the institution, to people with a nursing or care need. That provides more space for private initiative, hence for competition.

The individual budgets are being introduced in various areas. Not only for the purchase of physical care, but also for material care such as housing. Their introduction is still in very early stages of development. The present *PGB* scheme is rigid, as concludes the elderly people's union (*ANBO*, 2002), especially because it is still attuned to the specific sectors of nursing and care (home care, residential home, and nursing home care). Next to that, the present *PGB* schemes still carry along much administrative red tape, which renders the scheme attractive to only a limited number of people (*ANBO*, 2002). Therefore, the group of elderly with a socially or cognitively vulnerable position, has to rely on basic provisions in its own neighbourhood or place of residence, by means of accepting care in kind.

Recently, an interdepartmental policy study IBO (*Interdepartementaal Beleidsonderzoek*, 2002), has grappled with the introduction of individual budgets (PGBs) in the area of independent housing with care. These *PGBs* must enable elderly people with a greater care need to attune housing, care, and welfare facilities according to their own choice.

A number of conditions have to be realised if the introduction of *PGBs* really is to yield added value. For instance, consumers must have insight into the existent possibilities, whether on their own initiative or through the mediation of consultants. In other words: the supply must be transparent. Sufficient competition between providers is another important condition. After all, there is no real choice if all providers offer the same on equal conditions.

The introduction of truly and maximally integrated *PGBs* is still outstanding. It is a long-term issue, because more insight is required into the preconditions, and into issues concerning design and implementation (*IBO*, 2002). Also, more insight needs to be gained into the experiences of the clients themselves, and into the influence of individual budgets on their purchasing behaviour. There are still obscurities for instance about the size of the various individual budgets, and also about the question which "critical group" of care requesters shall be taken as a basis for the calculation of the cost price.

3.4   Housing, Welfare, Care

In the area of housing and care changes are occurring as well, not only as a result of the shift towards demand-oriented care, but also in the discourse on the elderly having to be able to function and be accommodated independently for as long as possible (*Ouderenzorg*, 2002).

National policies support this point of view with the concept of "care-friendly districts", i.e. areas in which explicit attention is paid to the improvement of the living surroundings, infrastructure, and facilities (*Ministerie van Volksgezondheid, Welzijn en Sport*, 2001c : 6).

As a result, there is cooperation at policy level too, for instance between the Ministries of Housing, Planning and Environment *(VROM)* and Health, Welfare and Sports (*VWS*). After all, the policy sectors welfare and (public) housing both come into the picture. From this cooperation, as from October 2000, "sheltered housing stimulation arrangements" have been issued. By means of these schemes, projects aiming at improving the interfaces between housing, care, and service are subsidised (*Ministerie van Volksgezondheid, Welzijn en Sport*, 2001c).

These schemes have found expression in many other initiatives. Care providers have begun operating across their sectors and offer intensive home care at ever more locations. Housing corporations are, in cooperation with municipalities and institutions for care and welfare, modernising existent residential and nursing homes into new care centres, and are also building new sheltered care centres where clients may remain living independently, with care. Also, housing corporations began to develop more sheltered care projects at medium prices, possibly in cooperation with private financiers (Aedes Arcares, 2002).

In January 1996, the Netherlands Centre for Housing of Old People (*NCHB*) and the Humanist Building Society for Old People (*HBB*) joined forces in order to achieve modern housing for senior citizens. They involved the housing corporation *Woonzorg Nederland* (Housing Care Netherlands), the largest national association for the housing of senior citizens. The main target was to bring their housing supply in line with the (modern) expectations of users by:

- installing information and communication technology, e.g. connection to the Internet;
- adaptable and adapted construction (building houses suitable for being lived in up to an advanced age, also in the case of functional limitations of the occupants; and
- application of the so-called *all-living concept*: the vision that senior citizens have to be able to call on a well-arranged package of services based on the client's requirements and desires.

Along this line, similar initiatives have led to the development of projects in lifetime housing (40 in 2001) and sheltered housing "complexes" (blocks) (700 in 2001). The projects in lifetime housing aim at creating such conditions in a district or village (with about 10,000 inhabitants), that elderly and disabled inhabitants can maintain their independence by staying in their own homes instead of moving into an institution. Sufficient adapted houses, an accessible environment and adequate care facilities are the main elements. Care is offered on a level that is comparable to that in residential homes and nursing homes. In the centre of the district a community care centre operates as the base for the various services, to be delivered at home or in the centre. Next to care and welfare functions, the centre also accommodates commercial services. The concrete arrangement of the community centre depends on the local context (Aedes Arcares, 2002).

A sheltered housing complex is a housing block of independent dwellings constructed in a manner geared to sheltered housing, including an agreed care and service arrangement. Sheltered housing complexes function as a replacement of residential homes and nursing homes. The houses meet adaptability standards. The greater part of the sheltered housing complexes have been built in the "social rented sector" and consist of three-room houses. Only 3% of the complexes has been realised in the owner-occupied property sector. There are some complexes (6%) with a combination of (expensive) rental and owner-occupied apartments. Well over half of the sheltered housing complexes are situated in the proximity of a care institution, 43% are detached houses in the district. Most sheltered housing complexes have communal rooms and/or care rooms (Aedes Arcares, 2002).

All these sheltered housing initiatives are not realised without struggle. The financial feasibility of projects constitutes one of the problems, as governmental contributions are low. At times, another bottleneck is presented by the limited number of services to be delivered, especially with respect to "well-being". Next, the legislation is still found to be lagging behind the demand. Neither do the procedures of the Ministries of *VROM* (Housing, Planning and Environment) and *VWS* (Health, Welfare and Sports) always match each other. Finally, insufficient cooperation between care providers may result in an inadequate care infrastructure (Aedes Arcares, 2002).

Not only do such initiatives by housing corporations form the basis of new projects, but also initiatives of the Board of Health Care Insurers lead to innovations. In 1999, the Board initiated an innovation programme, which was given shape in six pilot projects. Meanwhile, these projects have been evaluated. We will shed light on two of them as case-studies: the life time housing project in the rural municipality of Trynwalden (province of Friesland), and a project geared to a better connection of care and cure in the municipality of Woerden (from: Coolen et al., 2001).

3.4.1 Municipality of Trynwalden: The Sheltered Housing Zone

In the Frisian Trynwalden (10,000 inhabitants), the former residential home Heemstra State has been replaced by a complex of hundreds of apartments. With the support of the municipality, housing corporations, elderly people's organisations, and the regional administrative care office, a type of integrated care for the elderly has been developed. A coherent supply of provisions has been created, surrounding care, welfare, and adapted housing, which enables elderly people to opt for independent housing with suitable care-at-home. To that end, a collaboration structure has been formed, with participation of home care, the residential home, the nursing home, the welfare work for the elderly, the housing corporation, and the WVG window. The occupants rent a certain type of apartment and may there receive custom-made care within the boundaries of the needs assessment. The care network also supplies the required care to elderly people living independently elsewhere.

In Trynwalden the accent is placed on living independently with care, on the development of integrated care, and on working demand-oriented: individually attuning supply to demand.

Trynwalden wishes to support the elderly in directing their own lives. The so-called *omtinker* (consultant for the elderly) clarifies, together with the elderly person, the individual need for care and nursing, explores how and where the desired support can be acquired, and – when necessary – mediates between requester and provider.

438
Crucial here is a vision of support, which goes beyond the traditional notion of care. The emphasis is placed on connecting care and nursing, adapted housing, resources, and welfare services. Examples of the latter include nursing, housekeeping assistance, a linen service, provision of meals and a shopping service. Even education, clubs and associations providing a broad range of social-recreational activities are available.

In executing the Trynwalden experiment, various bottlenecks were encountered. As was found, the idea of custom-made care does not easily find expression in a standard supply of provisions, as it is (still) described by the assessment agency (*RIO*). In other words: The outcome of the needs assessment not solely reflects the perceived demands of the client but is also determined by the existing possibilities for services supply. Additionally, in order to offer integrated care, the old definitions of care need to be changed into integrated descriptions of care products, or care packages.

An evaluation amongst clients of Trynwalden shows that supply and demand are well attuned to each other. What the elderly receive in terms of types and contents of care, fits neatly with their request and the support they need regarding their disabilities. In terms of added value, the Trynwalden project offers an extension of options. The occupants are of the opinion that the care is better than before the start of the project (40% of them had previously been involved in "regular" care). Moreover, people were very satisfied with the mode of operation and the role of the *omtinker*. The elderly find it important to be able to discuss types and contents of their care arrangement, even if the *omtinker's* influence on the final result is not always as clear to them.

3.4.2 Woerden: Cure Plus Care Project

> In the region of Woerden, various initiatives have been put into motion, which have to promote custom-made care. 14 organisations were involved in the project (from the hospital to the Foundation Welfare for the Elderly) which aimed at: custom-made care for long-term care-dependent elderly people.

The Woerden experiment especially aimed at optimising the chain "needs assessment – care allocation – care delivery". Good supply of information is an essential precondition to this end. In the region of Woerden, people were struggling with problems surrounding the supply of information. It took elderly people too long to collect information about care, and the time span between care needs assessment and their delivery was too long. Also, the capacity of various service institutions in the region was found not to be utilised optimally.

    The Woerden experiment was supposed to result in an improved supply of information for, and about, the elderly. On the one hand, in order to accelerate the communication between institutions, for instance between hospital and home care or nursing home – via the *RIO* or the regional administrative care office. On the other hand, in order to increase the accessibility of the information to the clients – via one window – so that it would be clear to them which facilities and services exist in the area of care and welfare.

    Simultaneously, the experiment was required to offer elderly people with a care request the opportunity to be able to remain living in an own home or district for as long as possible.

    The objective of an integrated care supply was not achieved. It required more time in order for the parties involved to be able to solve, and overcome, impediments of a staffing, organisational and financial nature. Indeed, there appeared to be a basis for a better and non-ambiguous supply of information. The "failure" of the project can partially be attributed to the absence of a problem shared by all parties. The experiment, as it was, was forced onto the parties involved. The lesson is, that such an innovation only stands a chance of success if the initiative for the solution of problems comes from the bottom, and is carried by all concerned. This lesson is generally acknowl-

439

edged, since the objective of Woerden as a pilot study was to learn more about factors that hampered or promoted integrated care.

3.5 Individualisation of the Care System: Functions and One Window

In order to offer custom-made care, since 1990 service-providing institutions have worked to improve individual care plans. Sometimes, they proceeded to develop specific professions, such as case managers, assistants for independent housing, personal care consultants or "brokers", all of whom are supposed to further the attuning of supply and demand. An example is the previously mentioned *omtinker* of the Trynwalden project, who carries out his function on the basis of case management.

3.5.1 Case Management

In the region of Steenwijk and the North-East Polder, cooperating care institutions have set up a form of case management for the benefit of old people with a weak social network and decreasing self-direction. It mainly concerns elderly people over 75 to 80 years of age, living alone. With targeted, short-term guidance, i.e. case management, these elderly may be assisted in order to get more grip on their lives at home. Amongst other things, by means of agreements concerning better-arranged home care, suitable transportation, and meaningful day-time spending (Coolen et al., 2001).

3.5.2 Waiting List Management

In the region of Zwolle, care agencies and providers are developing a new approach to care for the disabled, specifically for persons on a waiting list for long-term care. Here, it is attempted to find a suitable response to a care request, by addressing a combination of existent categorical provisions (adapted housing, home care, supervised working, etc.). In doing so, an individual approach is maintained, which is supported by the application of an individual trailing budget (Coolen et al., 2001).

3.5.3 Consultant for the Elderly

In order to offer custom-made care, the function of a consultant for the elderly has been introduced and widely supported by Dutch policy. This rather new function fits neatly with the new idea of demand-steered care. The consultants are independent, well-trained professionals related to a municipality, and operate in welfare institutions, municipal information desks, but also at care providers and organisations for the elderly. At this moment 60% of the local welfare organisations have a consultant at their disposal. Upon request of a client, the consultant for the elderly (or "support worker") informs, advises, and mediates, in the areas of welfare, housing, and care. This occurs on the basis of a "working visit", or a referral. As an expert, the consultant is tasked with promoting the independent functioning of an elderly person, and with increasing his/her self-coping ability and well-being. His tasks also include signalling trends in the demand of the elderly, and of lacunas and bottlenecks in the supply (VOG, 2001).

3.5.4 The One-Window Idea

Partially, the above-mentioned functions constitute an overlap with so-called "windows" where the client may obtain information and advice about available services and facilities. The one-window idea meanwhile has become a true household notion in political Holland (*Congreskrant* OL2000, 2002). In various municipalities this has led to projects of integrated services, in which information and communication technology are essential. Municipalities are free in the manner in which to arrange the window. Indeed, the demand-oriented vision would prompt each municipality to adapt to the needs and questions of their residents.

441

In general, the one-window is a central service point for advise, information and help in clarifying the care need, sometimes located in a small-scale community centre. The *Vraagwijzer*-window (query-guide window) may serve as an example. This window aims at improving access to public information in the areas of both care and well-being. For the most part, physical windows (or telephonic windows) are created, sometimes they are established as an electronic window.

The physical window is a central point where people may go and address their questions to an adviser in the area of care and well-being. People are served immediately, or are brought into contact with bodies that can help them on their way. This may concern application of rent subsidy, or the arrangement of an intake-interview at the *RIO*. Sometimes these windows function as a gate of the RIOs: clients may apply for an assessment concerning home care or admission to a nursing home.

By the end of 2002, 125 municipalities are supposed to have such a window. In principle, each Dutch citizen should have a query-guide window in his/ her proximity in 2006. Meanwhile, an electronic window is being developed, where citizens may directly obtain their information by means of internet.

The central issue is whether the query-guide window, as a so-called "front-office", manages to make effective contacts with various provisions and functions in the "back-office": (in fact) the local service providers. The better the mutual cooperation between these providers, the better the chance that the query-guide window facility succeeds. And that is what finally constitutes both the field of tension and challenge (*Congreskrant* OL2000, 2002).

4   Conclusions

In the Netherlands, the modernisation of care for the elderly and disabled people is clearly in motion, in particular with regard to the replacement of large-scale institutions by small-scale facilities and community care.

Moreover, policy aims at the substitution of supply-driven care by a *demand-driven* system. Demand-driven care, in our view, simultaneously means *integrated care* since, when the requests and needs which the client may experience in various areas are met, integrated care is provided. Integration is realised when (s)he can dispose of the required care provisions, the adequate types, the accurate quantity, and delivered in the appropriate order and at the right moment in time. From the client perspective, this could be adopted as a definition of integrated care.

Another, related notion is *freedom of choice*. If the clients are offered the opportunity of choice, they are capable of arranging the package of provisions themselves, which fits with their needs.

In this report, we have described various attempts to accomplish integrated care systems in the Netherlands. Starting from the new system of needs assessment that is explicitly targeted at taking the entire living and needs situation of the client into consideration, independently of the available supply with all its boundaries. The development of sheltered housing zones is another expression of the idea of integration. In these projects, small-scale housing and care facilities are designed, which in the future are supposed to replace the huge large-scale institutions. In this area, the ambition is to integrate facilities in the sphere of housing, care and well-being. Finally, individual budgets were introduced to offer clients more freedom of choice, and thus the possibility to obtain the desired care according to their own wishes.

User choice and participation require that clients are well-informed. In practice, however, many frail elderly persons need support in finding their way in the complicated care system and its regulations, despite the striving to make it easier for them by creating "one window". Consultants, case managers and accessible information services are supposed to assist persons in articulating and expressing their care needs, and assist them in the procedures to acquire integrated care.

Especially people with dementia are unable to look after their own interests. In needs assessment and contacts with service providers, usually partners or relatives are consulted. The impact of dementia on health and social care is increasing. The expenditures for this condition already far exceed all other chronic diseases (De Klerk, 2001: 131). Furthermore, the trend towards "extramuralisation", expanding the opportunity for frail elderly persons to live in small-scale dwelling arrangements, is not yet realised for people with dementia. The statistical data show that the number of places for these people in nursing homes has increased during the last decade, while those for the elderly with physical disabilities and diseases were reduced in favour of housing conditions which offer more independence.

Despite the policy intentions to create a more demand-oriented system, the supply-oriented approach is still dominant in practice. Up to present, the care system was constructed highly sectorally and categorically, organised in various groups of professions and sectors, each with their own language, traditions, and cultures. Those cultural differences often impede co-operation and communication, and lead to interest conflicts. All that endangers the objective of policy-makers to obtain a system in which the client's demands determine which care (s)he receives. It could result in a half-hearted system, in which the client's demands are once again converted into the existing possibilities (Knapen, 2002). In particular the fact that the streams of money are still not sufficiently trailing the streams of care, is partially indebted to this state of affairs (Raad voor de Volksgezondheid en Zorg, 2001; Knapen, 2002). In sum, practice markedly lags behind intentions.

Besides these factors impeding integration in the care system, there are deficiencies in the quantitative supply of care for the elderly. Endeavours to reduce the waiting lists, which have been undertaken now for more than ten years, have largely failed. The scarcity of facilities impedes both inno-

443

vations in the care system and the client's freedom of choice. After all, a shortage of facilities in practice leaves little to choose from. The elderly concerned are sometimes allotted a temporary "bridging" provision, while others have to settle for a less desired solution.

In such cases it is especially the informal carer who often has to fill the gaps. Thus, the overburdening of these informal carers is an issue that increasingly demands attention. However, there still are only a few facilities to support the informal carer. This, too, can be labelled as an integration problem, if we widen the scope to the network of the elderly person in need.

Notes

1   The role of the RIOs is further discussed in section 3.
2   Horizontal substitution includes shifts between professions at equal levels (e.g. the different paramedical professions). Vertical substitution includes shifts between various groups of professions. At the "bottom" of their task list, performances and operations are transferred from specialists to general practitioners, from doctors to nurses and paramedics, from nurses to carers, and to patients themselves and their informal carers. For cost considerations, vertical substitution has been stimulated by the government and the insurers.

References

Aedes Arcares (2002) Kenniscentrum wonen-zorg. Retrieved from the World Wide Web in June 2002: http://www.kenniscentrumwonenzorg.nl

Algemene Rekenkamer (2002) *Zorgen voor toegankelijkheid in de ouderen- en gehandicapten-zorg*. Den Haag: Sdu Uitgevers.

ANBO (2002) Algemene Bond voor Ouderen. Retrieved from the World Wide Web in June 2002: http://www.anbo.nl

Berkhout, J.J. (2000) *Intergemeentelijk lokaal ouderenbeleid. Warmlopen voor ouderen*. Den Haag: VNG Uitgeverij.

Congreskrant OL2000 (2002) *Denken en werken vanuit de burger*. Den Haag: OL2000.

Coolen, J./Van Duren, M./Van der Hoeven, C./Meulemeester, M./Van Rossum, F./Van Rossum, H. (2001) *Over de grenzen van de AWBZ: evaluatie van innovatieprojecten*. Utrecht: Verwey-Jonker Instituut.

De Klerk, M.M.Y. (ed.) (2001) *Rapportage ouderen 2001. Veranderingen in de leefsituatie*. Den Haag: Sociaal en Cultureel Planbureau.

Delnoij, D.M.J./Kulu Glasgow, I./Klazinga N.S./Custers, T. (2001) *Gezondheid, zorg en stelsel. AMC/UvA-achtergrondstudie bij Vraag aan bod.* Den Haag: Ministerie van Volksgezondheid, Welzijn en Sport.

Dugteren, F. van (2001) 'Wonen', pp. 85-114 in: Klerk, M.M.Y. de (ed.), *Rapportage ouderen 2001. Veranderingen in de leefsituatie.* Den Haag: Sociaal en Cultureel Planbureau.

Ewijk, H. van/Kelder, T. (1999) *Who Cares? An Overview of the Dutch Systems of Health Care and Welfare.* Utrecht: Nederlands Instituut voor Zorg en Welzijn.

Goris, A./Brakenburg, H./Tielen, G./Berkhout, J. (2002*) Factsheet Senior Citizens in the Netherlands.* Utrecht: Nederlands Instituut voor Zorg en Welzijn, Nederlands Platform voor Ouderen in Europa.

Interdepartementaal Beleidsonderzoek Werkgroep IBO-RIO (2001) *Verzorgde toegang.* Den Haag: Ministerie van Volksgezondheid, Welzijn en Sport.

Interdepartementaal Beleidsonderzoek (2002) *Naar eigen smaak.* Den Haag: Ministerie van Volksgezondheid, Welzijn en Sport.

Jedeloo, S/De Witte, L.P./Schrijvers, A.J.P. (2001) Quality of Regional Individual Assessment Agencies Regulating Access to Long-term Care Services: A Client Perspective. Retrieved from the World Wide Web in June 2000: www.ijic.org/cgi-bin/pw.cgi-bin/pw.cgi/2002-3/000125/article_content.htm

Knapen, M. (2002) 'Sturing door de vraag of sturing van de vraag? De weg van behoeftes, via loketten, indicaties en zorgtoewijzing naar zorgrealisatie voor thuiswonenden', *TAP* 24 (1): 5-18.

Kodner, D.L./Kay Kyriacou, C. (2000) 'Fully Integrated Care for Elderly: Two American Models', *International Journal of Integrated Care* 1. Retrieved from the World Wide Web: http://www.ijic.org/cgi-bin/pw.cgi/2001-9/000088/index.html

Komp, K./Strümpel, C./Grilz-Wolf, M. (2002) *Working Paper no. 1. The Understanding of Integrated Care in an International Perspective and in Austria.* Unpublished paper Procare

Lammers, B./Driest, P. (2002) 'Zacht herstructureren', *Tijdschrift voor de Sociale Sector*, Jan/Febr: 4-9.

Ministerie van Volksgezondheid, Welzijn en Sport (1999) *Werken aan sociale kwaliteit. Welzijnsnota 1999-2002, deel B.* Den Haag: Ministerie van Volksgezondheid, Welzijn en Sport.

Ministerie van Volksgezondheid, Welzijn en Sport (2001a) *Modernisering AWBZ (26631) en persoonsgebonden budgetten (25657)*, 14, Den Haag: SDU-uitgevers.

Ministerie van Volksgezondheid, Welzijn en Sport (2001b) *Wat doet de rijksoverheid voor ouderen. Informatie over het beleid van de verschillende ministeries voor ouderen in 2001.* Den Haag: Ministerie van Volksgezondheid, Welzijn en Sport.

Ministerie van Volksgezondheid, Welzijn en Sport (2001c) *Wonen en zorg op maat.* Den Haag: beleidsnota VWS.

Ministerie van Volksgezondheid, Welzijn en Sport (2002) *Stand van Zaken. Uitvoering Programmalijnen. Welzijnsnota 1999-2002.* Den Haag: Ministerie van Volksgezondheid, Welzijn en Sport.

Ministerie van Volkshuisvesting, Ruimtelijke Ordening en Milieubeheer (2001) *Mensen, wensen, wonen.* Den Haag: Sdu Uitgevers.

Mosseveld, C.J.P.M. van/Smit, J.M. (2002) *Working paper zorgrekeningen 1998 – 2001.* Voorburg: Centraal Bureau voor de Statistiek.

Nationale Raad voor de Volksgezondheid (1994) *Tussen cure en care. Advies over een refe-rentiekader voor beleid.* Zoetermeer: Nationale Raad voor de Volksgezondheid.

445

Nispen, R.M.A. van/Sixma, H.J./Kerkstra, A. (2002) *Kwaliteit van de indicatiestelling door RI-O's vanuit cliëntenperspectief.* Utrecht: Nivel.

Nivel – Nederlands instituut voor onderzoek van de gezondheidszorg (2002) Thuiszorg aanbod: Hoe groot is het aanbod en neemt het toe of af? (http://www.nivel.nl/thuiszorg/aanbod1.shtml, 27-11-2002)

Ooms, I./Ras, M. (2002) *Intramurale AWBZ-voorzieningen. Achtergronden bij gebruik en eigen bijdragen.* Werkdocument 85. Den Haag: Sociaal en Cultureel Planbureau.

Ouderenzorg (2002) Magazine voor Management en Beleid, 2/3.

Raad voor de Volksgezondheid en Zorg (2001) *Care en cure.* Zoetermeer: Raad voor de Volksgezondheid en Zorg.

Rijkschroeff, R./Oudenampsen, D./Steketee, M. /van Vliet, K. (2002) *Toekomstverkenning modernisering AWBZ en de gevolgen voor de geestelijke gezondheidszorg. Een onderzoek in opdracht van het College voor zorgverzekeringen.* Amstelveen: College voor Zorgverzekeringen.

Schoenmakers-Salkinoja, I./Timmermans, J. (2001) 'Gezondheid', pp. 115-152 in: Klerk, M.M.Y. de (ed.), *Rapportage ouderen 2001. Veranderingen in de leefsituatie.* Den Haag: Sociaal en Cultureel Planbureau.

Schrijvers, A.J.P./Jedeloo, S./Jorg, F./Hoogerduin, J.G. (2001) *Rio, het jongste kind groeit op.* Utrecht: Julius Centrum /Universitair Medisch Centrum.

Schrijvers, A.J.P./Duursma, S.A./de Weert-van Oene, G.H./Jörg, F. (1997) 'Care for the Elderly', pp. 101-110 in: Schrijvers A.J.P. (ed.), *Health and Health Care in the Netherlands. A Critical Self-assesment of Dutch Experts in the Medical and Health Sciences.* Utrecht: De Tijdstroom.

Vliet, Katja van/Oudenampsen, Dick/Flikweert, Meta/Mak, Jodi (2003) *Mantelzorg in perspectief. Het betrekken van mantelzorg in het indicatieproces.* Utrecht: Verwey-Jonker Instituut.

VOG (2001) *Partners bij zelfstandigheid. Welzijnsdiensten voor ouderen. Een landelijk overzicht.* Utrecht: VOG.

Annex 1: List of Dutch (Statutory) Regulations and Agencies

ANBO (*Algemene Nederlandse Bond voor Ouderen*):
General Dutch Union for Elderly People

AWBZ (*Algemene Wet Bijzondere Ziektekosten*):
In the Netherlands, most long-term care is financed by special taxes under a social insurance law, called the Exceptional Medical Expenses Act.

Administrative care office (*zorgkantoor*):
These offices, which operate on a regional level, are responsible for all administrative tasks resulting from the AWBZ (e.g., the purchase of care and consultation between the parties involved).

First compartment in the health care:
The first compartment concerns the long-term care and the uninsurable risks (home care, care and nursing homes, care for the disabled, and a large part of the mental health care). Financing occurs from the AWBZ, and the execution is conducted by the regional administrative offices. Cure constitutes the second compartment, which is financed by premiums according to the *Ziekenfondswet* or private insurance.

Individual budget (*PGB – persoonsgebonden budget*):
A person receives a sum of money or a bond – a voucher – as a means for payment for public service (upon the consent of the RIO). With a PGB someone opts to negotiate himself with providers about the care arrangement and the related price.

Individual-trailing budget (*PVB* – persoonsvolgend budget):
In the case of an "individual-trailing budget" (*PVB*) a person receives the care in kind, whereas the payment "trails" the client: the administrative office pays the providers for the care they have delivered to the client.

"Leaning houses" (*aanleunwoningen*):
The lightest form of sheltered housing, where people live independently but next to (and if need be, lean on) the residential or nursing home, and may opt to use facilities thereof.

Regional Assessment Board (*RIO – Regionaal Indicatie Orgaan*):
Body responsible for determining type and amount of need in response to a request for care.

Second compartment in health care:
The second compartment contains those provisions, which are part of the "basic package" of the curative care (general practitioners, specialists, hospital care, and paramedics). Financing takes place under the ZFW (Ziekenfondswet) or private insurance. The execution is conducted by the (public) health insurance funds and private health cost insurers.

Substitution:
Substitution in care for the elderly aims at realising relative shifts in the utilisation of provisions. The direction of the contemplated shift moves from intramural to extramural provisions, from intensive to extensive care, from professional to informal care, and from expensive to cheap provisions.

WVG (*Wet Voorzieningen Gehandicapten*):
The Provisions for the Disabled Act covers provision of care facilities such as transportation, housing adjustments and wheelchairs.

ZFW (*Ziekenfondswet*):
Compulsory Health Insurance Act, applicable for those with income under a certain level, above which one should obtain private health insurance. Albeit with mentioned income restriction, the Dutch *ziekenfonds* (public health insurance fund) systematics best compare to the British NHS.

Annex 2: Model Ways of Working

A1 Regional Assessment Board (RIO)

Provider	Municipality
Objectives	The RIO attends to care requests of clients, which it may grant by needs assessment for relief in the area of care: nursing and (personal) care, care for the disabled, mental health care, wheelchair, living and transportation facilities.
Target group	Those who need care in the area of nursing and (personal) care, care for the disabled, mental health care, wheelchair, living and transportation facilities.
Practice domain	Clients' own homes
Staff involved	Persons (social workers, or nurses) that followed a higher vocational training as Assessment Consultant.
Methods used	Assessment on the basis of protocols and criteria, in dialogue with the client.
Related agencies	When the RIO deems the care need to be justified, the care request is passed on to the administrative care office in the region. Subsequently, this office is responsible for purchasing the required care.
Strengths	RIOs have been called into existence to enable the client to choose from various kinds of care through one window. RIOs are a first step on the way to care integration by rendering different sources of care accessible to a client. They constitute the starting point in the chain of needs assessment, care allocation, and delivery of care.
Weaknesses	Municipal differences in the provision of integrated care. The real care need (often) remains hidden by including the possible contributions of family members or other informal assistants in assessing the need. In practice, only to a limited extent does demand optimally direct supply.

449

A2 Personal Budgets (PGB)

Provider	Regional administrative care offices and National Insurance Institute (SVB)
Objectives	It is assumed that the introduction of individual budgets (PGB) is better geared to innovations in the care system. The administrative care office gives the person concerned a sum of money or a bond – a voucher – as a means to pay for public services instead of receiving care in kind.
Target group	A PGB has been introduced for those people who are in need of long-term care because of chronic illness, ageing, psychological problems, or a physical disability.
Practice domain	It is a financing system for clients.
Staff involved	Employees of administrative care offices and the National Insurance Institute (SVB)
Methods used	Individual approach
Related agencies	When the RIO deems the care need to be justified, the care allowance is passed on to the administrative care office in the region, which finally awards the care and the budget.
Strengths	It gives clients more individual autonomy and flexibility, and freedom of choice.
Weaknesses	The present PGB scheme is rigid, it is still attuned to the specific sectors of care and nursing. The present PGB schemes still carry along much administrative red tape, which renders the scheme unattractive to large numbers of people

A3 Sheltered Housing Complexes and Zones (e.g. *Trynwalden*)

Provider	Municipality, administrative care office, housing corporations, and service providers
Objectives	The main target is to bring the housing supply in line with the (modern) expectations of users. A sheltered housing zone is a normal district or village (with about 10,000 inhabitants), where care is offered in a manner that was once only supplied intramurally (e.g. in residential homes and nursing homes). A sheltered housing complex is a housing block of independent dwellings constructed in a manner geared to sheltered housing, including an agreed care and services arrangement. Sheltered housing complexes function as a replacement of residential homes and nursing homes, and may be part of a sheltered housing zone.
Target group	Elderly with care needs
Practice domain	Living areas in which explicit attention is paid to the improvement of the living surroundings, infrastructure, and facilities
Related agencies	The Netherlands Centre for Housing of Old People (NCHB) and the Humanist Building Society for Old People (HBB) joined forces in order to achieve modern housing for senior citizens. Not only do such initiatives by housing corporations form the basis of new projects, but also initiatives of the Board of Health Care Insurers lead to innovations. The municipality plays an active role as mediator: bringing the parties together.
Strengths	The supply and demand are well attuned to each other. There is an extension of options for clients: they are able to discuss types and contents of their care arrangement.
Weaknesses	The financial feasibility of projects constitutes one of the problems. The limited number of services to be delivered, especially with respect to "well-being". The legislation is still found to be lagging behind the demand.

A4 Optimising the Chain "Needs Assessment, Care Allocation and Care Delivery" (e.g. *Woerden*)

Provider	Regional administrative care offices, care providers, municipality
Objectives	An improved supply of information for, and about, the elderly. To offer elderly people with a care request the opportunity to be able to remain living in their own home or district for as long as possible • To accelerate the communication between institutions. • To increase the accessibility of the information to the clients – via one window • To accelerate the communication between institutions, for instance between hospital and home care or nursing home – via the RIO or the administrative care office.
Target group	Long-term care-dependent elderly people
Practice domain	Living arrangements for elderly in need of care
Staff involved	Staff of the different parties involved
Related agencies	14 organisations were involved in the project (from the hospital to the Foundation Welfare for the Elderly).
Strengths	Non-ambiguous supply of information to elderly from "one window".
Weaknesses	The objective of an integrated care supply was not fully achieved because the parties involved needed more time, and a more concrete aim (focus) to develop their strategy.

A5 Specific Professions, such as Case Managers, Assistants for Independent Housing, Personal Care Consultants, or "Brokers"

Provider	Social insurance agencies, welfare institutions, housing corporations
Objectives	The attuning of supply and demand to offer custom-made care for the elderly. The *consultant for the elderly* (or "support worker"): informs, advises, and mediates, in the areas of welfare, housing, and care. *Case managers* exist for the benefit of old people with a weak social network and decreasing abilities of self-direction. With targeted, short-term guidance these elderly may be assisted in order to get more grip on their lives at home. Amongst other things, by means of agreements concerning better arranged home care, suitable transportation, and meaningful time spending. *Waiting list managers* attempt to find a suitable response to a care request, by addressing a combination of existent categorial provisions (adapted housing, home care, supervised working, etc.)
Target group	Elderly clients in need of care
Practice domain	Care requests in the areas of welfare, housing, and care.
Staff involved	Consultants
Methods used	An individual approach
Strengths	To be able to consider types and contents of their care arrangement in mutual consultation with a professional.
Weaknesses	None

453

A6 Information Desks Constituting "One Window": The Query-Guide Window May Answer Their Questions

Provider	Municipalities and public service providers
Objectives	"Windows" where the client is served immediately, and may obtain information and advice about available services and facilities. Clients may also be brought into direct contact with bodies that can help them on their way.
Target group	(Elderly) clients in need of care
Practice domain	Care requests in the areas of welfare, housing, and care.
Staff involved	Employees of the information desks
Methods used	An individual approach
Related agencies	The local service providers
Strengths	The better the mutual cooperation between these providers, the higher the chance that the query-guide window facility succeeds.
Weaknesses	The central question is whether the query-guide window as a so-called "front-office" effectively realises contacts with various provisions and functions in the "back-office": the local service providers.

CHAPTER 11

Providing Integrated Health and Social Care for Older Persons in the United Kingdom

Kirstie Coxon, Jenny Billings, Andy Alaszewski

The Government has made it one of its top priorities since coming to office to bring down the "Berlin Wall" that can divide health and social care and create a system of integrated care that puts users at the centre of service provision (DoH, 1998, chapter 1, section 6.5).

Introduction

This report provides an overview of the development of integrated health and social care provision for older people in the UK. It explores why integration is important, identifies the main impediments to effective integration, considers failed past attempts and current initiatives designed to promote joined-up thinking and seamless care for older people, identifying the main models.

In the first two sections of this national report, we examine the national context within which health and social care provision has developed, and consider the extent to which recent policy changes encourage the move towards seamless health and social care. In the third section we review existing models that have evolved in response to the challenges facing these services today. In the annex we provide more detailed descriptions of specific initiatives that provide exemplars of the main models identified in the third section.

Defining "Integrated Care"

Section two of this report illustrates that increased "integration" of health and social services has been a policy objective of UK governments since the 1960s. A variety of terms have been used for this, including "joint working", "partnership" and "collaboration", but the actual meaning of "integrated care" has never been clearly defined within policy documents – there is a sense that understanding of this and other related terms is taken for granted or assumed. As part of their remit to support the modernisation process within public bodies in the UK, the Audit Commission has produced a paper on integrated care. Within this document, a "systems model" of organisational partnership is employed, and the following definition of partnership or "whole system working" is proposed:

"Whole system working takes place when:
- Services are organised around the user
- All of the players recognise that they are interdependent and understand that action in one part of the system has an impact elsewhere
- The following are shared:
  - Vision
  - Objectives
  - Action, including redesigning services
  - Resources, and
  - Risk
- Users experience services as seamless and the boundaries between organisations are not apparent to them" (Audit Commission, 2002: Section 1.2).

1 The National Context

In this section we will describe some relevant demographic issues, the main components of the service delivery system and consider the unique features of the political and policy-making system.

Demography of the UK – An "Aging Society" (DoH, 2001a: 1)

The current population of the UK is approximately 59 million. The most recent census in 2001 found that about 20% of the population is aged over

60, with about 1.1 million people aged 85+ (Summerfield/Babb, 2003) and the numbers of very elderly people (80 and above) is predicted to double by 2025 (DoH, 2001a). This increase will directly affect the health and social care services that provide care to vulnerable persons in this age group. In the UK, public funds pay for about 80% of health care (OECD, 2002). Already, about 40% of the health care budget and 50% of the social care budget is spent on older people, amounting to an annual cost in excess of £15 billion (about 21 billion EUR).

Table 1:   UK Demography and Health Expenditure

	1980	1990	2000
UK Population (millions)	55.9 (approx)	57.8	58.8
% UK population over 65 years	15%	16%	16%
Public Expenditure on health (as % of GDP)	5%	5%	5.9%
Total Expenditure on health (as % of GDP)	5.6%	6%	7.3%
Expenditure per capita £ (EUR)	£270	£590	£1,071
	(409 EUR)	(897 EUR)	(1,627 EUR)

Source: OECD, 2002 (4th Ed); Summerfield/Babb, 2003: 31-35.

1.1   Health and Social Care Service Delivery – Organisation and Process

In the UK, the state plays a key role in funding and providing health and social care. The state has delegated the prime responsibility for service planning and resource allocation to two discrete organisations, the National Health Service (NHS) and Local Authority Personal Social Services Departments. However, in contrast with much of the rest of Europe, both these agencies operate in the short term, within fixed, cash-limited budgets. That is to say, resources are supply-determined and not a function of demand. There are fundamental differences in the ways these two sets of agencies are funded and operate (see 1.2), and this has been a major contributory factor to the health and social care divide in the UK.

ACCESS TO HEALTH SERVICES

Individuals may refer themselves to their own general practitioner (GP), a community-based doctor who specialises in all aspects of family health. The

457

GP will assess their medical needs and should also recognise where social needs are becoming an issue, and is obliged to refer a patient to acute hospital services, where necessary. The GP is effectively a gatekeeper for acute medical services, and screens individuals according to clinical criteria before making a referral to secondary services (Ham, 1997). All health services including GP consultation and hospital treatment are free to the patient, and secondary services are effectively "accessed" by the GP on the patient's behalf. In emergencies older people or their carers can bypass their GPs and gain direct access to more specialist services through A & E (Accident and Emergency departments in hospitals) or through direct contact with a social services team.

UK PROVISION OF HEALTH CARE

As Table 2 suggests, there is a trend in the UK for a reduction of acute care beds, and also in hospital "length of stay", despite an overall rising admission rate for chronically-ill elderly people. In common with the rest of Europe, this has led to increasing pressure on acute care beds with concomitant cost increases (Saltman, 1998), and policies directed towards greater provision of community and social care resources. Recognition of these challenges has led to many initiatives, such as intermediate care (DoH, 2001a), pooled funding (Health Act 1999) and "partnership proposals" (DoH, 2003b), all of which are designed to reduce the use of in-patient services and increase the availability of ongoing care in the community, and these services are discussed more fully in Section 3 of this report. These new and developing services necessarily involve closer working between health and social care professionals at every organisational level, and it is perhaps worth commenting that their genesis is a result of financial and service pressures upon the health service rather than a desire on the part of these professions to work in a collaborative manner.

Table 2:   Health Care Provision (UK), 1980-2000

	1980	1990	2000
Physicians per 1000 people	0.9	1.4	1.8
Acute beds available	3.5	2.8	3.3
Average (acute care) length of stay (days)	8.5	5.7	6.2

Source: OECD, 2002.

Access to Social Services

Recent statistics suggest that about 13% of social services referrals are generated to the community by GPs or district nurses. Individuals or their carers can also contact social services directly, and about 31% of referrals to social services comprise either self-referrals or referrals made by families (or informal carers) of vulnerable clients (DoH, 2000b). This means that the majority of social services referrals are actually generated by acute hospitals, and therefore occur after some crisis event, such as a fall or a period of illness, has led to hospitalisation.

Thus, the need for integrated services is often first identified in the health setting. In cases where the physical and mental condition of an older person worsens gradually, then the general practitioner should recognise that immediate carers are no longer able to cope and refer the older person for an assessment of care needs. When there is an emergency such as a fall, then hospital plays a key role. In a hospital setting, a multidisciplinary team comprising nurses, doctors, physiotherapists, occupational therapists and social workers should start discharge planning as soon as an older person is admitted and in consultation with the older person and their carers, assess the person's need for continuing care and agree a package of care. The main aim is to identify a package of community health service (district nursing), social care and adaptations to the home, which will enable the older person to return home and maintain independent living.

A key factor in achieving this is of course the availability of suitable housing for older people with increasing needs. This issue leads to a further need for integration between local housing providers (often local authorities, but many "social housing" and "sheltered housing" schemes are privately funded and managed) and both health and social care providers. The importance of housing within integrated care has been highlighted within current government policy statement (DoH/DETR, 2001), with a view to improving both provision of appropriate housing and increased information to users, carers and professionals about what is available. This is particularly important because when the risks of discharge home to existing accommodation, or simply remaining at home, are considered to be too high then a temporary, or permanent, residential placement may be recommended.

The decision to implement a package of community care, or residential placement, is generally achieved by conducting a "joint assessment".

These are one-off meetings held either in the hospital or community setting (depending on where the patient is), specifically to assess care requirements and plan provision accordingly. The key professional members present at these meetings are a qualified nurse (ideally the named nurse for that patient), a care manager, occupational therapist/physiotherapist (depending on the need for input from either profession), the patients themselves and very often their immediate family or informal carers. This group considers the professional assessments of the multidisciplinary team together with the thoughts and wishes of the patient as part of the process of care planning.

Once agreement is reached, the resulting package of care is accessed in a fragmented way. The nurse refers to district or community services, and any services provided by this professional group will be free to the service user. The care manager accesses the domiciliary care services, and the therapists will liase with their own bureau to effect adaptations or request equipment – for both of these groups, the provision of care is means-tested, and the recipient may have to contribute to the cost or even pay the full cost, depending on income and level of savings. Rehabilitation care becomes even more confusing – if the service is provided by health (for example a "hospital at home" scheme or community hospital "step down" bed) it will be free to the patient, but if social services are the provider (e.g. residential rehabilitation beds) then the client may be means-tested – and this is in turn dependent on local funding and commissioning agreements. This fragmentation of service provision is compounded by the restriction of information. The record of the assessment is usually held as a hard copy in the patient's hospital notes rather than being held by the patient, (and hence not accessible to any community practitioner at a later stage). The government is committed to the development of electronic records which users and health professionals can access to enable health professionals "maintain continuity of care and knowledge of their patients" (DoH, 2000a: 19).

The different definition of and approach to individuals in receipt of services is one of the key observable differences in culture between health and social services. Social services refer to their users as "service users" or "clients" (O'Hagan, 2001), and have tended to develop models of service provision that attempt to involve the user as an autonomous person (Davies, 2000). Whilst health services have also become increasingly aware of the disempowering nature of medical jargon, even health policy documents continue to refer to "patients" (e.g. DoH, 2000a).

In addition, the relationship between health and social services is asymmetrical, with the NHS being the senior and dominant partner (Hudson, 2002; Roberts, 2002). The NHS enjoys considerable public and political support, created as it was in 1948 as one of the major pillars of the welfare state in the UK. Its main service providers, doctors and nurses, continue, despite some high profile disasters, to enjoy high public esteem and trust (Finlay, 2000). In contrast social services have, since their formation in the 1970s, been subject to a continued media and political criticism. In part this relates to the "residual" nature of the services provided to vulnerable groups who can be victimised and portrayed as "welfare scroungers" (Finlay, 2000). It is also connected to highly visible failures, especially the failure to protect vulnerable children from abuse for which social services and social workers take the main responsibility and blame. The relatively low standing and status of key service providers including social workers, home helps and care staff at residential units further demonstrate the unequal power balance between these two agencies.

This asymmetrical relationship between health and social services is one of the major impediments to effective collaboration between the two agencies. It is a source of tension, even mutual antagonism between the two agencies. Long-standing inter-professional "turf wars" have led to what might be considered mutual incomprehension between health and social care workers, a situation which in Hudson's view is mediated by the extent of disagreement between two or more professional groups (Hudson, 2002). This type of environment is not conducive to effective collaboration and provides one of the major impediments to the development of joint working.

A further significant difference is that the level of funding for the NHS and for Social Services is not equal (see Table 1). The health service currently receives 70% of the £35 million total budget for health and social care. About half of all social service expenditure is likewise spent on older people (DoH, 2003). The health service is therefore perceived as being both better funded and a relatively more deserving recipient of public funds (DoH, 2001a: 1).

UK Provision of Social Care

Table 3 (below) suggests there has been a 50% increase in social services expenditure since 1990, and also an increase in the number of individuals receiving social services assistance, and Table 4 illustrates the shift from public to independent provision of social care that has occurred in the UK.

Table 3:   Social Services Expenditure 1990-2000

	1990	2000
LA personal social services expenditure	£5.3 billion	£10.1 billion
Expenditure on residential care (elderly)		£3.45 billion
Expenditure on non-residential care (elderly)		£1.72 billion
Number of households receiving domiciliary social care		400,000
No. of individuals in LA supported residential care (nb: all care groups – elderly account for 80% of bed usage)	125,000 (approx)	261,800 (approx)

Source: DoH, 2003.

Table 4:   Increased Use of Independent Sector for Personal Social Services 1997-2001

	1997	2001
Contact hours		
Provided by Local Authority	1.5 million (56%)	1.16 million (44%)
Provided by Independent sector	1.1 million (39%)	1.7 million (61%)
Total Contact Hours	2.6 million	2.86 million
No. of households receiving home help/personal care		
Provided by Local Authority	335,100	194,300
Provided by Independent Sector	144,000	205,300
Total no. of households receiving support	479,100	399,600

Source: DoH, 2003.

1.2   Government and Policy-Making in the UK

In relation to health, policy-making for older people has been largely influenced by a "policy community" or "iron triangle" (Haywood/Hunter, 1982) centred on the Department of Health. This involves ministers and professional expertise within the department, as well as national groups such as the British Geriatric Society. The use of professional expertise in developing policy can be clearly seen in the development of the National Services Framework for Older People, a recent document setting out national standards of care (DoH, 2001a). The Department used ten reference and task groups to provide expertise for the development of the framework. These groups were chaired by senior professionals or academics and included experts with diverse backgrounds and institutional affiliations (DoH, 2001a: 161-171).

With respect to fiscal policy, the UK has a highly centralised system. While there is some devolution to national assemblies in Scotland, Wales and Northern Ireland, the control of the Treasury over fiscal policy and allocation of public expenditure means that effective decision-making is concentrated in the so-called "Whitehall Village". Within this village there is fragmentation and competition between the major spending departments, for example between the Department of Health and the Department of Education.

The NHS is a centrally directed service accountable to the Secretary of State for Health who sets the budget. It is "universalistic", providing a service for all citizens who have a health need (mainly) free at the point of delivery funded from the central exchequer. Under current service provision arrangements, health care is "commissioned" or bought, by local Primary Care Trusts (PCTs). These are groups of health and social care professionals (e.g. G.Ps, nurses, social workers) with responsibility for identifying health needs for a given population (between 46,000-257,000). PCTs are freestanding organisations accountable for both commissioning and providing community health care for local populations. These trusts must identify the health care needs of the population they serve, recognise local inequality issues and purchase appropriate services, mainly from NHS bodies such as Hospital Trusts or from community based general practices (DoH, 2001c).

463

Social services form part of local government and there is accountability to locally elected councillors as well as to the Secretary of State for Health. Councillors set budgets for the social services, predominantly based on central funding but using some resources from local taxation and charges. This service is not "universalistic" but means-tested (Lewis, 2002). While social services provide assessment and care management as needed, users usually have to make a contribution to some of the services they receive if they have the financial resources to do so. There is strong managerial control within social services of resource allocation through the nationally and locally set eligibility criteria, but care managers also play a role through assessing individual need and agreeing packages of care to meet those needs within available budgets. Care managers are individuals who take on a case management role, and who may hold a social work qualification or alternatively a professional qualification in either nursing or occupational therapy. Social services are responsible for commissioning social care but unlike NHS fund-holding bodies, commission domiciliary support and residential care mainly from the private sector (Stanley et al, 1998).

The different organisation and roles of the NHS and social services give the UK a distinctive character. While the main objectives are to provide older people with services that maintain their dignity, security and independence (DoH, 2000a) there is particular concern with deprivation and inequalities creating socially excluded deprived groups. In contrast with most other European countries, the central direction of policy and allocation of funding of health and social care provision means that there is a strong emphasis on "best value". Where new services are created, these must be capable of demonstrating their strengths and efficacy against existing models, in order to secure ongoing funding. The combination of a finite budget with such clinical uncertainty has perhaps contributed to the speed and breadth of recent health care reform in the UK, culminating in comparatively radical changes to health and social care policy (Koko et al., 1998). This will be expanded upon in the following section.

2 The Development of Health and Social Care Integration

The boundary between health and social care has been disputed since the 1940s (Lewis, 2002). Since then there have been repeated attempts by central government to overcome this boundary but few of the resulting initiatives have achieved effective action. Many of these attempts have been characterised by rhetoric and exhortation rather than action (Griffiths, 1988). In this section we place the various initiatives in context.

2.1 The "Health and Social Care Integration Problem" and Structural Reform

When the welfare state in the UK was set up in the 1940s, it had a highly fragmented structure. While it was possible to identify broad services such as the health service, personal social services and social security, there was little coherence between and within these services. The NHS was internally divided into a hospital service, primary care service and community health services. Personal social services were fragmented between client-based departments in local authorities, children's" departments, welfare depart- ments for older people and health departments for maternity services and people with mental illness and learning disability (Lewis 2002).

In the early 1960s central government initiated a programme of wel- fare reforms requiring improved coordination. For example the successful implementation of 10-year plans for hospital and social services, especially the closure of long stay or "chronic" hospitals, depended on the develop- ment of alternative services for vulnerable adults within local authorities and community care (Ministry of Health, 1962; 1963). However the Minis- try had neither the means nor the inclination to ensure that the two sets of plans were brought together at a local level and the initiative was short-lived (Challis et al., 1988).

By the end of the 1960s fragmentation both within and between serv- ices was recognised as a major defect of the welfare state and the govern- ment undertook a radical programme of reform involving both a restruc- turing of the health services and social services and improved collaboration within and between services. In England, social services departments were established in 1971 bringing together services for a range of vulnerable us- ers and fostering a new conception of a generic social work profession. In 1974 the NHS was reorganised and new Area Health Authorities (AHA) were created with responsibility for planning, delivering and coordinating serv- ices. The AHAs brought together health professionals responsible for de- livering primary care, community health services and hospital services. There was a strong emphasis on coordination between health and social services. Not only did AHAs and social services departments share the same boundaries (co-terminosity), they had to create Joint Consultative Commit- tees to coordinate their activities, and share membership (one third of the AHA members were local authority councillors). Also, there was a legal duty on AHAs to collaborate and the new planning system brought together inter- disciplinary joint care planning teams to create integrated plans. While AHAs and social service departments maintained separate budgets, some resources were ring-fenced as joint finance to provide an incentive for collaborative and integrated services for older people (Hudson, 1998).

465

2.2 Funding and Economic Incentives

By the 1980s it was generally acknowledged that the structural reform pro-gramme of the 1970s had not improved the integration of health and social care. The coordinating mechanisms were not sufficiently robust to overcome the increased gap between health and social care, as well as other services that contributed towards the health and well-being of older people (Ottewill/ Wall, 1990). Initial reports of the effectiveness of joint planning were disap-pointing, due in part to complex processes that were difficult to navigate and the small amounts of money ultimately handled by joint finance (Nocon, 1994).

The government response to these perceived failures was to initiate a number of reviews and develop new policies. A common theme can be iden-tified in these reviews and initiatives, the centrality of finance and the im-portance of using monies to create incentive for more effective collabora-tion and service provision. In 1990, the "NHS and Community Care Act" (DoH, 1990) introduced the principle of "government by the market". This involved administratively separating the responsibilities for funding or "purchasing" health and social care, from the responsibility of provision. The responsibility for "purchasing" was given to health authorities and fund-holding GPs (for health care) and social service authorities and care manag-ers (for social care). For those agencies that provided the care, the notion of competition entered the arena, providing an incentive for increasing respon-siveness to the needs of service users and attending to cost and quality. It was anticipated that for users who needed both health and social care such as older people, purchasers would coordinate their activities through "joint commissioning" (Hudson, 1998).

For older people the principles underlying the 1990 Act were actually not implemented until 1993 (Lock, 1996). In practical terms, this Act was designed to ensure that older people should remain in their own homes for as long as possible, funded if necessary by money which was previously used to fund residential, nursing home or hospital care (Lock, 1996). Serv-ice provision therefore was to become needs-led rather than service-led and resulted in some flexible initiatives, such as the "out of normal hours" car-ing service, and evening "meals on wheels" deliveries (Dobson, 1994).

The introduction of competitive markets posed many challenges to the effective integration of services. The competitive dimension injected con-siderable rivalry between agencies supplying care (Wistow et al., 1996). This had the effect of reducing inter-agency communication as organisations became reluctant to share information, and made the management of complex networks essential to effective collaboration difficult (Wistow/Hardy, 1996). In the absence of a single health and social care budget, managers were not able to commit resources for a unified package of care and there was a lack of clarity in relation to the purchasing of "continuing care" for patients with long-term support needs (Hudson, 1998). At the same time, acute hospitals were under pressure from the Department of Health to reduce waiting lists and increase throughput. Tensions between acute hospitals and other services rose over "bed-blocking" in patient discharges arising from delays in assessments, development of care packages and funding of social care support (Hudson/Henwood, 2002). Even if agencies were prepared to work more closely together, there were many legal ambiguities around contracts and data protection that could prevent them.

There emerged particular issues in relation to the professional demarcation of work. The 1990 Act distinguished between "health care" and "social care" (Lock, 1996). Social services were given the lead role in assessing need and funding packages of care and some health care agencies challenged their competence to assess health care needs (Duggan, 1995). In addition, health authorities became reluctant to continue to pay for the social care they had been providing (Lock, 1996). As a consequence, the boundary between health and social care was characterised by conflict between agencies and professions, rather than cooperation and collaboration (Hudson/Henwood, 2002).

Paying for Community Care

Under current arrangements, health services are provided free to clients wherever these are provided. This includes district nursing services, "day-hospitals" and support from mental health specialists for older people with cognitive impairment. Prior to the 1990 Act, district nursing services were able to provide personal care services to chronically disabled clients, but this is now entirely the domain of Local Authority social services departments. If a client requires help with personal care, such as washing or dressing, or help with shopping or housework, the care is provided by mainly private agencies. The client makes a contribution to the cost, and this can extend to the full cost of care if the client's income and savings are above a particular threshold. The average cost of this service is about £10 per hour, and "care packages" tend to range between 4 to 14 hours per week, depending on the dependency of the client, and the availability of "informal" support from family and friends.

BENEFITS FOR DISABLED INDIVIDUALS

"Attendance Allowance" is a tax-free social security benefit, available to people over 65 years of age who are living in their own homes, who need help with personal care, and have needed such help for at least six months. It is intended to help the client afford the care required. There are two rates payable, the lower rate (£37.65, 54 EUR per week) and the higher rate (£56.25, 81 EUR), depending on the extent of help an individual needs, and whether they need support during the night as well as the day. At present, about 1.3 million people claim Attendance Allowance, and just under 50% receive the higher rate (DWP, 2003). There is also an allowance called Disabled Living Allowance, which assists with mobility costs.

BENEFITS FOR INFORMAL CARERS

A slightly different allowance is the "Invalid Care Allowance", which is intended for carers and may be claimed by people who are caring for a relative or friend for more than 35 hours a week. This benefit is means-tested, and payable at £42.45 (61 EUR) per week. It is intended to recompense the carer for loss of paid employment, but the amount is really quite small – working the same hours even at the minimum wage would generate an income of about £ 160 (230 EUR) per week.

3   Current Models of Health and Social Care Collaboration

When the Labour government came to power in 1997, the government recognised that the development of public services in Britain had not kept pace with public expectations and that there was a need for a major programme of modernisation. This programme has involved additional allocation of funding, including from 2003 an increase in direct taxation and a major new ideology, the so-called "Third Way" (Means et al., 2002). In health and social care the third way involves replacing the competitive relations of internal or managed markets with collaborative partnerships both within the public sector and between the public and private sectors (Hudson/Henwood, 2002). In the NHS the major visible sign of this new approach was a shift from purchasing by health authorities and GP fund-holders to "commissioning" by newly created Primary Care Trusts (DoH, 1997). In this section we will focus on the main elements of the reform programme as they affect joint working. We will start with a brief overview and then provide more detailed consideration of each aspect of joint working.

3.1 Current Initiatives

When the Labour Party was elected in 1997 it followed a long period in opposition and it was committed to making its mark. There followed a rapid programme of reform and modernisation, which has had major implications for the health and social care divide. *The New NHS: Modern, Dependable* policy document (DoH, 1997) outlined a raft of key partnership initiatives. The NHS Plan published in 2000 (DoH, 2000a) was a major stock-taking exercise summarising the achievement of the government's first term in office and outlining the aims for its second term. The chapter on "Changes between health and social services" outlines the main framework of the modernisation programme, with innovations in structure, incentives, audit and service delivery.

469

STRUCTURE

The NHS Plan outlines the legal changes which the government had introduced in the 1999 Health Act (DoH, 1999) to facilitate "Partnership Working" and looks forward to new integrated structures, "Care Trusts", which will be elaborated upon later.

The NHS Plan notes that the 1999 Act is designed to enable the NHS and local authorities work more closely and has reduced the impediments to joint working by allowing:
- pooled budgets: this involves local health and social services putting money into a single dedicated budget to fund a wide range of care services
- lead commissioning: either the local authority or the health authority/primary care group takes the lead in commissioning services on behalf of both bodies

- integrated providers: local authorities and health authorities merge their services to deliver a one-stop package of care (DoH, 2000a: 70).

The Plan notes that these changes create the conditions for more innovative collaboration, such as social care staff working in GPs surgeries alongside GPs and other health care staff (DoH, 2000a).

AUDIT

Long-standing central government concerns about the cost and performance of the public sector have underpinned the development of an audit culture in the UK. The Treasury as the major funding of the public sector is only willing to increase allocation to health and social services if it receives evidence that these resources achieve agreed service aims. Thus the Treasury has created "service agreements" with major spending departments. These Departments have to produce evidence that they have indeed achieved the aims and have created systems for measuring performance including performance indicators and inspectorates as well as demonstrating that spending will be limited within the government's budgetary planning. The Department of Health uses a combination of three overlapping inspectorates, the Audit Commission that assesses performance of all the public sector, the Commission for Health Improvement for the health care and the Social Services Inspectorate for social care. In the NHS Plan, the Department indicates that these three inspectorates will jointly inspect health and social care organisations to assess their joint working and the performance measurements will include:

- reducing the number of cases where an older patient's discharge is delayed from hospital
- reducing preventable emergency admissions and readmissions of older people and those with mental health problems
- increasing the speed at which the needs of older people are assessed (DoH, 2000a: 72).

NEW SERVICE DELIVERY STRUCTURES: INTERMEDIATE CARE

Central to the government's strategy for improving health and social care services for older people, is a new type of service, intermediate care. In October 1997 the government made available £300 million for hospital trusts to develop services to ease "winter pressures" and "bed-blocking" through innovative schemes to either reduce "unnecessary" hospital admissions or to facilitate early discharge of mainly older people who no longer required acute hospital care (Scrivens et al., 1998; Doran, 1997). Many of the resulting initiatives have matured into "Intermediate Care".

Intermediate care is designed to "promote independence and improve quality of care for older people" (DoH, 2000a: 71) by either preventing their admission to acute hospital or by facilitating their discharge. Intermediate care is a generic name used to describe a range of different services that may include primary care (e.g. rapid response teams), secondary care (e.g. intensive rehabilitation) or social care (e.g. integrated home care teams). There is no prescribed format for intermediate care rather a menu of possible services that health and social services can use. The NHS Plan describes the menu in the following way:

- *rapid response teams*: made up of nurses, care workers, therapists and GPs working to provide emergency care for people at home and helping to prevent unnecessary hospital admissions
- *intensive rehabilitation services:* to help older people regain their health and independence after a stroke or major surgery, normally situated in hospitals
- *recuperative facilities:* many patients do not always need hospital care but may not be quite fit enough to go home; short-term care in a nursing home or other special accommodation eases the passage
- *arrangements at GP practice or social work level to ensure that older people receive a one-stop service:* this might involve employing or designating key workers or link workers, or basing case managers in GP surgeries
- *integrated home care teams:* so that people receive the care they need when they are discharged from hospital to help them live independently at home (DoH, 2000a: 71-72).

The development of intermediate care represents the greatest investment of resources. The NHS Plan indicates that the government is committed to investing £900 million in the development of intermediate care by 2003/04 (DoH, 2000a: 71).

It is clear that the government in Britain sees the health and social care divide as a major impediment to the development of integrated seamless care for older people. The major programme of reform initially outlined in 1997 and restated in 2000 has major implications for the health and social care interface. Some of the proposed reforms involve changes to financial systems and monitoring arrangements and will therefore only have an indirect effect on joint working. Others such as intermediate care are having a direct impact on joint working and we will explore these developments in more detail in the next section.

3.2   Development of Current Models

Some of the developments outlined in the NHS Plan (DoH, 2000a) and National Service Framework for Older People (DoH, 2001a) build on and develop established initiatives. For example the various intermediate care initiatives developed in response to funding criteria for "Winter Pressures" money. Such schemes tend to be relatively well-established and it is possible to explore their implications for joint working and we discuss these schemes in the first part of this section. Other schemes are more recent, for example the Single Assessment Process and the "Care Trusts". It is likely that they will stimulate joint working but since there are only limited pilot schemes, it is at this stage difficult to explore the full implications of these initiatives for joint working. We will consider the ways in which these schemes are developing in the second part of this section.

3.2.1 Intermediate Care and Joint Working

While intermediate care in England has been developed to meet specific service needs, especially those of acute hospitals experiencing "bed-blocking" problems, they represent a major investment in and development of joint working between health and social care. A review of intermediate care published in 1999 identified examples in over 70 trusts in England and this was only a sample of existing schemes (Vaughan/Lathlean, 1999). To date there has been no comprehensive survey of intermediate care provision, although a national survey is in progress at present (DoH, 2002a). Given the Department of Health's expectations that all agencies will participate in intermediate care, it seems likely that intermediate care will become established as a major component of service provision for older people.

JOINT WORKING

While there are several different models of intermediate care, these share one common feature in that they all involve joint working to some extent. Early definitions of intermediate care tended to emphasise the function or purpose of intermediate care, such as reduced pressure on acute hospitals, rather than joint working. For example in 1997 Steiner defined intermediate care as:

> That range of services designed to facilitate the transition from hospital to home, and from medical dependence to functional independence, where the objectives of care are not primarily medical, the patient's discharge destination is anticipated, and a clinical outcome of recovery (or restoration of health) is desired (Steiner, 1997: 18).

The Department of Health has developed Steiner's objective, making it clear that joint or "cross-professional" working is a key feature of intermediate care. The National Service Framework for Older People (DoH, 2001a) specifies that intermediate care services should:

- be targeted at people who would otherwise face unnecessary prolonged hospital care stays or avoidable admission to acute in-patient care, long-term residential care or continuing NHS inpatient care
- be provided on the basis of a comprehensive assessment, resulting in a structured individual care plan that involves active treatment and rehabilitation
- be designed to maximise independence and to enable patients/users to remain or resume living at home
- involve short-term interventions, typically lasting no longer than 6 weeks and frequently as little as 1-2 weeks or less
- involve cross-professional working, within the framework of the single assessment process, a single professional record and shared protocols (DoH, 2001b: 43).

The Department emphasised the importance of joint-working and inter-agency collaboration in the following way:

> An essential component of intermediate care services is that they should be integrated within a whole system of care including primary and secondary health care, health and social care, the statutory and independent sectors. This creates challenges for the commissioning, management and provision of care entailing complex multi-sectoral working (DoH, 2001b: 43).

3.2.2 Diversity of Approach in Intermediate Care Service Models

While joint working was a feature of intermediate care from the start, it tended to be joint working within the context of and led by acute hospitals. This is reflected both in the prime purpose and funding of early schemes.

473

Vaughan and Lathlean's (1999) sample of schemes identified three main types, early discharge, community-based rehabilitation and hospital at home. These schemes were designed to reduce pressure on acute hospitals by increasing discharges or reducing admissions of older people.

With the focus of intermediate care being mainly around the shortening of hospital stays after an acute episode (and of course expediting discharge where the cause of admission is lack of social support coupled with loss of self-care abilities), or preventing admission and re-admission in the first place, it is perhaps not surprising that many of these schemes originated in acute hospitals. Drawing on the examples listed in a directory of intermediate care schemes (Vaughan/Lathlean, 1999) of 30 early discharge/ discharge prevention schemes, 19 were funded entirely by health agencies, 10 jointly funded and only 1 was funded by social services alone. Of 27 community-based rehabilitation projects, 12 were funded by health alone, 13 by joint finances and 2 by social services. The 7 "hospital at home" schemes mentioned were all funded by health trusts. This sample was selected by the authors to represent the range of services available at that time, but it does not necessarily follow that the above figures are truly representative, partly because much has changed since this directory was published. However, the picture that emerges is one of multi-disciplinary team development within the established hospital workforce.

There has therefore been a demonstrable policy shift towards expanding rehabilitation service provision in the UK, accompanied by a substantial funding investment into "intermediate care". However, it should be recognised that such services to a large extent exclude older people with complex medical needs, cognitive impairment or dementia and chronic, long-term conditions which are not amenable to short-term input. This means that this policy only addresses one particular aspect of older people's health and social care – perhaps to the detriment of more dependent individuals.

A further, as yet unacknowledged issue is the "knock-on" effect on family and informal carers when an older person is discharged as soon as possible from hospital, or maintained at home with increased support. Such carers frequently provide the mainstay of daily support and assistance to older persons, and an assumption underlying the current policy is that these carers can maintain (or even increase) a high level of input, often including being available overnight to their relatives for an unspecified amount of time.

MODELS IN PRACTICE

There are a number of intermediate care models across the UK, but the types of services provided tend to be fairly similar. What the following examples demonstrate is that while intermediate care is an important and significant development, it does not necessarily mean that "joint working" in its full sense is taking place. The extent of joint working and the creation of a "seamless" service would appear to depend upon the practicalities of geographical location, such as whether teams work in the same building, and the budgetary arrangements with respect to the financial leadership and accountability within the services. Although there is a drive towards "pooled budgets", financial organisation has tended to be more loosely arranged within joint finance schemes funded through NHS or social services budgets. Ongoing access to funds for service requirements can become a lengthy bureaucratic process, and particularly in the NHS, budgets can become vulnerable to diversion into other more resource intensive areas. Increasingly however, financial management of joint-working schemes is being done through newly formed Primary Care Trusts, which may limit these potential difficulties.

475

EARLY DISCHARGE OR "HOSPITAL AT HOME" SCHEMES

As would be expected, these schemes are targeted at individuals who are already in hospital, but who have recovered from their immediate "acute" phase. Social service packages of care are initiated and funded by hospital care managers using NHS money in order to expedite the patient's discharge, instead of waiting for social service initiated assessments to take place. The details of care packages are agreed with professionals, patients and carers following joint assessments pre-discharge. Some care packages offer mainly social support for discharged patients – such as help with personal care, assistance with shopping, or emotional support. Others offer therapeutic intervention, especially after orthopaedic admissions, with occupational therapists or physiotherapists visiting the patients at home and instigating a rehabilitation programme, which may then be maintained by rehabilitation assistants. A third variation is to offer community nursing services, perhaps with GP backup. There is normally collaborative professional involvement, and all schemes are time-limited, from 2-6 weeks.

ADMISSION PREVENTION/RAPID RESPONSE TEAMS (EXAMPLE – SEE ANNEX A3)

These teams are designed to prevent admission to hospital or residential homes. Teams are comprised of nurses and social workers, with nurses responsible for the initial assessment and referral. Overall management of the teams can be either through the NHS or social services, but workers have separate professional line management. Again, the service delivery is variable within areas, but a common pattern is referral to a rapid response team, either from A&E staff, or from GPs or other community sources, and a fast-track assessment and implementation of health or therapies and social care which is delivered in the person's own home. The time frame within which help is offered is normally up to 3 days, therefore quick responsive referral to other agencies is a vital component of this service. With nurse and social worker roles intrinsic to the team and funding being increasingly managed through Primary Care Trusts, the conditions for joint working to occur would appear to be in place. However, teams tend to be "virtual" and with nurses and social workers housed in different geographical locations, the implications for communication are clear. In addition, for seamless care to be effected, quick referral response from agencies outside of the rapid response team (such as therapies) must come about.

Unlike other schemes where joint working is intrinsic to the service delivery by virtue of the multi-agency team development, this method maintains a degree of professional separatism. The financing of the care packages through the NHS also creates further "rifts" in professional collaboration in care and can cause considerable disruption for clients. Once the period of intervention is over (2 to 6 weeks depending on the scheme), the responsibility for financing and providing care is passed back to the community social services or health services who operate independently from the acute hospital, necessitating another round of assessment and intervention for the client. Cornes and Clough (1999) have identified this as a problem, and suggest that rather than contributing to joint working, there is a risk that intermediate care can simply add another layer to an increasingly complex assortment of services and providers, causing confusion and disruption to the client and actually moving away from what joint working is supposed to achieve.

COMMUNITY ASSESSMENT AND REHABILITATION TEAMS (CART) (EXAMPLE – SEE ANNEX A1)

This service model was one of the earliest developments in intermediate care, with many schemes set up during the mid-1990s, prior to the "winter pressures" funding (Vaughan/Lathlean 1999). With respect to joint working, the important difference is that a multi-professional team is central to the service design and is housed in one location, usually in a health service setting. CARTs take referrals both from hospital and community settings, both pre-admission and post-discharge. The intention is that the intervention be available before a point of crisis requiring hospital admission is reached. The teams are usually made up of nurses, occupational therapists and physiotherapists, and should conduct an integrated assessment of the individual. One professional will take the lead role, depending on which therapy is most needed – for example, if the person has had a number of falls, and the assessment suggests that physiotherapy would be the most appropriate intervention, the physiotherapist will take on the lead role of assessment and evaluation. Other specialities such as speech therapy or a dietician may be either on the team, or available to them. Social services care managers form part of some teams, and liaise externally with others. Although variable, these are jointly-funded schemes managed either through the NHS or social services.

RESIDENTIAL REHABILITATION UNITS (EXAMPLE – SEE ANNEX A2)

The provision of residential rehabilitation is a service that can be difficult to differentiate from traditional rehabilitation wards within hospitals, although this type of care may be offered by community hospitals, residential or nursing homes, in nurse-led units, or within social services residential units. A number of regions have started to provide such a service. In order to fit in to the policy definition of intermediate care, such units should be offering time-limited rehabilitative (enabling) care, with discharge home being a feasible and anticipated objective.

This is also a service area which has suffered from the different charging arrangements for health and social services – health-based units are able to offer rehabilitation programmes free at the point of delivery, whilst social services units and residential/nursing homes have, until recently, had to charge the individual in accordance with the normal means-testing criteria.

477

This is currently subject to regional variation, and also subject to negotiation with local social services authorities.

Residential rehabilitation programmes are most appropriate for older people who are medically stable, but need intensive therapeutic input to regain their functional independence. Most units specify the need for "24 hour supervision" as part of their admission criteria, reflecting that this client group is likely to be at high risk of either hospital or residential home admission. Where such a service is provided, it is normally part of a wide spectrum of intermediate care provision, and tends to be accessed by the most heavily dependent clients.

FUTURE DIRECTIONS – THE SINGLE ASSESSMENT PROCESS AND THE NEW "CARE TRUSTS"

This section provides an account of new areas of development, namely single assessment and Care Trusts. Potentially these schemes will have a major impact on the quality of support received by older people and joint working. However given the early stage of these developments it is only possible at this stage to outline their likely impact.

SHARING INFORMATION: TOWARDS A SINGLE ASSESSMENT PROCESS

A major impediment to the development of seamless care has been the separate collection and storage of information. Currently, each professional group involved in older person's care has its own method of assessment and record keeping. This means that not only is information not shared but also that older people are subject to repeated assessment and questioning. To improve coordination, the Department of Health is committed to the development of a single assessment process whereby agreed information is collected and shared between all the main caregivers:

> By April 2002, we will introduce a single assessment process for health and social care, with protocols to be agreed locally between health and social care. Initially this will be introduced for those older people who are the most vulnerable, for example, those who live alone or those who are recently bereaved or those discharged from hospital or entering residential or nursing homes (DoH, 2000a: 125).

The planned development of a single assessment process is perhaps one of the most ambitious areas of current policy. The government's guidance describes a record of core needs assessment that is carried out once, on behalf of all the health and social care providers involved, with a particular client. Ideally, this should be an electronic record (DoH, 2002e). However, there is a question around whether the necessary infrastructure exists for such an undertaking. John Hudson (2002) comments that both the health service and social services have multiple information technology problems, including poor resources, limited financial support and cultural negativity within the workforce towards IT systems. Such factors, together with other issues such as the cost of training a workforce in an IT system and the financial implications of developing a universally accessible database, may explain why the current guidelines are fairly low-key on the subject of an electronic system.

A further practical (and legal) issue is that the consent of the client must be secured, because the information gathered will be shared across the traditional boundaries of care provision – that is, between hospital trusts, community (primary health) teams, and social services providers. Local arrangements must also be made to agree an assessment format, clarify which professional should make the main assessment, and ensure that the information is subsequently available "around the clock" to any other agency which requires it (DoH, 2002e: 34). In addition, a written record of any resulting care plan should be copied to the client. To achieve such an ideal seems far from possible at present, as the practical problems it presents mean that how professionals from numerous organisations communicate at every level needs to be completely re-thought.

In 2003, the Department of Health accredited the "MDS" single assessment tool for use with older people in the UK. The government has also published an extensive list of domains and sub-domains for assessment, together with guidance on involving clients and carers in the assessment.

The development of a single assessment format has attracted the attention of researchers, particularly in the medical domain, and several studies have been undertaken to validate the various data-gathering instruments that are being developed to meet the Department of Health criteria for a single assessment tool (DoH, 2002c; Carpenter/Challis, in press; see also www.interrai-uk.org). The government has set out a timetable for achieving a single assessment process, commencing in April 2002, with a projected date of April 2005 by which time all localities are expected to have assessment systems which are compliant with the single assessment guidelines (DoH, 2002e).

The current situation is that no region has managed to achieve consensus on a single assessment process, although a number of localities have begun moving towards this goal. Three regions have been suggested as resource points for other agencies due to their progress on this area of practice. Cambridgeshire agencies are ready to pilot an electronic data collection tool, which, it is anticipated, will eventually be used across the whole region (see Annex A4). In Leeds, five Primary Care Trusts (PCTs) have established "Joint Care Management Teams (JCMTs), which work with a "whole systems" approach. One of these teams is developing and piloting an electronic record system to improve information sharing and documentation. In Surrey, an initiative from primary care agencies (GPs, district nurses, practice nurses, health visitors and care managers) established a basic assessment by drawing on the common areas used by both health and social care practitioners. This initiative is being expanded across the county of Surrey, and an electronic version is being developed concurrently.

Commenting on these evolving schemes, the Department of Health (DoH, 2002c) identifies a number of lessons that other agencies can learn from the experience of these "trailblazers". In Cambridge, the key areas were IT training, and addressing the cultural changes necessary for the IT to be acceptable to the workforce. The Leeds project highlighted the process of obtaining consent, and includes work on joint consent and confidentiality protocols. In West Byfleet (Surrey), issues of professional culture were addressed, and this area offers the following guidance:

> Professionals have to understand and respect each other's roles and responsibilities. They must be prepared to lose individual ownership of processes and information, and replace it with joint ownership of the responsibility to meet the needs of service users/patients (DoH, 2002c: 22).

It would seem that there are a number of hurdles to be overcome on the road to achieving a single assessment process. The above comments refer to issues of professional identity and accountability, which are construed by social scientists to explain why the professions (and "semi-professions") display territorial behaviour when working within a multi-disciplinary framework (Hudson, 2002). It is unclear whether health and social care professionals are ready to lose individual ownership of information and assessment processes.

There is also a perceived lack of financial resource for this policy – no grants or funds have been made available specifically for funding the single assessment process. Despite this perception, the funding issue has partly been addressed by the Department of Health, which announced a new national strategy for IT within the NHS (DoH, 2002f) with earmarked funds to assist in the development of electronic records (Dodson, 2002). However, what this initiative does not address is the resources required for each region to develop inter-agency teams to reach consensus on single assessment, develop the appropriate documentation and practice protocols, obtain the informed consent and cooperation of service users (many of whom have sensory and/or cognitive impairment) and train the relevant professionals and support staff. At present, it cannot be assumed that the "single assessment process" is universally viewed as an achievable goal by key health and social care professionals.

481

MOVING TOWARDS CARE TRUSTS

The NHS plan (DoH, 2000a) provides a structural joint working framework for the development of "Primary Care Trusts", which are stand-alone units, capable of both commissioning and providing integrated primary and community care for the designated local population. Many of these are now in place. The NHS Plan also outlines the structure of a new type of organisation, the Care Trust (see Annex A5). These are "new single multi-purpose legal bodies ... to commission and deliver primary and community healthcare as well as social care for older people and other client groups ..." (DoH, 2000a: 73). While the Department of Health sees the introduction of these new Trusts as essentially voluntary, presenting them as a vehicle that local agencies can choose to use, it also reserves the right to impose such structures where it has evidence that collaboration is not taking place:

> Where local health and social care organisations have failed to establish effective joint partnerships – or where inspection or joint reviews have shown that services are failing – the Government will take powers to establish integrated arrangements through the new Care Trust (DoH, 2000a: 73).

The creation of new structures provides the opportunity for pooling resources. Indeed the NHS Plan acknowledges that the 1999 Health Act initiatives have created joint schemes with budgets of over £200 million (DoH, 2000a: 71). In addition the Department has set aside or "ring fenced" a budget to provide "incentive payments to encourage and reward joint working" (DoH, 2000a: 72). In the NHS this budget will be allocated through a National Performance Fund, while local authorities will be rewarded through a separate fund with £50 million allocated for 2002/3 and £100 million for 2003/4.

Given the chequered history between health and social services, it is however this reform that has been the source of much critical debate, especially from social service quarters who fear that Care Trusts are an NHS "takeover" and may be unsympathetic to social service priorities (Hudson/Henwood, 2002). This NHS "takeover" may be increased if the management of Care Trusts is linked to the hospital bed and waiting list agendas. In addition to this, the development of National Service Frameworks for Older People (DoH, 2001a) may also lock local government into an NHS-led system. Others have expressed concerns in relation to the upheaval of yet more major structural change, the consequences for service users, and the potential for "empire building" of whichever care-giving agency dominates. However, these proposals are still evolving, and in the meantime the move to Primary Care Trusts is seen as a suitable means for potentially bringing about integrated services (Hudson/Henwood, 2002).

3.3 Comment on Models of Joint Working in the UK

The current Labour Government in the United Kingdom is committed to reforming public services. It has accepted that the development of public services has lagged behind public expectations and a government priority is increased investment in public services. However if such investment is not to be wasted, it must be accompanied by a programme of reform and modernisation involving the development of greater cooperation and collaboration within and between sectors and joint working practices. There have been a range of initiatives such as intermediate care for older people and while most of these initiatives are at a relatively early stage in their development, some preliminary evidence is beginning to emerge about the impact on joint working and the quality of services received by older people.

482

4   Conclusion

4.1   *The Development of Joint Working in the UK*

In this final section we highlight the factors that have shaped the development of joint working in the UK and consider the current state of play.

THE POLICY CONTEXT

The distinctive features of the British political and welfare system have heavily influenced the development of services for older people in the UK. The British polity is highly centralised both in terms of policy-making and financial allocation. Policy-making tends to be dominated by a "policy community" or triangle of key decision-makers, ministers, civil servants and major pressure/expert groups. The Treasury forms a part of this community, as it is the source of responsibility for ensuring that public funds are properly allocated and effectively used. It has developed a system of formal service agreements with spending departments such as the Department of Health, which subsequently form the basis of the audit process.

At a local level, services for older people are predominantly funded and delivered by public agencies such as the NHS and social services, though Governments since the 1980s have encouraged the independent sector to take on the delivery of health and especially social care. However, the majority of community care is provided free by informal carers (relatives and friends) and the UK government could be said to rely heavily on family provision of care. Given the dominant position of the public sector within "formal" care provision, mechanisms for managing the private sector such as regulatory frameworks established by law have historically played a relatively minor role in the UK, although the recent development of new inspection and regulatory bodies under the Care Standards Act (2000) appears to be impacting significantly on the private sector. Instead, the main mechanism for providing direction and therefore the main source of evidence for reviews are central government policy statements such as the NHS Plan (DoH, 2000a) and the National Service Framework for Older People (DoH, 2001a). It is important to note that central government in the UK not only controls the policy agenda, but also has a major influence on evaluative research as it is the main source of funding for this type of research.

THE HEALTH/SOCIAL CARE DIVIDE

In the United Kingdom there is a long-standing problem of coordination between health and social care services. The government is partially responsible for the creation of the "Berlin Wall" between health and social services. In restructuring the welfare state at the end of the 1960s, the government fostered health and social care professions and provided them with dominant positions at the core of the major agencies designed to plan, fund and deliver health and social care. Differences of status, ideology, funding, and at times mutual hostility between professions have tended to reinforce the competitive elements in the system and have provided little incentive for collaboration or joint working.

Since the 1970s there have been repeated attempts to overcome this divide. In the 1960s the emphasis was on the development of plans that were mutually adjusted. When there was little evidence of mutual adjustment, the emphasis shifted to structural reforms. The divisive tendencies of the restructuring of the 1970s were to be counteracted by a range of collaborative initiatives, co-terminosity, common membership, joint planning and joint finances. When in turn these initiatives failed to deliver improved collaboration and joint working, increased emphasis was placed on financial incentives. In the 1980s and 1990s there was an ideological commitment to the "invisible" hand of the market, and internal markets in which "money followed patients" were adopted as a panacea. Again there was little evidence that "internal markets" improved collaboration and joint working and in 1997 a new government identified them as the problem and placed collaboration and partnership at the centre of its commitment to modernise health and social care services.

MODERNISATION, COLLABORATION AND JOINT WORKING

Following repeated failure to create a seamless health and social care system in the UK, the current government has initiated a major programme of reform. It has indicated that it will not tolerate resistance to reform and is willing to reconfigure both welfare agencies and the professions that work in them to ensure that older people and other users receive continuity of care.

The current reform programme does not rely on one single approach but brings together a number of different changes. It includes:

- *structural changes* to services creating the opportunities for new integrated "Care Trusts",
- *improved financial incentives* with monies being used to facilitate and reward collaboration and joint working,
- *audit* with joint audits by the Audit Commission, Commission for Health Improvement and the Social Services Inspectorate to ensure closer collaboration and joint working,
- *shared information* with the introduction of a single assessment system facilitating the sharing of information between agencies and professionals,
- *new service models* with intermediate care combining features of social care, primary care and hospital care and enhancing joint working.

4.2   The Current Position of Joint Working in the UK

The current government in the UK is committed to a major programme of modernisation at the core of which is a commitment to the development of joint working between public services and especially between health and social services. It is already possible to see the impact of this programme on services for older people especially in the development of intermediate care. Intermediate care is an umbrella term, which includes different models of support. The government expects joint working and collaboration to form a prominent feature of all models of intermediate care. In some models joint working between health and social care is an intrinsic element, for example community assessment and rehabilitation teams. However in other models it is less central and joint working takes place amongst health care workers rather than between health and social care, for example early discharge schemes and hospital at home. Other parts of the reform programme, such as the single assessment process and Care Trust are at an earlier stage in their development and as yet it is difficult to assess their full implications for joint working. These initiatives are more recent than intermediate care. However it is also possible that their slow pace on developments is a reflection of both the intrinsic complexity of the proposed changes, especially in the case of joint assessment where key components of the infrastructure are not in place, and resistance, especially in the case of Care Trusts where local government is concerned about an NHS take-over.

485

Since this modernisation programme is at a relatively early stage of its development it is perhaps too early to assess the extent to which it will enhance collaboration and create joint working. It is not clear whether the current labour government will succeed in breaking out of the historical cycle. Since the 1950s all governments in the UK have sought to enhance collaboration and create joint working in services providing support for older people. However to date there is very little evidence that any of the initiatives have successfully overcome the divisive and competitive tendencies within the public sector.

References

Audit Commission (2002) *Integrated Services for Older People: Building a Whole System Approach in England.* London: Audit Commission.

Carpenter, I./Challis, D. (In Press) 'A Thread from Many Strands', *The Milbank Quarterly (special report).* New York: Milbank Memorial Fund.

Challis, L. et al. (1988) *Joint Approaches to Social Policy; Rationality and Practice.* Cambridge: Cambridge University Press.

Cornes, M.L./Clough, R. (1999) 'Trailblazers and Trouble shooters. Report of External Evaluation of four Intermediate Community Care Projects in Cumbria'. Lancaster University.

Davies, C. (2000) 'Improving the Quality of Services', in: Brechin, A./Brown, H./Eby, M.A. (eds.), *Critical Practice in Health and Social Care.* London: Sage Publications/The Open University.

Department of Health (1990) *The NHS and Community Care Act.* London: Her Majesty's Stationery Office (HMSO).

Department of Health (1997) *The New NHS: Modern, Dependable.* London: The Stationery Office.

Department of Health (1998) *Modernising Social Services: Promoting Independence, Improving Protection, Raising Standards.* Cmnd 4169. London: The Stationery Office.

Department of Health (1999) *National Health Service Act.* London: The Stationery Office.

Department of Health (2000a) *The NHS Plan: A Plan for Investment. A Plan for Reform.* London: Department of Health.

Department of Health (2000b) *Community Care Statistics 1999/2000.* www.doh.gov.uk/public/comcare2000/r3.xls

Department of Health (2001a) *National Service Framework for Older People.* London: Department of Health.

Department of Health (2001b) 'Intermediate Care', Health Service Circular Local Authority Circular HSC 2001/01 : LAC 2001/01 dated 19th January 2001 (available at http://www.doh.gov.uk/coinh.htm)

Department of Health (2001c) *Primary Care Groups.* http://www.doh.gov.uk/pricare/pcgs.htm

Department of Health (2002a) *National Service Framework for Older People: Supporting Implementation: Intermediate Care: Moving Forward.* London Department of Health.

Department of Health (2002c) *The Single Assessment Process: Assessment Tools and Scales* (version dated 29th March 2002). London: Department of Health.

Department of Health (2002e) *The Single Assessment Process – Guidance for Local Implementation.* London Department of Health.

Department of Health (2002f) *Delivering 21st Century IT: Support for the NHS.* London: Department of Health.

Department of Health (2003) *Community Care Statistics 2001.* London Department of Health http://www.goh.gov.uk/public/comcare2001

Department of Health (2003b) *Partnership in Action: New Opportunities for Joint Working between Health and Social Care.* London: Department of Health.

Department of Health/Department of Environment, Transport and Regions (2001) *Better Care, Higher Standards: A Charter for Long Term Care.* London: Department of Health.

Department of Work and Pensions (2003) *Disability Care and Mobility Benefits November 2002 Quarterly Statistics Enquiry* http://www.dwp.gov.uk

Dobson, R. (1994) 'Valley of Care', *Community Care* 1031: 10.

Dodson, S. (2002) 'Where IT Matters Most', *NHS Magazine* September: 24-25.

Doran, A (1997) *Emergency Services Action Team (ESAT) Report to the Chief Executive on Winter Pressures.* London: Department of Health http://www.doh.gov.uk/pub/doh/winter.pdf

Duggan, M. (1995) *Primary Health Care – A Prognosis.* London: Institute for Public Policy Research.

Finlay, L. (2000) 'The Challenge of Professionalism', in: Brechin, A./Brown, H./Eby, M. (eds.), *Critical Practice in Health and Social Care.* London: Sage Productions (for The Open University).

Gloucestershire Health Authority/Gloucester Social Services/East Gloucester NHS Trust/ Severn NHS Trust (1999) *Final Evaluation Report of the Rapid Response Community Rehabilitation Team Pilots in Cheltenham, Gloucester and Stroud* (unpublished report).

Griffiths, R. (1988) *Community Care: Agenda for Action. A Report to the Secretary of State for Social Services.* London: The Stationery Office.

Ham, C. (1997) *Health Care Reform: Learning from International Experience,* 1st ed. Buckingham: Open University Press.

Haywood, S./Hunter, D. (1982) 'Consultative Processes in Health Policy in the United Kingdom: A View from the Centre', *Public Administration* 69: 143-162.

Hudson, B. (1998) 'Circumstances Change Cases: Local Government and the NHS', *Social Policy and Administration* 32 (1): 71-86.

Hudson, B. (2002) 'Interprofessionality in Health and Social Care: The Achilles' Heel of Partnership?', *Journal of Interprofessional Care* 16 (1): 8-17.

Hudson, B./Henwood, M. (2002) 'The NHS and Social Care: the Final Countdown?', *Policy and Politics* 30 (2): 153-166.

Hudson, J. (2002) 'Community Care in the Information Age', in: Bytheway, B./Bacigalupo, V./ Bornat, J./Johnson, J./Spurr, S., *Understanding Care, Welfare and Community – a Reader.* London: Routledge/Open University.

Kodner, D.L./Spreeuwenberg, C. (2002) 'Integrated Care: Meaning, Logic, Applications and Implications: A Discussion Paper', *International Journal of Integrated Care* 2 (November), www.ijic.org

Koko,S./Hava, P./Ortun, V./Leppo. K. (1998) 'The Role of the State in Healthcare Reform', in: Saltman, R./Figueras, J./Sakellarides, C. (eds.), *Critical Challenges for Healthcare Reform in Europe.* Buckingham: Open University Press.

Lewis, J. (2002) 'The Boundary Between Health and Social Care', in: Bytheway, et al., *Understanding Care, Welfare and Community: A Reader*. London: Routledge OUP.

Lock, K. (1996) 'The Changing Organisation of Health Care: Setting the Scene', in: Twinn, S./ Roberts,B./Andrews, S., *Community Health Care Nursing: Principles for Practice*. Oxford: Butterworth-Heinemann.

Means, R./Morbey, H./Smith, R. (2002) *From Community Care to Market Care?* Bristol: The Policy Press.

Ministry of Health (1962) *A Hospital Plan for England and Wales*, Cmnd 1604. London: HMSO.

Ministry of Health (1963) *The Development of Community Care*, Cmnd 1973. London: HMSO.

Nocon, A. (1994) *Collaboration in Community Care in the 1990's*. Sunderland: Business Education Publishers.

OECD (2002) *OECD Health Data 2002* – "frequently asked data", http://www.oecd.org

O'Hagan, G. (2001) *Improving Older People's Services: Inspection of Social Care Services for Older People*. London: Department of Health.

Ottewill, R./Wall, A. (1990) *The Growth and Development of the Community Health Services*. Sunderland: Business Education Publishers.

Roberts, Y. (2002) 'Power Imbalance May Affect Joint Work', *Community Care* 25 (April-May): 23.

Saltman, R.B. (Ed.) (1998) *Critical Challenges for Health Care Reform in Europe*. Buckingham: Open University Press.

Scrivens, E./Cropper, S./Beech, R. (1998) *Making Winter Monies Work: A Review of Locally Used Methods for Selecting and Evaluating supply-side Interventions*. Keele University: Centre for Health Planning and Management.

Stanley, N./Manthorpe, J./Bradley, G./Alaszewski, A. (1998) 'Researching Community Assessments: A Pluralistic Approach', pp. 69-84 in: Cheetham, J./Kazi, M.A.F. (eds.), *The Working of Social Work*. London: Jessica Kingsley Publishers.

Steiner, A. (1997) *Intermediate Care: A Conceptual Framework and Review of the Literature*. London: King's Fund.

Summerfield, C./Babb, P. (Eds.) (2003) *Social Trends*, No. 33. London, The Stationery Office.

Vaughan, B./Lathlean, J. (1999) *Intermediate Care: Models in Practice*. London: King's Fund Publishing.

Wistow, G./Hardy, B. (1996) 'Competition, Collaboration and Markets', *Journal of Interprofessional Care* 10 (1): 5-10.

Wistow, G./Knapp, M./Hardy, B./Forder, J./Kendall, J./Manning, R. (1996) *Social Care Markets: Problems and Prospects*. Buckingham: Open University Press.

488

Annex: Model Ways of Working

A1 Model "Community Assessment and Rehabilitation Teams"

Name of the exemplar	Gloucester Community Rehabilitation Team (South-west England)
Provider	Jointly funded by Gloucestershire Health Authority and Gloucestershire Social Services
Objectives	• To improve health and social care through partnership working • To avoid inappropriate admissions to hospital • To reduce admissions to residential and nursing homes • To slow the rate of complex community care packages • To reduce length of stay for medically stable in-patients
Target group	Hospital patients in need of home rehabilitation. Clients at home with a crisis (e.g. fall, chest infection), or short-term rehabilitation need
Practice Domain	Acute hospitals/clients' own homes
Joint Working Initiatives	Qualified nursing staff and occupational and physiotherapists (from health sector) work alongside social services care manager Specialist generic rehabilitation assistants also employed (care assistants trained to give rehabilitative care using an enabling/social care model)
Methods	Provide rapid intervention for clients at home, or support after hospital discharge, with rehabilitation/therapy input (for up to 6 weeks) Interdisciplinary approach, with shared work-base for whole team Overnight on-call care provision Individualised assessment, care planning and evaluation Timely, smooth and seamless discharge from team Ongoing service-user evaluation and audit
Strengths and Weaknesses	*Strengths:* • A positive approach to joint working between health and social services personnel. Protocols, admission criteria, intervention and evaluation all jointly agreed • Service available over 24 hours, and discharge planned to provide "seamless" care • Reflective approach allowed changes in service provision to be made in response to service user and provider needs • Continued evaluation of outcomes and user satisfaction

489

	Weaknesses: • Pilot scheme – therefore long-term funding uncertain, causing initial recruitment problems • No external evaluation
Evaluation Results (Local Audit)	Community Rehabilitation Teams have prevented admissions (78% of referrals "could have been admitted to hospital" but only 11% required hospital admission) Dependency improved in 40% of those on the scheme A small rise in formal care (i.e. social services care at home) was documented following discharge from the team Treatment given by CRT's has been well received by users. Although hospital admissions fell during the study period, there were no measurable differences between admission rates for areas with or without CRT's Source of Information: Gloucestershire Health Authority/Gloucester Social Services/ East Gloucester NHS Trust/Severn NHS Trust (1999) "Final Evaluation Report of the Rapid Response Community Rehabilitation Team Pilots in Cheltenham, Gloucester and Stroud" (unpublished report)

A2 Model: An Integration Project (Intermediate Care)

Name of the exemplar	The Limes and Livingstone Integration Project (Dartford, Kent, South-East England) – Community and Recuperative Care Beds
Provider	A partnership agreement (pooled funding and integrated working) between Kent County Council and Dartford, Gravesham and Swanley Primary Care Trust
Objectives	• To work in partnership and develop a seamless service to promote independence for older people • To decrease preventable hospital admissions and reduce length of hospital stay • To promote rehabilitative care on a short-term basis and enable people to resume living at home by maximising their independence
Target group	Clients over 65 years who are medically stable, in need of rehabilitation or recuperative care, and who are expected to return home, given appropriate support
Practice Domain	Residential beds – community hospital and social services rehabilitation unit, housed on same site

Joint Working Initiatives	Health Services nursing staff work alongside Social Services therapists and care assistants. A new post of "Generic Rehabilitation Worker" has been developed so that support staff can work in both settings Joint management of all staff
Methods	Integration of "The Limes" recuperative care centre and The Livingstone Community hospital (which co-exist next door to each other), under one management structure, with pooled budget development Provision of a full range of social and health rehabilitation, either as a "step down" intermediate care facility or a "step up" from home, avoiding acute hospital admission Provide inter-professional working with a single assessment framework, single professional records, shared protocols and shared admission and discharge criteria
Strengths and weaknesses	*Strengths:* • Positive "can-do" management approach to joint working • Commitment to meeting the practical challenges of collaborative working • Involvement and training of staff to facilitate "enabling" culture with a clear training and development pathway • Able to expand the "entry gate" for rehabilitative care, by drawing on the combined skills of nursing and therapy staff, so that higher dependency clients can be taken on *Weaknesses:* • This project is still being established, and is a "trailblazer" in the sense that it uses innovative funding and management approaches. Its true impact on the local target population is as yet unknown • The above information could not have been included without the assistance of Christine Ballard, Development Manager for Partnerships and Project Manager for the "Limes/Livingstone" development

491

A3 Model: Rapid Response Teams

Name of the exemplar	Community Care in Cumbria: Rapid Response Teams (Cumbria, North-West England)
Provider	Morecambe Bay Health Authority
Objectives	• Promote user independence • Reduce dependency on continuing health and social services

	• Prevent inappropriate admission to hospital • Facilitate early, safe discharge from hospital • To work in partnership with existing services and agencies in a collaborative and integrated manner
Target group	Patients medically fit for hospital discharge but awaiting "social care" arrangements, or patients at home experiencing an acute illness episode
Practice Domain	Acute NHS hospital wards, clients' own homes
Joint Working Initiative	Teams of qualified nurses assess care needs, and purchase "social care" from local agencies on behalf of service users
Methods	Facilitate hospital discharge (or prevent hospital admission) by offering home-based personal or social care for up to 2 weeks Liaise with mainstream Social Services agencies to establish continued care after this period
Strengths and weaknesses	*Strengths:* Qualified nursing staff able to assess care needs and organise a package of care quickly, circumventing delays in "mainstream" system Evaluation study suggests that early discharge may have been facilitated, and that unnecessary hospital admissions (particularly for clients "at risk" with social care needs) prevented, although the methodology did not permit a true comparison with existing care methods *Weaknesses:* Scheme operated in addition to existing social services framework, rather than in collaboration with this. Intervention time limited to 2 weeks – carers were not able to remain involved throughout the recovery period, and transferring care to social services after this time meant that users had to adjust to a different team of carers. Interventions concentrated on giving supportive personal care rather than enabling a return to independence – described as a "stop-gap" measure to address the organisational problem of providing community support quickly rather than a client-centred approach to maximise independence at home. (The above comments are derived from a descriptive evaluation study commissioned by the scheme providers [Cornes/Clough, 1999]. The "Rapid Response" model was only one of three models involved in the study. It is not the intention to suggest that all Rapid Response Teams have the same problems, but for the purposes of the "Procare" study, it seems useful that these issues were identified.)

A4 Model: Single Assessment Process (electronic database)

Name of the exemplar	Cambridgeshire Common Assessment Tool (CAT) (Cambridgeshire, South England)
Provider	Cambridgeshire Social Services Department Cambridgeshire Health Authority
Objectives	• Collaboration amongst health and social care providers, to develop a single comprehensive assessment for older persons • Establish a shared, person-centred approach to care provision • Ensure that assessment format would be useful and acceptable to different professionals, and explore user views on information sharing
Target group	Older people in Cambridgeshire requiring comprehensive assessment of social and health care needs
Joint Working Initiatives	IT departments from health and social care agencies work together to create and test a single assessment form
Methods	• Collaboration between health and social care agencies to develop a common assessment tool • "Action Learning Approach" used, to test acceptability across different professional groups • Explore user views on information sharing, and establish procedure for obtaining consent and maintaining confidentiality • Electronic version of "CAT" now ready to be piloted
Strengths and Weaknesses	*Strengths:* • A nationally recognised unit, leading the field of single assessment • Able to advise other areas on the process of achieving single assessment *Weaknesses:* • At present, this project has not been evaluated

493

A5 Model: Strategic Development

Name of the exemplar	Bradford District Care Trust (near Leeds, North East England)
Provider	Bradford Health Partnership (Bradford Metropolitan Council and Bradford Health Authority)
Objectives	• Creation of a "Care Trust", to meet the health and social care needs for a defined population • Improved, client-centred services, sensitive to the ethnic and cultural diversity of the population • Improved use of resources and facilities, with increased flexibility and pooling of expertise • An enhanced, stable working environment • An integrated information system
Target group	The Care Trust has four directorates, and provides services for users with mental health needs (including elderly mental health services) and learning disabilities. The target population is within the Bradford District (approximately 500,000 people)
Joint Working Initiatives	Existing community mental health services to be merged with Social Services, to create the new organisation
Methods	• Formation of Care Trust (2nd September 2002) • Build on history of collaborative working • Extend availability of "home treatment model" for mental health users (a service which has NHS beacon status) • Quality assurance through multidisciplinary clinical governance groups and user focus groups
Strengths and weaknesses	*Strengths:* • Organisational power – the "Care Trust" model has been developed specifically to enhance collaborative working between health and social care services • Built on a successful history of joint working • Realistic time frame in place, to allow planned programme of integration • Application for "Care Trust" status based on "an extensive consultation process involving public, staff, users and relatives/carers" (Bradford District Care Trust, 2002: 1)

Weaknesses:
- Whilst elderly mental health services are to be provided by the Care Trust, the "social care" component for this particular client group will remain external to the new organisation. The reasons for this decision are unclear, but it suggests that even within an organisation designed to promote joint working at regional level, the boundary between health and social care provision may remain intact

Source of Information	Bradford District Care Trust (2002) Application and Prospectus for the New Organisation

List of Contributors

Austria

Margit Grilz-Wolf, Researcher at the European Centre for Social Welfare Policy and Research, Vienna

Charlotte Strümpel, Psychologist, Researcher at the European Centre for Social Welfare Policy and Research, Head of the Programme "Ageing, Care Policies and Social Services"

Kai Leichsenring, Political Scientist and Consultant in Organisational Development, Research Associate at the European Centre for Social Welfare Policy and Research

Kathrin Komp, studied Home Economics and European Studies at the Universities of Giessen and Leipzig (Germany) and contributed to the Austrian country report during an internship at the European Centre for Social Welfare Policy and Research

Denmark

Ellinor Colmorten, Sociologist, Head of Department at the Ministry of Social Affairs, contributed to the Danish country report while working as a Researcher at the Danish National Institute of Social Research, Copenhagen

Thomas Clausen, Political Scientist, Researcher at the Danish National Institute of Social Research

Steen Bengtsson, Sociologist, Senior Researcher at the Danish National Institute of Social Research

Finland

Paula Salonen, free-lance Social Researcher, collaborating with the National Research and Development Centre for Welfare and Health (STAKES), Helsinki

Riitta Haverinen, Development Manager, Head of the Evaluation of Social Services Group at the National Research and Development Centre for Welfare and Health (STAKES), Helsinki

France

Michel Frossard †, died during his contribution to the French national report in 2002; as a Professor of Economics he had been Director of the "Centre Pluridisciplinaire de Gérontologie" at the University Pierre Mendès France of Grenoble. He was one of the pioneers in analysing the political economy of ageing, and widely recognized both in French and international gerontology

Nathalie Genin, Researcher at the University Pierre Mendès France of Grenoble, "Centre Pluridisciplinaire de Gérontologie"

Marie-Jo Guisset, Gerontologist, Consultant for the "Union nationale interfédérale des oeuvres et organismes privés sanitaires et sociaux" (UNIOPSS) and at the "Fondation Médéric Alzheimer", Paris

Alain Villez, Technical Advisor concerning services and policies for older persons at the "Union nationale interfédérale des oeuvres et organismes privés sanitaires et sociaux" (UNIOPSS), Paris

Germany

Günter Roth, Chair in Social Management at the University of Applied Science of the German Red Cross, Göttingen, "Forschungsgesellschaft für Gerontologie e.V.", Institute of Gerontology at the University of Dortmund e.V.

Monika Reichert, Psychologist, Professor at the Institute of Gerontology at the University of Dortmund, "Forschungsgesellschaft für Gerontologie e.V."

Greece

Aris Sissouras, Professor of Operational Research at the University of Patras and Scientific Manager of PROCARE at the Institute of Social Policy at the National Centre for Social Research (EKKE), Athens

Maria Ketsetzopoulou, Sociologist and Economist, Senior Researcher at the National Centre for Social Research (EKKE), Athens

Nikos Bouzas, Economist, Senior Researcher at the National Centre for Social Research (EKKE), Athens

Evi Fagadaki, Political Scientist, Researcher at the National Centre for Social Research (EKKE), Athens

Olga Papaliou, Legal Expert, Researcher at the National Centre for Social Research (EKKE), Athens

Aliki Fakoura, Sociologist, contributed to the Greek country report as an external collaborator at the National Centre for Social Research (EKKE), Athens

Italy

Giorgia Nesti, Political Scientist, Researcher at emmeerre S.p.A., Padua

Stefano Campostrini, Professor of Social Statistics at the Universities of Padua and Pavia; Partner of emmeerre S.p.A., Padua

Stefano Garbin, Economist, Partner of emmeerre S.p.A., Padua

Paola Piva, Sociologist, Scientific Director of Studio Come s.r.l. Rome, Consultant for the Ministry of Equal Opportunities

Patrizia Di Santo, Sociologist, Managing Director and Expert Consultant of Studio Come s.r.l., Rome

Filomena Tunzi, Sociologist, Senior Researcher and Consultant of Studio Come s.r.l., Rome

The Netherlands

Carine Ex, Psychologist, Researcher at Verwey-Jonker Institute, Utrecht

Klaas Gorter, Social Psychologist, Researcher at Verwey-Jonker Institute, Institute for Research into Social Issues, Utrecht

Uschi Janssen, Human Geographer, Researcher at Verwey-Jonker Institute, Utrecht

United Kingdom

Andy Alaszewski, Professor of Health Studies at the Centre for Health Service Studies at the University of Kent in Canterbury

Jenny Billings, Research Fellow at the Centre for Health Service Studies at the University of Kent in Canterbury

Kirstie Coxon, Research Associate at the Centre for Health Service Studies at the University of Kent in Canterbury

Wohlfahrtspolitik und Sozialforschung
Herausgegeben vom Europäischen Zentrum Wien
mit dem Campus Verlag, Frankfurt am Main/New York

Band 1: DE SWAAN, A. (1993)
Der sorgende Staat. Wohlfahrt, Gesundheit
und Bildung in Europa und den USA der Neuzeit
345 S., *vergriffen*

Band 2: KENIS, P., SCHNEIDER, V. (Hg.) (1996)
Organisation und Netzwerk.
Institutionelle Steuerung in Wirtschaft und Politik
566 S., *vergriffen*

Band 3: FRIEDBERG, E. (1995)
Ordnung und Macht.
Dynamiken organisierten Handelns
419 S., EUR 45,-

Band 4: CATTACIN, S. (1994)
Stadtentwicklungspolitik zwischen
Demokratie und Komplexität.
Zur politischen Organisation der Stadtentwicklung:
Florenz, Wien und Zürich im Vergleich
237 S., EUR 34,90

Band 5: KRÄNZL-NAGL, R., RIEPL, B.,
WINTERSBERGER, H. (Hg.) (1998)
Kindheit in Gesellschaft und Politik.
Eine multidisziplinäre Analyse am Beispiel Österreichs
536 S., EUR 51,-

Band 6: FEHÉR, F., HELLER, A. (1995)
Biopolitik
110 S., EUR 29,90

Band 7: HELLER, A. (1995)
Ist die Moderne lebensfähig?
229 S., EUR 24,90

Band 8: PRINZ, CH., MARIN, B. (1999)
Pensionsreformen.
Nachhaltiger Sozialumbau am Beispiel Österreichs
500 S., EUR 45,-

Campus Verlag, Postfach 90 02 63, D-60442 Frankfurt am Main
Tel: (069) 97 65 16-0; Fax: (069) 97 65 16
www.campus.de, info@campus.de, vertrieb@campus.de

Wohlfahrtspolitik und Sozialforschung
Herausgegeben vom Europäischen Zentrum Wien
mit dem Campus Verlag, Frankfurt am Main/New York

Campus Verlag, Postfach 90 02 63, D-60442 Frankfurt am Main
Tel: (069) 97 65 16-0; Fax: (069) 97 65 16
www.campus.de, info@campus.de, vertrieb@campus.de

Behindertenpolitik zwischen Beschäftigung und Versorgung. Ein internationaler Vergleich
OECD

Noch immer steht eine Antwort auf die Frage aus, wie OECD-Länder die beiden eng verknüpften, potentiell aber gegensätzlichen Anliegen der Behindertenpolitik miteinander in Einklang bringen können. Zum einen soll sichergestellt sein, dass behinderte Mitbürger nicht ausgegrenzt werden: dass sie zu größtmöglicher Teilhabe am Wirtschafts- und Gesellschaftsleben ermutigt und befähigt werden, insbesondere zur Aufnahme einer entgeltlichen Beschäftigung, und dass sie nicht zu leicht oder zu früh aus dem Arbeitsmarkt gedrängt werden. Zum anderen soll gewährleistet werden, dass jene Personen, die behindert sind oder es werden, über sichere Einkommen verfügen: dass sie nicht auf Grund von Behinderungen, die ihr Verdienstpotential einschränken, der Mittel für ein menschenwürdiges Leben beraubt werden.

Der vorliegende Bericht liefert eine systematische Analyse eines breiten Spektrums an Arbeitsmarktmaßnahmen und Programmen zur sozialen Sicherung für Menschen mit Behinderungen. Durch die Untersuchung der Zusammenhänge zwischen den ergriffenen Maßnahmen und den erzielten Ergebnissen in zwanzig OECD-Ländern sollen dem Leser die Probleme der Behindertenpolitik klarer vor Augen geführt und erfolgreiche Maßnahmen bzw. Maßnahmenpakete vorgestellt werden. Der Bericht gelangt zu der Schlussfolgerung, dass sich ein vielversprechendes neues Konzept der Behindertenpolitik stärker an der Philosophie der Programme für Arbeitslose orientieren sollte, und zwar durch:

* eine Betonung von Aktivierungsmaßnahmen,
* die Förderung von auf den Einzelnen zugeschnittenen Frühinterventionen,
* die Beseitigung von Negativanreizen zur Aufnahme einer Beschäftigung,
* die Einführung einer Kultur der gegenseitigen Verpflichtungen,
* die Einbeziehung der Arbeitgeber.

Der Bericht zeigt auch, dass sich in der Behindertenpolitik vieler Länder bereits Elemente finden, die in einem solchen neuen Konzept eine wichtige Rolle spielen.

Frankfurt am Main: Campus, 2003. ISBN 3-593-37420-X, 408 S., € 34,90, www.campus.de

Public Policy and Social Welfare
A Series Edited by the European Centre Vienna
vols. 1-10 with Campus Verlag/Westview Press, Frankfurt am Main/Boulder, Co.

Publications Officer, European Centre, Berggasse 17, A-1090 Wien
Tel: (01) 319 45 05-27; Fax: (01) 319 45 05-19
www.euro.centre.org, stamatiou@euro.centre.org

Public Policy and Social Welfare
A Series Edited by the European Centre Vienna with
Ashgate, Aldershot, Brookfield USA, Singapore, Sydney

Public Policy and Social Welfare
A Series Edited by the European Centre Vienna with
Ashgate, Aldershot, Brookfield USA, Singapore, Sydney

www.ashgate.com

European Disability Pension Policies
11 Country Trends 1970-2002
With an Introduction by Bernd Marin
Christopher Prinz (Ed.)

This book is the result of an extension of the European Centre's research on disability benefit policies which has been partly funded by the Swiss Federal Office of Social Insurance. It contains an introduction and theoretical overviews by Bernd Marin and Philip R. de Jong, respectively, as well as chapters on the following 11 European countries: Austria, Denmark, Finland, Germany, Italy, the Netherlands, Norway, Poland, Slovenia, Sweden, and Switzerland.

During the last twenty years, the longer-term sustainability of social insurance systems has become a major issue in all European countries. The debate is generally dominated by a focus on the rising costs of old-age pensions, driven by rapidly changing population age structures. In recent years, however, analysts and governments increasingly started to worry about the growth in the number of disability benefit recipients – a growth with significant variations in the composition of new recipients in terms of age, gender and health conditions.

After a long phase of expansion of disability benefit schemes via increasing benefits, broading coverage and easing access (in particular for elderly unemployed people), since the late 1980s and the beginning 1990s more and more countries have started to reform their systems – ranging from piecemeal changes (e.g. in Switzerland) to more far-reaching reorientation (e.g. in Germany) or even fundamental reconstruction (e.g. in the Netherlands). While policy measures differ widely, policy goals tend to converge. Some policy elements, such as the identification of and benefit provision for partial disability, seem particularly controversial.

The purpose of this book is to analyse and compare disability benefit policies in eleven European countries in the last two or three decades, and to examine the outcome of these policies. Often policies appear to have immediate short-term effects, while being much less effective in a longer perspective, thus asking for continual reform. For some of the newer challenges, such as the rapidly increasing number of benefit claims on psychological grounds, responses have yet to be found.

Christopher Prinz is Administrator at the OECD Social Policy Division, Paris.

Aldershot (UK): Ashgate, 2003. ISBN 0-7546-1972-9, pp. 430, £ 25, www.ashgate.com

Transforming Disability Welfare Policies
Towards Work and Equal Opportunities
Bernd Marin, Christopher Prinz, Monika Queisser (Eds.)

On the occasion of "The European Year of People with Disabilities 2003", the OECD and the European Centre for Social Welfare Policy and Research organised an international conference at the UNOV in Vienna on "Transforming Disability into Ability". The purpose of this event was to discuss disability policies for the working-age population. The conference addressed key challenges in disability policy, and discussed policy recommendations as outlined in the recent OECD report. The main policy conclusions from the report formed the basis for the thematic sessions. The conference was organised around five themes:

- What do we mean by "being disabled"?
- What rights and responsibilities for society and for persons with disabilities?
- Who needs activation, how, and when?
- How should disability benefits be structured?
- What should and what can employers do?

More than 40 invited speakers discussed proposals for more effective disability policies and the improvement of existing institutions and measures in light of best practices in international comparison. Particular emphasis was placed on the implementation of the report's policy conclusions. One session of the conference was devoted to the discussion of "Barriers to Participation" from the perspective of disabled people; it was organized by an international association of organisations representing disabled people.

This book is a follow-up of the OECD report on "Transforming Disability into Ability" (2003) as well as a twin publication to the recent Ashgate volume on "European Disability Pension Policies" (Prinz Ed. 2003) and to the companion booklet on "Facts and Figures on Disability Welfare. A Pictographic Portrait of an OECD Report" (Marin / Prinz 2003). It brings together contributions from inter-governmental institutions such as the OECD, the European Centre, the WHO, the World Bank, from several former and acting government representatives, ministries concerned with disability issues, the business community, the European Disability Forum and from experts from national, regional and local NGOs, as well as authors from universities and research centres.

Bernd Marin is Executive Director of the European Centre for Social Welfare Policy and Research in Vienna. *Christopher Prinz* is Administrator at the OECD Social Policy Division in Paris. *Monika Queisser* is Principal Administrator at the OECD Social Policy Division in Paris.

Aldershot (UK): Ashgate, 2004. ISBN 0-7546-4284-4, pp. 392, £ 35.00, www.ashgate.com

Facts and Figures on Disability Welfare
A Pictographic Portrait of an OECD Report
Bernd Marin, Christopher Prinz

Displays new data on up to 20 OECD countries, trying to answer puzzles as ...

What share of the population is defined as (severely) disabled in which OECD countries? And how many people are awarded what disability benefits – with what trends over time? Where are men and where are women more affected by work incapacity – and who is granted what entitlements? What are the main determinants of disability prevalence? Are expenditures still rising? Is disability welfare more costly than unemployment, and if so, how much more expensive? What about personal and household income sources and income security of disabled persons? How many disabled persons are without income? For whom – disabled or not – does work pay? Is income maintenance or job discrimination the main problem for people with disabilities? How much employment exclusion of persons with (severe) disabilities exists in which countries? How much less employment opportunities and how much more unemployment risk is there for people with what degree of disabilities, of what age, and with what education? How many recipients of a disability benefit actually work? How can great country differences be explained? To what an extent is non-employment and not unemployment the main joblessness problem of disabled persons? Are there gaps between shares of disabled people and disability beneficiaries – and how big are they? Where does a (great) majority of (severely) disabled people not receive a disability benefit? How many disability benefit recipients do not classify themselves as "disabled"? And in which OECD countries do these inclusion and exclusion errors amount to what scale? What determines the employment rates of disabled persons? And how protected or regular are employment relations of disabled people? How do benefit inflow and outflow rates compare over the life cycle? Where are country divergences widest? What incapacity levels qualify where for what benefit entitlements? What differences are there in benefit rejection rates – and in appeals to benefit rejection and their probability of success? How much does early retirement coincide with age bias in disability benefit inflows – and where? How many more people are awarded a disability benefit than receiving vocational rehabilitation or other special employment services – and what are the extra costs of social exclusion? Do those most in need participate in active programmes; and if not, then who else does? Do participation in employment programmes or cash benefits raise employment rates of persons with disabilities? What is the employment value for active programme money? How do benefit coverage and generosity determine recipient numbers? How has the direction of disability policy changed during the last decades?

Bernd Marin is Executive Director of the European Centre for Social Welfare Policy and Research in Vienna. *Christopher Prinz* is Administrator at the OECD Social Policy Division in Paris.

Vienna: European Centre, 2003. ISBN 3-900376-98-0, pp. 104, € 15, www.euro.centre.org

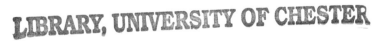